Textbook of FORENSIC ODONTOLOGY

Textbook of FORENSIC ODONTOLOGY

Editor

Nitul Jain MDS

Assistant Professor
Department of Oral and Maxillofacial Pathology
Eklavya Dental College and Hospital
Kotputli, Rajasthan, India

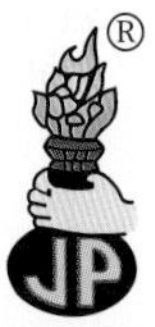

JAYPEE BROTHERS MEDICAL PUBLISHERS (P) LTD

New Delhi • Panama City • London • Dhaka • Kathmandu

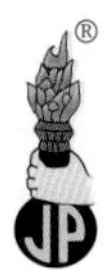

Jaypee Brothers Medical Publishers (P) Ltd

Headquarters

Jaypee Brothers Medical Publishers (P) Ltd
4838/24, Ansari Road, Daryaganj
New Delhi 110 002, India
Phone: +91-11-43574357
Fax: +91-11-43574314
Email: jaypee@jaypeebrothers.com

Overseas Offices

J.P. Medical Ltd.
83, Victoria Street, London
SW1H 0HW (UK)
Phone: +44-2031708910
Fax: +02-03-0086180
Email: info@jpmedpub.com

Jaypee-Highlights Medical Publishers Inc.
City of Knowledge, Bld. 237, Clayton
Panama City, Panama
Phone: Phone: + 507-301-0496
Fax: +507-301-0499
Email: cservice@jphmedical.com

Jaypee Brothers Medical Publishers (P) Ltd
17/1-B Babar Road, Block-B, Shaymali
Mohammadpur, Dhaka-1207
Bangladesh
Mobile: +08801912003485
Email: jaypeedhaka@gmail.com

Jaypee Brothers Medical Publishers (P) Ltd
Shorakhute, Kathmandu
Nepal
Phone: +00977-9841528578
Email: jaypee.nepal@gmail.com

Website: www.jaypeebrothers.com
Website: www.jaypeedigital.com

Inquiries for bulk sales may be solicited at: jaypee@jaypeebrothers.com

Textbook of Forensic Odontology

First Edition : **2013**

ISBN 978-93-5025-722-7

Printed at Replika Press Pvt. Ltd.

Dedicated to

Remembrance of my grandparents
Late Mrs and Mr Parmanand Jain
and
My humble, lovely and ever-supporting family members
My parents, Mrs and Mr Naresh Jain
My wife, Monika
My sisters, Nidhi and Dr Anjali
and
Our one year old little darling, Tim-Tim

Contributors

Abhishek Singhania MDS
Department of Conservative Dentistry and Endodontics, Eklavya Dental College and Hospital
Kotputli, Rajasthan, India

Ajay Telang MDS
Department of Oral Pathology
Penang International Dental College
Penang, Malaysia

Anil Pandey MDS
Department of Oral Pathology
Maharana Pratap Dental College and Research Centre, Gwalior
Madhya Pradesh, India

Gaurav Atreja MDS
Department of Prosthodontics
MM Mullana Institute of Dental Sciences
Mullana, Ambala, Haryana, India

Hemanth M MDS
Department of Oral Pathology
Malabar Dental College and Research Centre
Edappal, Kerala, India

Nitul Jain MDS
Department of Oral and Maxillofacial Pathology
Eklavya Dental College and Hospital
Kotputli, Rajasthan, India

Shikha Atreja MDS
Department of Pedodontics
MM Mullana Institute of Dental Sciences
Mullana, Ambala, Haryana, India

Sohail Lattoo MDS
Department of Oral Pathology
Government Dental College
Srinagar, Jammu and Kashmir, India

Soniya Adyanthaya MDS
Department of Oral Pathology
Yenepoya Dental College and Hospital
Deralakatte, Mangalore, Karnataka, India

Vishal Saxena MDS
Department of Oral Medicine and Radiology
Eklavya Dental College and Hospital
Kotputli, Rajasthan, India

Vishwas Bhatia MDS
Department of Prosthodontics
Eklavya Dental College and Hospital
Kotputli, Rajasthan, India

Preface

Generally the dentists are better known for pulling, drilling and filling the teeth. However, largely the general people and even dentists themselves have limited conceptions regarding the potential of this 32-member strong, hardest natural arsenal of human body, known as human dentition, which render them to survive various thermal, chemical and physical assaults where all other body tissues may not survive to enable identification.

Around the globe, since decades, forensic dentists have been credited for solving multiple mysterious cases involving human identifications or age estimations and facial reconstructions for both high-profile cases and even in mass fatality disasters.

Forensic Odontology is the study of dental applications in legal proceedings. Human identification is a mainstay of civilization and the identification of unknown individuals always has been of paramount importance to the society. Forensic Odontology plays an important role in the retrieval of evidence and identification, having a high degree of reliability and simplicity.

The science of Forensic Odontology is comparatively new in India and is still struggling to establish itself as a known specialty amongst its citizens. Lack of subject teaching at undergraduate level and simultaneously no specialization or postgraduate course in this discipline may be the two main factors for general lack of interest in this subject, which is having a promising future and bright prospects, both in India and abroad.

Textbook of Forensic Odontology, in its first edition, has been tailored to make the subject interesting and easy-to-understand for undergraduates and has also included the requisite details needed for postgraduate students in the subject of oral pathology, oral medicine and forensic medicine.

Various disciplines like identification, age estimation, bite marks have been presented as separate chapters, supplemented with concerned historical cases and color photographs.

Importance of dental record keeping and guildelines involving forensic photography has been well emphasized.

In this very first endeavor of ours, we have utilized our efforts in best possible way to bring out to students a simple and concise volume of this book, which we promise will be interesting to readers, yet errors may have been incorporated inadvertently. Readers are always welcome for their suggestions and constructive criticism to make the title more authentic.

Nitul Jain

Acknowledgments

As popularly said, no dream is too big. To author a book on my name had been a long awaited dream for me for the last many years. Thanks to Almighty God for listening and fulfilling my dream. This dream would have remained dream only, if I had not got support from my friends, colleagues and my family members.

I am immensely thankful to Prof Dr Pushparaja Shetty, Head, Department of Oral Pathology, AB Shetty Memorial Institute of Dental Sciences, Mangalore, India, for his valuable guidance throughout my postgraduation. With his vast knowledge, he has always been a constant source of inspiration for me.

It is with great honor and pride that I convey my honest gratitude to my honorable sir, Prof Dr VS Sabane, Ex-Principal, Bharati Vidya Peeth Dental College and Hospital, Pune, and Head, Department of Oral Pathology, Eklavya Dental College and Hospital, Kotputli, for his able guidance and help. I thank him for the personal concern he has shown throughout preparation of the manuscript.

I especially wish to say thanks to Mr Tarun Duneja, Director-Publishing, Jaypee Brothers Medical Publishers (P) Ltd, New Delhi, for showing utmost belief in new authors and giving me an opportunity to fulfill my dream. I also need to say thanks to Mr KK Raman (Production Manager), Ms Samina Khan (PA to Director-Publishing), Mr Ashutosh Srivastava (Asstt. Editor), Mr Manoj Pahuja (Graphic Designer), Mr Rakesh Kumar (DTP Operator) and entire staff of Jaypee Brothers Medical Publishers, for patiently answering all my queries and making this title published.

Contents

Chapter 1

Forensic Sciences: The Historical Perspective and Branches

Nitul Jain

Chapter Overview

- Identification parameters
- Historical aspects
- Events and advances
- Most famous contributors to Forensic Sciences
- What is a forensic dentist?

INTRODUCTION

Bodies may remain undiscovered until they are wholly or partially skeletonized for a number of reasons. Some bodies are deliberately concealed after death, whereas for others, death occurs in isolated or inaccessible areas. However, a proportion of severely decomposed bodies are found in the deceased's own home months, or even years after death **(Fig. 1.1)**. Sometimes, these cases receive extensive media coverage and the sadness of the circumstances may be seen as an indictment on society and on responsible authorities. Long delays in the discovery of bodies in houses often occur because the deceased was socially isolated in life. Factors such as mental and physical illness or disability, drug and alcohol addiction, or trauma from previous abuse can contribute to, or accompany, a person's disengagement from society.

Modern conveniences, such as telephone banking, 24 hours shopping and internet access, can also help to eliminate the need for physical interaction with others. Additionally, automated payment systems can allow rent and bill paying to continue long after death. The discovery of skeletonized or partially skeletonized remains in dwellings raises numerous social and legal questions that must be addressed as part of a coronial investigation.

However, the effects of decomposition can complicate the autopsy and render some routine procedures, such as organ histology, less useful.

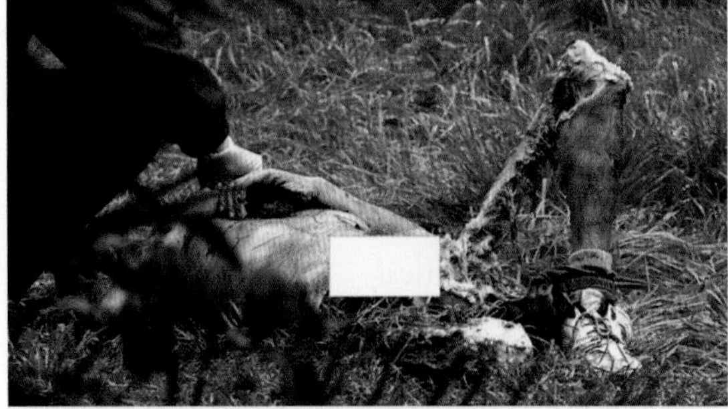

Fig. 1.1: Decomposed body showing human remains after a catastrophe

The passage of time can also cause difficulties at other levels of the investigation since the recollections of witnesses potentially fade, and death scenes may become contaminated and altered.

Given the complexity of the medicolegal investigation required of these cases, it is preferable for a combination of specialists to address the major questions raised by the coroner or other relevant authority. There are a variety of techniques available from forensic pathology, anthropology, odontology and entomology that may help to establish the deceased's identity, cause of death, factors contributing to death and the timing of death.

Forensic identifications by their nature are multidisciplinary team efforts relying on positive identification methodologies as well as presumptive or exclusionary methodologies. Typically, this effort involves the cooperation and coordination of law enforcement officials, forensic pathologists, forensic odontologists, forensic anthropologists, serologists, criminalists, and other specialists as deemed necessary. In each discipline, there is the need to develop scientific evidence relative to the questions of fact regarding identification in a defensible manner grounded on general rules of acceptance, reliability and relevance.

Most techniques applied are used by all or most of the disciplines, often for slightly different purposes. In the forensic sciences, a great deal of effort is spent on the identity or confirmation of identity of the victim(s) and perpetrator(s). This labor intensive aspect of a medicolegal investigation focuses on the six major questions, asked in any such forensic investigation:

1. Who is the victim?
2. What are the injuries?
3. How were the injuries sustained?
4. Where did the injuries occur?
5. When did the injuries occur?
6. If the injuries were caused by another person, by whom?

Each of the questions are correlated. Most investigations involve several "autopsies", one of the victim(s), one of the scene, and one of the circumstances of injury and/or death. These "autopsies" are designed to discover and preserve evidence, document that evidence, analyze that evidence, and apply that evidence towards reconstructing the events leading to the injury and/or death. Most such investigations focus on physical evidence that is deposited or transferred from victim to perpetrator and vice versa. This presumed relationship is known as Locard's principle and is the basis for much of what is attempted in the fields of criminalistics and forensic chemistry.

The development and application of molecular biology techniques, especially DNA profiling, reflects this principle and the current reliance on technology in medicolegal investigations.

Identification Parameters

Legal certification of an individual's identity is based on a number of parameters most of which are centered about the individual's appearance and personal effects. As such, many persons are buried or cremated based on a visual identification or other presumptive identification methods. Where possible, a positive identification is preferred to a presumptive identification in such medicolegal cases. Positive identifications traditionally involve a comparison of pre and postmortem data which are considered unique to the individual. These methods include **(Figs 1.2A to C)**:

1. Dental comparisons,
2. Fingerprints, palm prints, and footprints,
3. DNA identifications, and
4. Radiographic superimpositions (vertebrae, cranial structures including frontal sinuses, pelvic structures, bone trabeculae and prosthesis).

Presumptive identifications, which include visual recognition, personal effects, serology, anthropometric data, and medical history do not

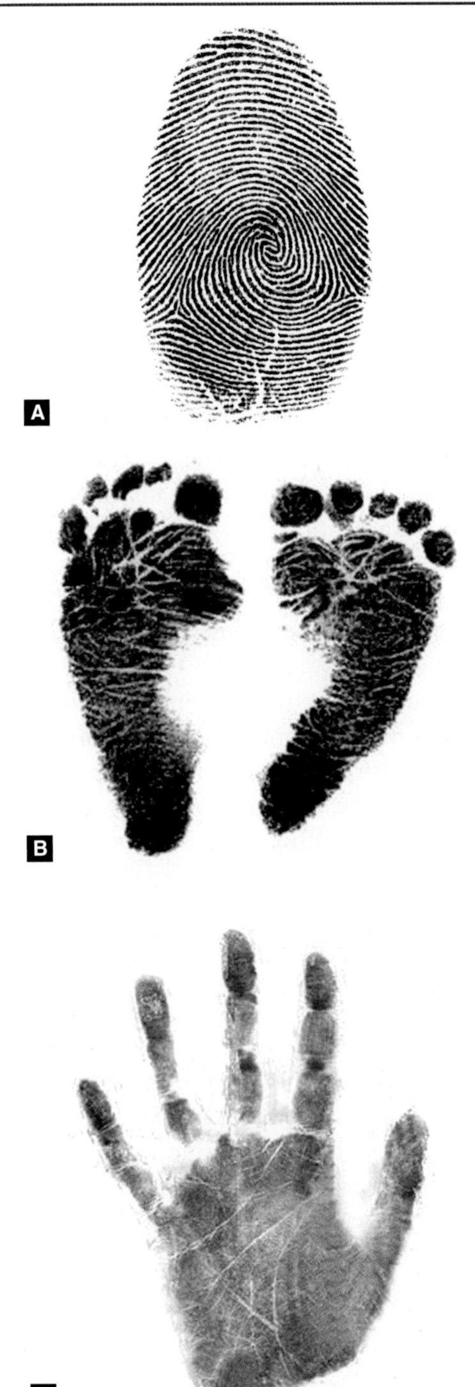

Figs 1.2A to C: One of the identification parameters used for human identification, (A) Fingerprints, (B) Foot prints, (C) Palm prints

usually identify unique characteristics of the individual but rather present a series of general or class characteristics which may exclude others based on race, sex, build, age, blood group, etc. Most positive identifications today are based on dental examinations and fingerprints and are fundamental procedures in medicolegal death investigations including mass disasters. The development of DNA analysis is providing investigators with yet another very important tool in the identification process.

The identification of unknown deceased persons is the primary focus of the forensic odontologist. This is usually achieved by comparison of the antemortem dental records and postmortem dental charts. There is usually copious circumstantial evidence to suggest identity when people are found deceased in their homes; however, formal confirmation is still required to eliminate doubt. Locating the treating dentist can be time consuming and sometimes impossible in cases involving socially isolated people, as they may not have visited a dentist for many years (if at all). Also, the dentist may be located far from where now they live, either interstate or overseas. However, despite the inherent difficulties, a search for treating dentists should always be attempted. This is especially true where no relatives can be located to provide a DNA sample for comparative analysis.

Odontologists may also examine the teeth and orofacial skeleton for trauma. They may potentially identify chips, breaks or recent tooth loss that can indicate antemortem trauma to the mouth. Such injuries could be sustained either as a result of non-accidental or accidental trauma. Odontologists can also examine the structure of the teeth and jaws, and degree of dental attrition for clues that may support anthropological age estimates.

Historical Aspects

The word Forensic is derived from the Latin forens(is): of or belonging to the forum, public, equivalent to for(um) forum + ens — of, belonging to + ic. By extension it came to also mean disputative, argumentative, rhetorical, belonging to debate or discussion. From there it is but a small step to the modern definition of forensic as pertaining to, connected with, or used in courts of judicature or public discussion and debate. Thus the forensic sciences encompass the application of specialized scientific and/or technical knowledge to questions of civil and criminal law, especially in court proceedings. Forensic Medicine has come to be recognized as a special science or discipline that deals with relationships and applications of medical facts and knowledge to legal problems. Some prefer to call it legal medicine or medical jurisprudence.

Evidence of the origin of legal or forensic medicine can be found in records of ancient people some thousands of years ago, when occasionally a law appears to influence medicine or medicine is found to influence or modify a law. The Egyptian, Imhotep, may have been the first to apply both the law and medicine to his surroundings. Hammurabi codified medical law circa 2200 BC, and medicolegal issues were covered in early Jewish law. Later, other civilizations — the Greeks, ancient India, the Roman Empire—evolved jurisprudential standards involving medical fact or opinion. Early cultures recognized the desirability of controlling the organization, duties, and liabilities of the medical profession. They also were acquainted with the importance of the knowledge and opinion of the medical person in the legal consideration of issues of great moment such as the use of drugs or poisons, the duration of pregnancy, virginity, superfetation, the prognosis of wounds in different body locations (a physician determined that only one of Caesar's 23 stab wounds was fatal), sterility and impotence, sexual deviation, and suspicious death. Early in the sixteenth century a separate discipline of forensic medicine began to emerge. New codes of law required expert medical testimony in trials of certain types of crime or civil action. The first medicolegal books appeared in the late sixteenth and early seventeenth centuries and, after 1650, lectures on legal medicine were given in Germany and France. The first book on medical jurisprudence in the English language appeared in 1788 and 19 years later the first Regius Chair in Forensic Medicine was recognized by the Crown at the University of Edinburgh. The English coroner's system was imported to the colonies in North America in 1607, and it was not until 1871 that Massachusetts, later followed by New York and other jurisdictions, established a medical examiner system. Upon this base of professionalism in death investigation, supported by the framework of solid scientific and technical advances during the twentieth century, was erected the modern structure of forensic medicine which covers a heterogeneous, sometimes loosely related, family of numerous disciplines or subspecialties sharing a common interest.

Forensic dentistry can be defined in many ways. One of the more elegant definitions is simply that forensic dentistry represents the overlap between the dental and the legal professions.

There is an extensive history of the distinctive nature of tooth arrangement with legal implications. As no two fingers are identical, neither two mouth nor two teeth are exactly identical. Identification of human remains by dental characteristics is a long standing and well established component of forensic science.

Right through history, the human dentition has been used numerous times in identifying individuals. Harvey (1973) has traced one of the earliest recorded incidences of dental identification to 66 AD, when the severed head of the wife of Roman emperor Nero was identified by a rival from her black anterior tooth. In (1193) AD, the Maharaja of Kannauj, Jai Chandra Rathor was identified by his false teeth following his death in a battle. The English king Charles 'the bold', who also died in battle in 1477, was identified from his dental features, courtesy the court physician who identified his two recently extracted teeth (Furness, 1972).

Paul Revere is credited as being the first dentist to identify a person from dental features (Luntz, 1970). He identified his friend Joseph Warren, a victim in the American Revolution in 1775 from a silver and ivory bridge which he had prepared.

Gustafson (1962) suggests that the role of forensic odontology in human identification came to prominence only towards the end of the 19th century, after two major fires in Europe. The first occurred in 1881, when the 'Ring Theatre' in Vienna was destroyed during a performance, with 449 casualties. The second, the Charity Bazaar fire in Paris in 1897, resulted in the deaths of 127 people. In both these events, dental features were used for identification.

According to Harvey (1973), one of the dentists who assisted the identifications in Paris was a Cuban named Oscar Amoedo. In 1898, he wrote one of the first books on forensic odontology, *L'art Dentaire en Medicine Legale*, and is considered a pioneer of modern forensic dentistry.

According to Suzuki however, the first course in forensic dentistry was probably conducted by Professor Sadanori Mita of Japan as early as 1903. The correspondence course outlined "methods of examination, evaluation and classification of bite marks and the differences between ante- and post-mortem appearances". This course subsequently formed the basis of his lectures at Tokyo Dental College between 1922 and 1936.

Forensic dentists in the 20th century have made major contributions in identification: notable among the cases are **(Figs 1.3A and B)** Adolph Hilter (1945), Zia–ul–Haq (1988) and Rajiv Gandhi (1991).

Apart from dental identification, forensic odontology is also applied in the investigation of crimes caused by the dentition, such as bite marks **(Fig. 1.4)**. Bite marks are a common feature of sex crimes and violent fights. They may also occur on objects such as chewing gum or chocolate that may be found at a crime scene.

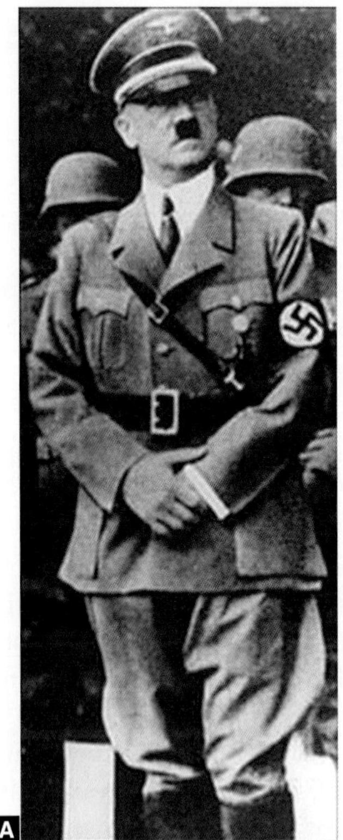

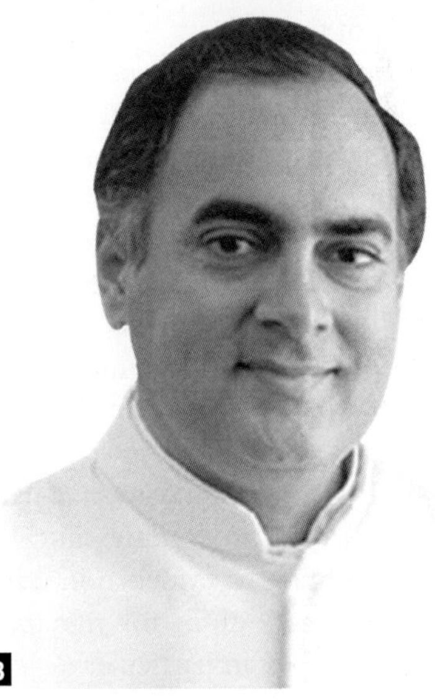

Figs 1.3A and B: (A) German ruler Adolf Hitler, whose identification was done because of his dental prosthesis, (B) Rajiv Gandhi

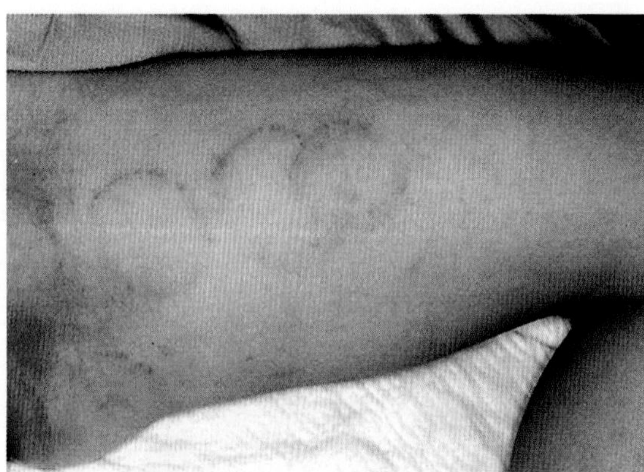

Fig. 1.4: Multiple bite marks on a victim's leg showing an important parameter of identification for the culprit

Bite marks, however, are not a recent discovery. As early as the 6th century AD, the Indian sage Vatsyayana had devoted an entire chapter on 'love bites,' with a detailed classification in the book Kama Sutra (Harvey, 1973).

In medieval Britain, during the reign of William I (1027–1087 AD), green wax seals with the impression of the king's teeth were implanted on state documents to avoid falsification and indicate the authenticity of the seal.

The use of bite marks as evidence in court can be traced back to 1692 in the United States.

Harvey (1973) cites a 1906 case where, a burglar was convicted in Britain because his dental models matched the marks left on cheese found at the crime scene. Subsequently there have been numerous cases that made use of bite marks with varying degrees of success. Therefore, bite marks remained a contentious area of forensic sciences. However, over the later half of the 20th century, bite mark procedures have greatly advanced and it is now routinely used in court proceedings in the West. Its objective application as evidence in crime can have far reaching implications for the society in general and criminology in particular.

Forensic dentists also handle bite marks caused by animals. This requires a basic knowledge of various animal dentitions, the study of which is known as comparative anatomy.

As a result of its versatile use, forensic dentists are considered an integral part of the forensic team of experts.

Events and Advances

Keiser-Nielsen assessed the uniqueness of teeth mathematically.

Sognnaes et al (1982), demonstrated the uniqueness of bite marks even in identical twins by computer comparison.

Vale et al (1976) indicated at least 6 possible positions of each tooth to demonstrate individuality. Fellingham and coworkers have calculated that there are 1.8×10^{19} possible combinations of the 32 teeth being intact, decayed, missing or filled.

Sweet and Pretty considered the size, shape and pattern of the incisal or biting edges of upper and lower anterior teeth to be specific to an individual.

In the past, bite mark evidence was analyzed by the use of the transparent overlay technique. This method uses a clear thin sheet of acetate paper laid over a photographic transparency or print of the inflicted area. The marks of the bite are traced on paper and compared with the tracing of the incisal and cutting edges of the teeth of a suspect. By this method persons could be included or excluded as possible suspects.

Transilluminating the tissue and intensification of the image have produced sharp image details of damage to the tissue caused by biting forces. Transillumination is easily adopted for use with a cadaver but is of limited value with the living victim of a bite.

The xeroradiographic enhancement of the incisal edge is apparent. The impression left by the incisal edges can be accurately compared with the dentition producing the original bite.

Videotape analysis of bite mark evidence was introduced in a California court. Photography and videotaping of the evidence at right angles are absolutely necessary. Many hours of editing are needed to achieve results from the videotape.

David TJ et al have used scanning electron microscopy in bite mark analysis. With the use of SEM, what appeared to be class characteristics were clearly identified as individual characteristics.

David Sweet proposed a computer-based technique for the production of life sized bite mark comparison overlays. This method allows objective selection of the biting surfaces of a suspect's teeth from dental study casts, which can be used in bite mark analysis.

Over the later half of the 20th century, bite mark procedures have greatly advanced and are now routinely used in court proceedings in the West. Its objective application as evidence in crime can have far reaching implications for the society in general and criminology in particular.

Most Famous Contributors to Forensic Sciences

1813, Mathiew Orfila: Father of modern toxicology, made significant contributions to the development of tests for the presence of blood in a forensic context and is credited as the first to attempt the use of a microscope in the assessment of blood and semen stains.

1835, Henry Goddard, of Scotland Yard's Police, first used bullet comparison to catch a murderer.

1879, Bertillon began to develop the science of anthropometry

1891, Hans Gross, **(Fig. 1.5A)** coined the word Criminalistics

1900, Karl Landsteiner **(Fig. 1.5B)** first discovered human blood groups and was awarded the Nobel Prize for his work in 1930. Formed the basis of all subsequent work.

1928, Locard's Exchange Principle **(Fig. 1.6)**, according to which whenever two objects come into contact there is always a transfer of material.

1977, Masato Soba, a latent print examiner was the first to develop latent prints intentionally by "Super glue (r)" fuming.

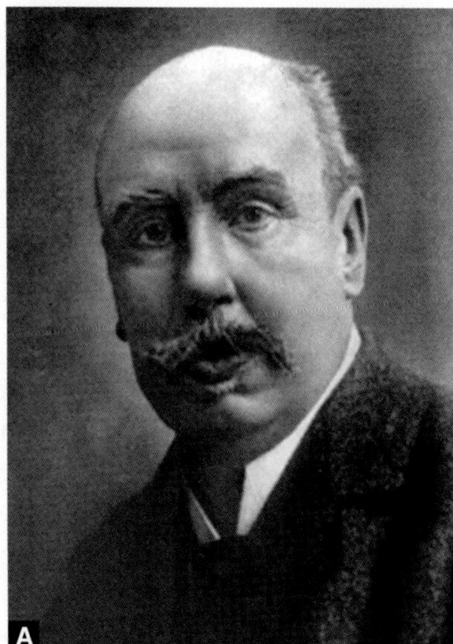

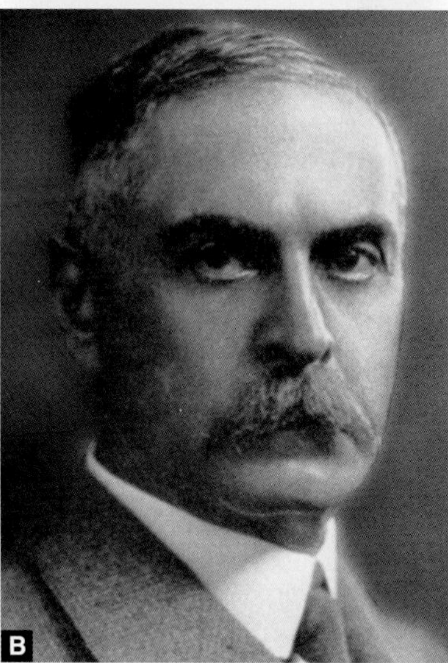

Figs 1.5A and B: (A) Hans Gross, the important contributor to the field of forensic sciences. (B) Karl Landsteiner, who discovered the most commonly used blood grouping system

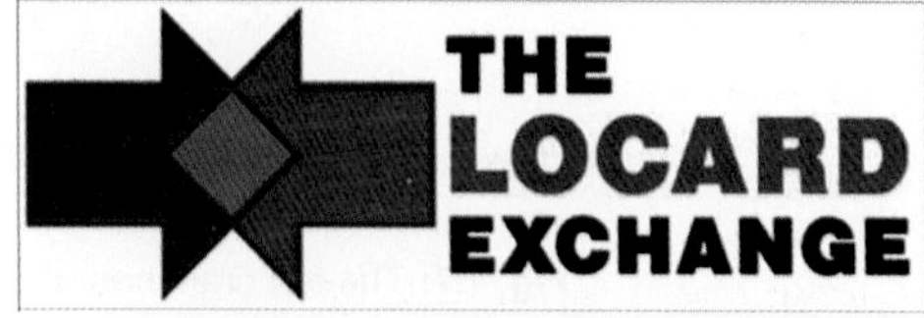

Fig. 1.6: The Locard exchange principle

1998, FBI DNA database—NIDIS, enabling interstate cooperation in linking crimes, was put into practice.

2000, CODIS (Combined DNA Index System) Identification system used tracking suspects by DNA profiling

What is a Forensic Dentist?

A forensic dentist is first a scientist. When he applies his scientific knowledge to assist juries, attorneys, and judges in understanding science, he is a forensic dentist. Forensic scientists are thinkers, good with details, good with putting pieces of a puzzle together, and curious. They may work in laboratories, go out to crime scenes or teach in colleges and universities.

Importance

Primarily deals with identification based on recognition of unique features present in an individual's dental structures. Forensic odontology plays a major role in identification on man made or natural disasters events that result in fatalities that may not be identifiable through conventional means as fingerprints. Relies on sound knowledge of teeth, jaws and incorporates dental anatomy, histology, radiography, pathology, dental material and developmental anatomy.

It delves into:

1. Identifying unknown human remains through dental records
2. Assisting at the location of the mass disaster
3. Eliciting the ethnicity and assisting in building up a picture of lifestyle and diet of skeletal remains
4. Determining the gender of unidentified
5. Age estimation of both the living and deceased
6. Recognition and analysis of bite marks found on victims of attack
7. Presenting evidence in court as an expert witness.

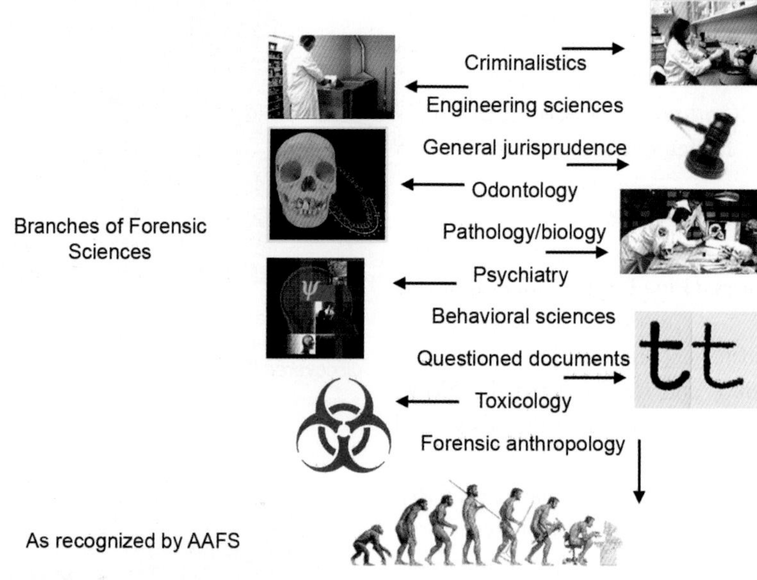

Fig. 1.7: The ten branches of Forensic Sciences, as recognized by AAFS

The American academy of forensic sciences recognizes 10 areas of forensic endeavor (**Fig. 1.7**):

1. Criminalistics
2. Engineering science
3. General jurisprudence
4. Odontology
5. Pathology/biology
6. Psychiatry
7. Behavior science
8. Questioned documents
9. Toxicology
10. Physical anthropology

Criminalistics: Analyze, compare, identify, and interpret physical evidence. Involved in area of laboratory testing of various types of physical evidence, including biologic fluids, DNA and suspicious chemicals.

Engineering science: Structural aspects of crime/accident scene. Applies the principles of mathematics and science for to the purpose of the law. How could the accident have happened? Why did the airplane crash?

General jurisprudence: Application of science to assist courts in resolving questions of fact in criminal and civil trials.

Forensic dentistry (odontology): A vital branch of forensic science that involves the application of dental science to the identification of unknown human remains and bite marks, using both physical and biological dental evidence.

Pathology: The study of disease: Pathologists study disease by performing an autopsy and examining the tissues removed, Analysis of fluids taken from the body, such as blood or urine.

Forensic anthropologists: Identify individuals killed in disasters resulting in the death and mutilation of bodies

Forensic psychiatry and behavior sciences: Address a broad range of legal issues. In criminal law, such issues as competence (e.g. competency to stand trial and to testify) and the assessment of mental illness or innocence by reason of mental illness or defect are the focus.

Questioned documents: The document examiner discovers and proves the facts concerning documents and related material, such as ink, paper, toner from a copier or fax, and ribbons, such as from a typewriter. Questions such as: Who wrote this? Is this a true signature? Has this document been altered? Are there additions and/or erasures on this check?

Toxicology: the study of harmful effects of chemicals or drugs on living systems. It primarily deals with the medicolegal aspects of toxicology.

BIBLIOGRAPHY

1. Archer MS, et al. Social isolation and delayed discovery of bodies in houses: The value of forensic pathology, anthropology, odontology and entomology in the medicolegal investigation. Forensic Science International 2005;151:259-65.
2. Fairgrieve SI, SEM Analysis of incinerated teeth as an aid to positive identification. J Forensic Sci. 1994;39(2):557-65.
3. Melissa N. The role of the dentist at crime scenes. Dent Clin N Am 2007;51:837-56.
4. Pretty IA, Sweet. A look at forensic dentistry—Part 1: The role of teeth in the determination of human identity. British Dental Journal 2001;190:359-66.

Chapter 2

Forensic Odontology and its Applications

Hemanth M, Anil Pandey

Chapter Overview

- Definition
- Dental identification
- Bite marks
- Identification
- Comparative dental identification
- Principles and phases of dental identification
- Reconstructive postmortem: Dental profiling
- Opinion from forensic anthropologists
- Role of DNA molecule in identification

As we enter a new millennium, society is faced with fresh challenges in every conceivable area. Despite leaps in modern technology, medical breakthroughs and the geographical changes that the last century has brought, crime still persists in all aspects of our lives. Violent and heinous activities that shatter the lives of victims, their friends and families occur everyday. Often, little can be done to repair such damage. The apprehension and subsequent prosecution of the perpetrator(s) is essential to maintain law and order. Through the specialty of forensic odontology, dentistry plays a small but significant role in this process. By identifying the victims of crime and disaster through dental records, dentists assist those involved in crime investigation. Always part of a bigger team, such personnel are dedicated to the common principles of all those involved in forensic casework: the rights of the dead and those who survive them. The most common role of the forensic dentist is the identification of deceased individuals.

Definition

"That branch of dentistry which, in interest of justice deals with proper handling and examination of dental evidence, and with the proper evaluation and presentation of dental findings".

—FDI recognizes two distinct areas, identification and bite marks

Dental Identification

Based on theory that all individuals are unique

All humans are born with anomalies or acquire artifacts.

- An anomaly is a unique congenital condition (e.g. mesiodens, missing lateral incisor, spina bifida)
- An artifact is man made alteration (dental restorations, extracted tooth, scar, tattoo, appendectomy).

Types of Identification

The identification is of two basic types: Unknown and Confirmation

BITE MARKS

This is also based on the fact that no two dentitions are identical.

Bite mark has traditionally been defined as "a pattern injury": That is any injury in which the instrument of injury can be determined and possibly may be individualized as the weapon making the injury.

A bite mark is an injury to skin in which the instruments of the injury are teeth. The injury is a contusion caused by the rupture of small blood vessels as the individual teeth compress the tissue. In contrast to finger prints, which leave a definite ridge marks, bite marks leave blurred contusions, which tend to leak in surrounding tissues.

IDENTIFICATION

Why a Dentist for Identification?

A dentist is the best person to solve the mysteries of crime because of the following reasons, which he can deal in a better way than others. As all of us know that teeth are the hardest substance in body and these may be only tissue available to identify after surviving most of insults and consequences encountered at death and during decomposition (explosions, accidental trauma, aircraft crashes). Various authors have said tooth to be more unique than the DNA. Identification, using dental impressions is an invaluable tool. Most scientists agree that bite marks are even more unique than DNA—Identical twins share the same genetic makeup, but their dental impressions will differ.

Tooth has been used as the cornerstone in positive identification of living/deceased persons using the unique traits and characteristics of teeth and jaw. Also, using the forensic techniques in dental tissue are the most challenging aspect of this discipline.

"There are 28 teeth, plus four wisdom teeth, in an adult's dentition," Delattre says, "each tooth has five surfaces, for a possible total of 160 surfaces. Each surface has its own characteristics and may have fillings, crowns, extractions, bridges, etc. In addition to the teeth we see in our mouths, the roots and bone around them are specific to each person." Given all of these parameters, it is safe to say that the physical make-up of each person's dentition is unique.

That's why of all the above mentioned reasons that a dentist, possessing the vast knowledge of oro-facial tissues may be better able to answer the questions arising during a death investigation, where all other forensic ancilliary techniques have been failed to conclude on an unknown identity.

Three types of personal identification circumstances that use teeth, jaws and oro-facial characteristics exist in forensic odontology.

1. Comparative dental identification: The most frequently performed examination is a comparative identification that is used to establish (to a high degree of certainty) that the remains of a decedent and a person represented by antemortem (before death) dental records are the same individual. Information from the body or circumstances usually contains clues as to who has died.
2. Reconstructive postmortem dental profiling: In those cases where antemortem records are not available, and no clues to the possible identity exist, a postmortem (after death) dental profile is completed by the forensic dentist suggesting characteristics of the individual likely to narrow the search for the antemortem materials.
3. Others (mainly DNA profiling methods) when no other evidence remains apart form a small tissue fragments.

COMPARATIVE DENTAL IDENTIFICATION

When body is too fragmented/mutilated/ incinerated, identification by next of kin i.e. (visual recognition) may give false positive or false negative results. **(Figs 2.1A to C)**. Circumstantial evidences including personal possessions (wallets, jewelry) and context of scene may suggest who it is that has died. Antemortem records for this person is sought for. Intra/extra oral radiographs, clinical photographs, study casts, ortho/prostho appliances, mouth guards all can be used. Congenital/acquired characteristics are compared. Discrepancies may also be seen, but should be explainable.

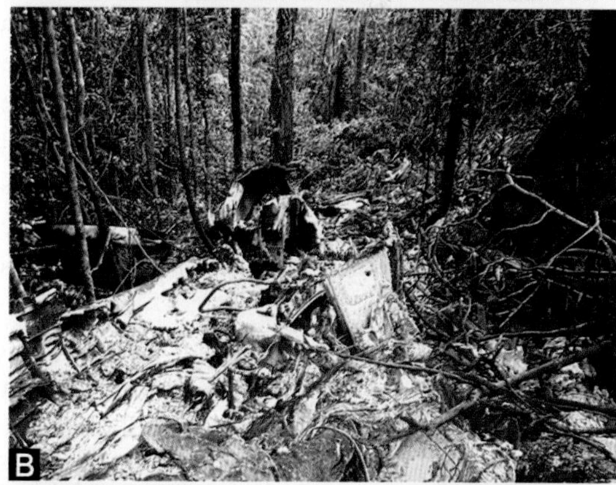

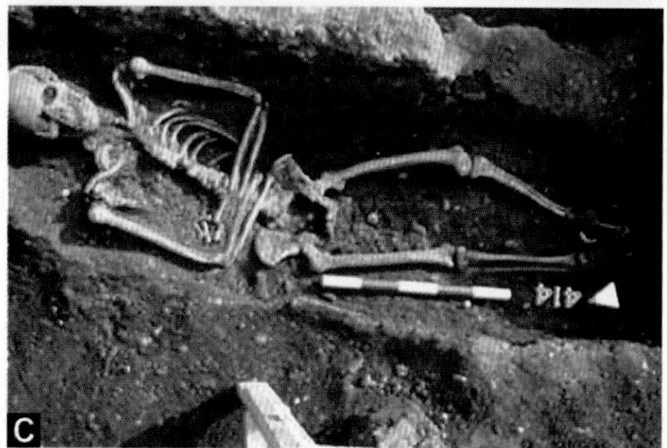

Figs 2.1A to C: (A and B) Decomposed human remains in various kind of assaults making identification almost impossible, (C) Skeltonized human remains found in a grave

Dental identification of humans occurs for a number of different reasons and in a number of different situations (see **Table 2.1**).

a. The bodies of victims of violent crimes, fires, motor vehicle accidents and work place accidents, can be disfigured to such an extent that identification by a family member is neither reliable nor desirable.
b. Persons who have been deceased for some time prior to discovery and those found in water also present unpleasant and difficult visual identifications.
c. Dental identifications have always played a key role in natural and manmade disaster situations and in particular the mass casualties normally associated with aviation
d. Because of the lack of a comprehensive fingerprint database, dental identification continues to be crucial in the United Kingdom.

An overarching principle is recognition and evaluation of certain changes over time like radiological comparisons of progression of carious lesions, changes in alveolar bone contours (see **Table 2.2**).

Principles and Phases of Dental Identification

Typically, human remains are found and reported to the police who then initiate a request for dental identification. Often a presumptive or tentative identification is available (i.e. wallet or driving license may be found on the body) and this will enable antemortem records to be located. In other instances, the geographical location in which the body is found or other physical characteristics and circumstantial evidence, may enable a putative identification to be made, frequently using data

Table 2.1: Common reasons for identification of found human remains

Criminal	Typically an investigation to a criminal death cannot begin until the victim has been positively identified
Marriage	Individuals from many religious backgrounds cannot remarry unless their partners are confirmed decreased
Monetary	The payment of pensions, life assurance and other benefits relies upon positive confirmation of death
Burial	Many religions require that a positive identification be made prior to burial in geographical sites
Social	Society's duty to preserve human rights and dignity beyond life begins with the basic premise of an identity
Closure	The identification of individuals missing for prolonged periods can bring sorrowful relief to family members

Source: IA Pretty, Sweet. A look of forensic dentistry—Part 1: The role of teeth in the determination of human identity. British Dental Journal 2001;190:359-66.

Table 2.2: Features examined during the comparative dental identification. This extensive list represents the complexity of these cases, particularly in those instances in which restorative treatment is absent or minimal

Teeth

Teeth present
a. Erupted
b. Unerupted
c. Impacted

Missing teeth
a. Congenitally
b. Lost antemortem
c. Lost postmortem

Tooth type
a. Permanent
b. Deciduous
c. Mixed
d. Retained primary
e. Supernumerary

Tooth position
a. Malposition

Crown morphology
a. Size and shape
b. Enamel thickness
c. Contact points
d. Racial variatlons

Crown pathology
a. Caries
b. Attrition, abrasion, erosion
c. Atypical variations, enamel pearls, peg laterals etc.
d. Dentigerous cyst

Root morphology
a. Size
b. Shape
c. Number
d. Divergence of roots

Root morphology
a. Dilaceration
b. Root fracture
c. Hypercementosis
d. Root resorption
e. Root hemisections

Pulp chamber/root canal morphology
a. Size, shape and number
b. Secondary dentine

Pulp chamber/root canal pathology
a. Pulp stones, dystrophic calcification
b. Root canal therapy
c. Retrofills
d. Apicectomy

Periapical pathology
a. Abscess, granuloma or cysts
b. Cementomas
c. Condensing osteitis

Dental restorations
1. Metallic
   a. Non-full coverage
   b. Full coverage
2. Non-metallic
   a. Non-full coverage
   b. Laminates
   c. Full coverage
3. Dental implants
4. Bridges
5. Partial and full removable prosthesis

Periodontal tissues

Gingival morphology and pathology
a. Contour, recession, focal/ diffuse, enlargements, inter-proximal craters
b. Color – inflammatory changes, physiological (racial) or patho-logical pigmentations
c. Plaque and calculus deposits

Contd...

Contd...

Periodontal ligament morphology and pathology a. Thickness b. Widening c. Lateral periodontal cysts and similar *Alveolar process and lamina dura* a. Height, contour, density of crestal bone b. Thickness of interradicular bone c. Exostoses, tori d. Pattern of lamina dura e. Bone loss (horizontal/vertical) f. Trabecular bone pattern and bone islands g. Residual root fragments	**Anatomical features** *Maxillary sinus* a. Size, shape, cysts b. Foreign bodies, fistula c. Relationship to teeth *Anterior nasal spine* a. Incisive canal (size, shape, cyst) b. Median palatal suture *Mandibular canal* a. Mental foramen b. Diameter, anomalous c. Relationship to adjacent structures *Coronoid and condylar processes* a. Size and shape	b. Pathology *Temperomandibular joint* a. Size, shape b. Hypertrophy/atrophy c. Ankylosis, fracture d. Arthritic changes *Other pathologies* a. Developmental cysts b. Salivary gland pathology c. Reactive/neoplastic d. Metabolic bone disease e. Focal or dilfuse radiopacities f. Evidence of surgery g. Trauma – wires, surgical pins etc.

Source: IA Pretty, Sweet. A look of forensic dentistry—Part 1: The role of teeth in the determination of human identity. British Dental Journal 2001;190:359-66.

from the missing persons' database. Antemortem records are then obtained from the dentist of record.

Dental comparisons have high degree of reliability and simplicity. Teeth are most durable organ in body that can be heated to temperatures of 1600°C without appreciable loss of microstructure **(Figs 2.2A to E)**.

The dentist acts as a consultant to the medical examiner only when requested by the certifying official. He should always consider necessary armamentarium before proceeding. Excision of facial tissues when necessary to remove maxilla/mandible should occur with expressed concurrence of pathologist. The entire process should take place in following phased manners.

Phases

1. *Comprehensive consultation:* This is done in order to fulfill the need to establish characteristics of situation, and also to begin making appropriate arrangement for next steps.

2. *Preliminary evaluation:* After comprehensive consultation, the forensic odontologist should
   a. Establish exactly what is being requested
   b. Parameters of postmortem examination
   c. Ascertain nature of death and reason for dental input.

Because most of corpses are unidentifiable by other means, they are likely to be decomposed/burned/completely skeltonized. Knowing situation in advance can help to prepare for the type of disfigurement. One must also, ensure that antemortem records are being obtained for comparison at later stage. The examiner should also make necessary arrangement for suitable radiographs of corpse.

3. *Postmortem examination:* Typically done after pathologist completes autopsy and possibly after other experts, such as forensic anthropologists, radiologists. It is prudent to initiate examination of corpse before viewing ante-mortem information. It is in many ways similar to living person's examination except for limited access because of rigidity of corpse (rigor mortis, refrigeration or decomposition). If excision of jaws is necessary,

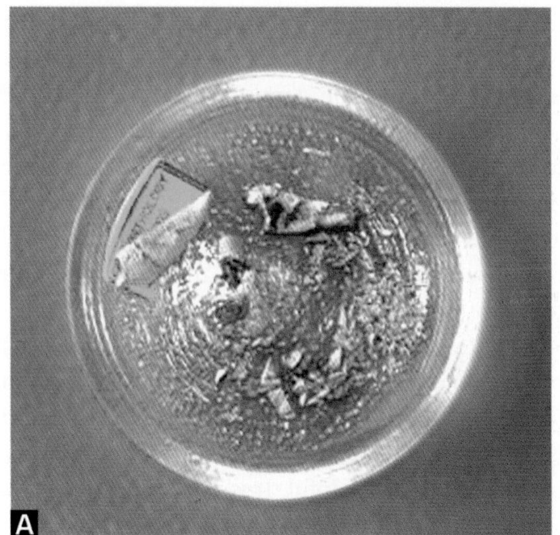

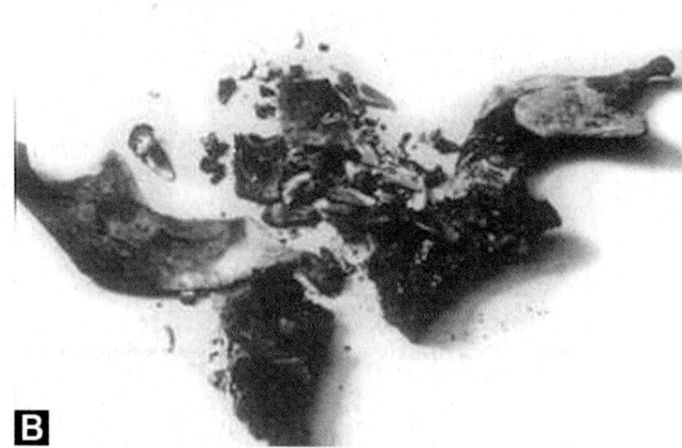

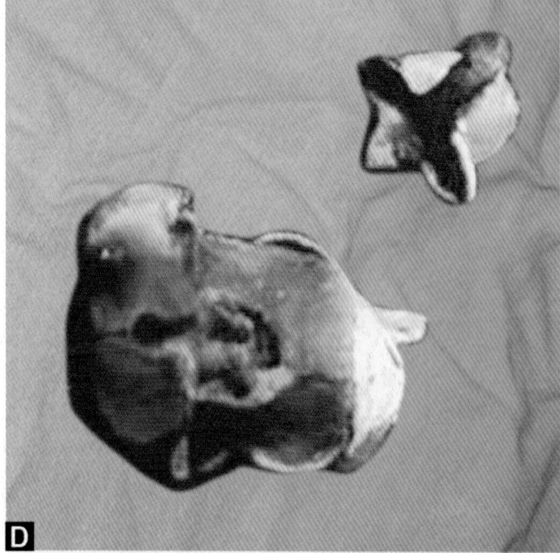

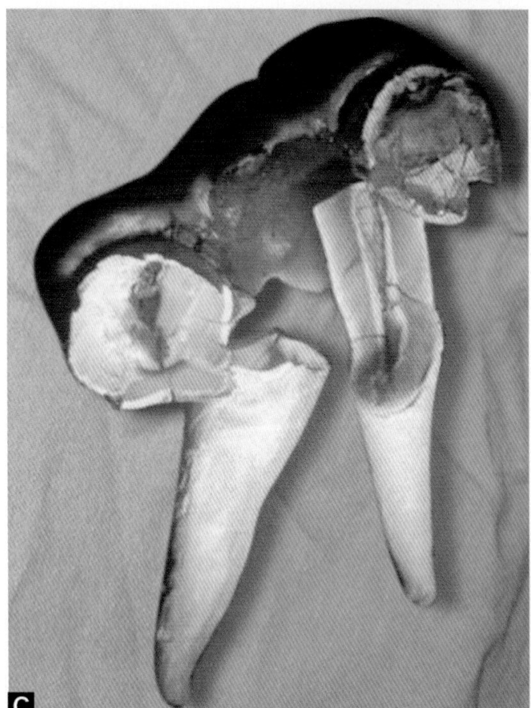

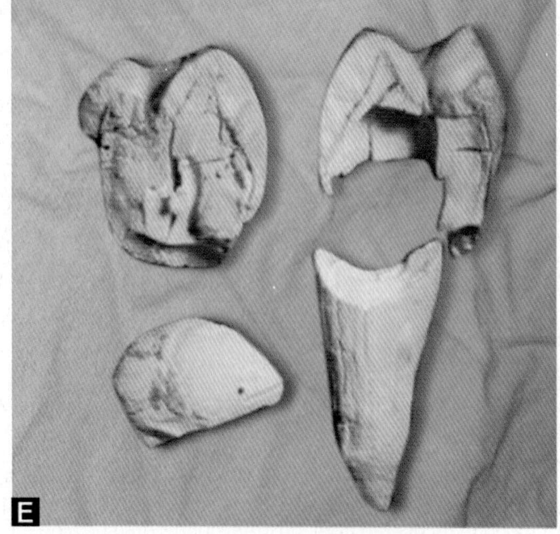

Figs 2.2A to E: (A) Tooth fragments recovered after a burn episode, (B) Jaw fragments form a burnt corpse, (C to E) Tooth remains after an experimental exposure of teeth to a temperature of approximately 1000°C

Le-fort osteotomy of maxilla and a horizontal or tangential osteotomy of ascending ramus of mandible posterior to the last molar tooth is preferred. Since teeth may be brittle in burned cases, they need to be reinforced with cyanoacrylate cement, polyvinyl cement, or clear acrylic spray paint prior to examination.

Radiographic examination: Charting of dental/soft tissues/hard tissues findings are then completed on standardized forms.

4. *Antemortem investigation and data collection:* Often clues from personal effects, **(Figs 2.3A and B)** history, tattoos, scars, ethnicity, sex or other features may point out to some one's identity that is who it is most likely to be? Then after proper legal proceedings the dentist whom the deceased most likely might have visited before death is located, and any information pertaining to the deceased is sought after (antemortem records). All available materials from all the dentists, medical records, hospitals is charted and translated on forms.

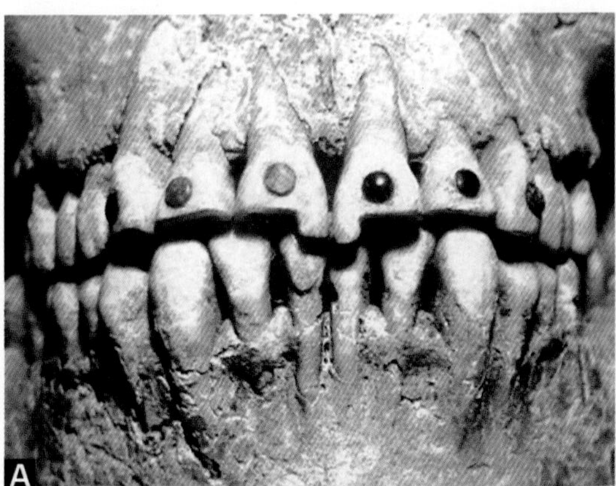

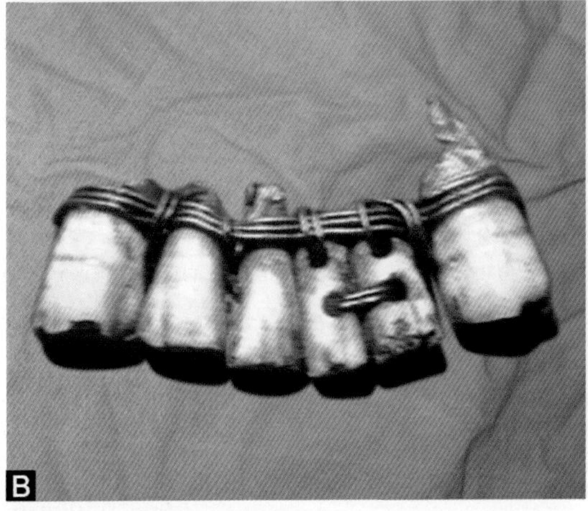

Figs 2.3A and B: (A) An ancient file photo showing various kind of traits of that particular era embedded in the dentition, (B) A bridge recovered from the prehistorical era showing the splinting of the teeth by wire

Universal system is **(Figs 2.4A and B)** predominantly used in USA, while FDI system **(Fig. 2.5)** is followed in the rest of the world and is also recommended by WHO. Bitewing views are particularly more helpful. It is important to always ask for original records. Other types of records-casts, prosthesis, photographs, appliances, digital records are also investigated.

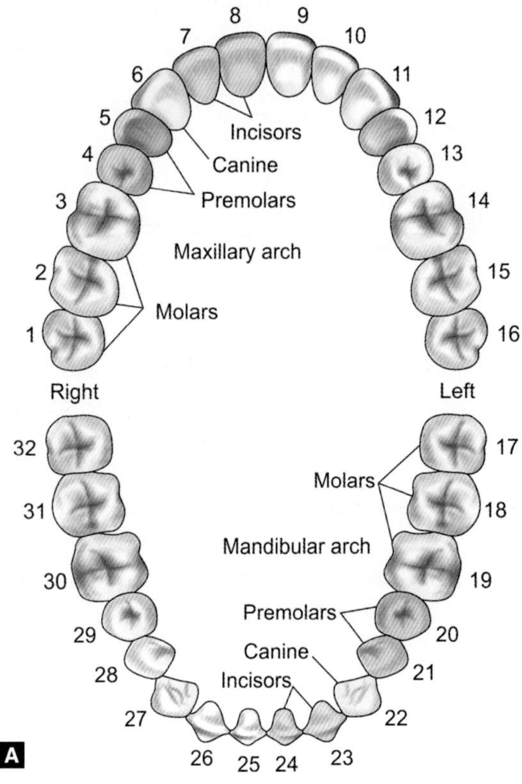

Fig. 2.4A

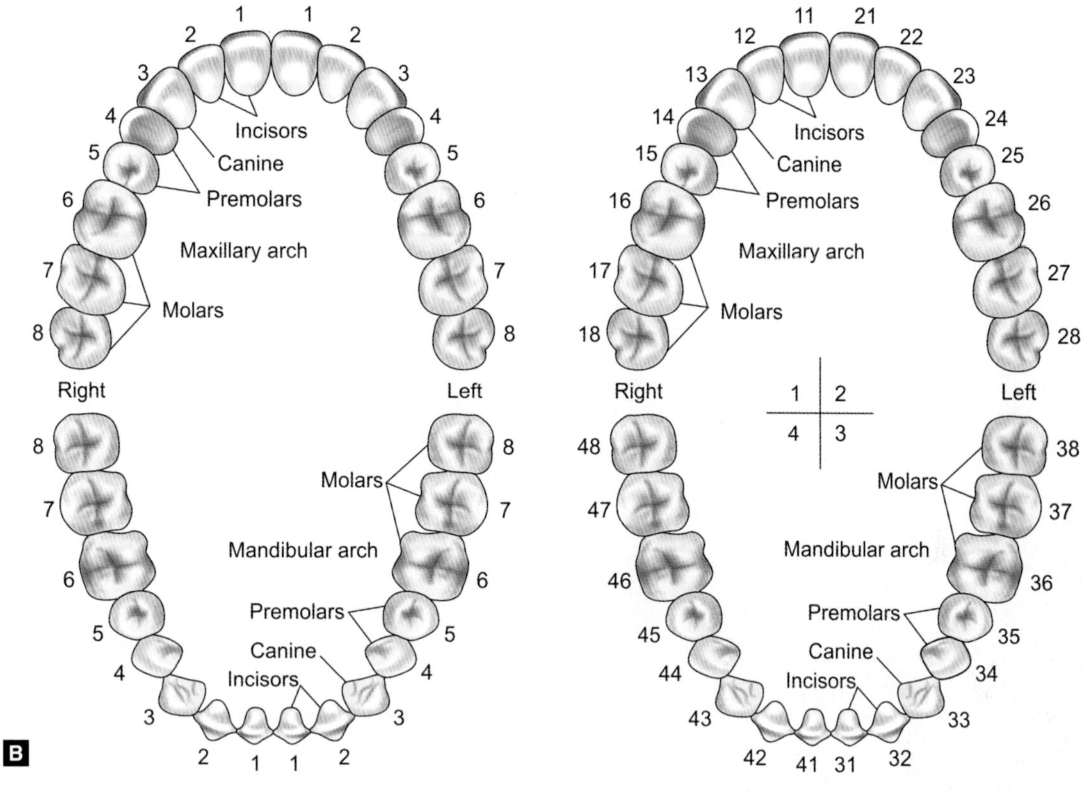

Fig. 2.4B

Figs 2.4A and B: (A) Universal system for nomenclature of permanent dentition, (B) Palmar system for nomenclature of permanent dentition

Fig. 2.5: FDI system of nomenclature for permanent dentition

5. *Comparison and conclusion:* Once all the AM/PM records are obtained and charted, results can be compared and a conclusion **(Figs 2.6A and B)** can be reached. It is vital to complete all identification procedures before the body is cremated. Note any potential discrepancies and develop suitable explanation for the same. Cases in which dentists/dental staff can fraud by billing for the procedures that were not performed should also be kept in mind.

Most commonly comparisons are made based on individual teeth and dental restorations encompassed along with presence/absence of teeth, tooth positions, recent extractions and eruption conditions. If there are no sufficient above mentioned comparisons, then the morphology of coronal/root portions of teeth, size/shape of pulp chamber along with any pathosis, size/location of nerve canals, foramina, sinuses and TMJ can compared. But rarely these are definitive solitary features to make an identity.

The forensic dentist produces the postmortem record by careful charting and written descriptions of the dental structures and radiographs. If the ante-mortem records are available at this time, postmortem radiographs should be taken to replicate the type and angle of these. Radiographs should be marked with a rubber-dam punch to indicate antemortem and postmortem to prevent confusion—one hole for antemortem films and two holes for postmortem films.

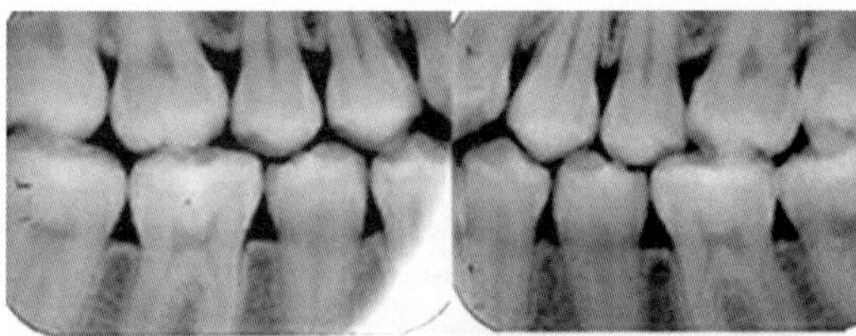

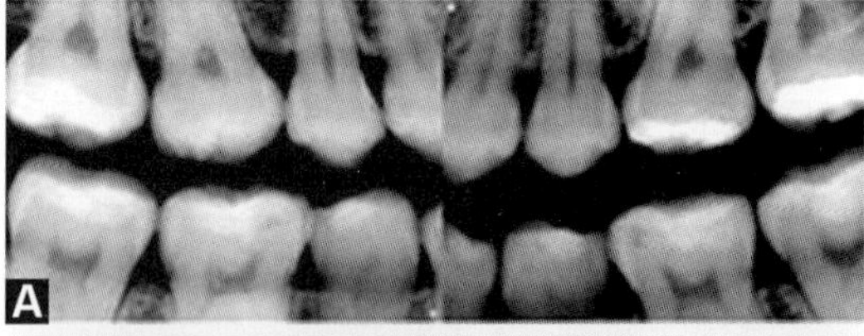

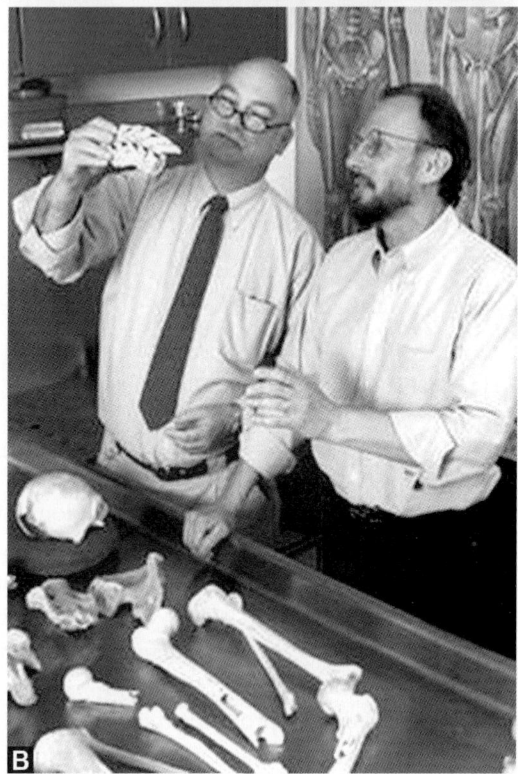

Figs 2.6A and B: (A) Radiograph showing the comparisons of ante-mortem and postmortem bite wing radiographs, (B) Picture showing the anthropological comparisons of human remains

A range of conclusions can be reached when reporting a dental identification. The American Board of Forensic Odontology recommends that these be limited to the following four conclusions:

1. *Positive identification:* The antemortem and postmortem data match in sufficient detail, with no unexplainable discrepancies, to establish that they are from the same individual.
2. *Possible identification:* The antemortem and postmortem data have consistent features but, because of the quality of either the postmortem remains or the antemortem evidence, it is not possible to establish identity positively.
3. *Insufficient evidence:* The available information is insufficient to form the basis for a conclusion.
4. *Exclusion:* The antemortem and postmortem data are clearly inconsistent.

It is important to note that there is no minimum number of concordant points or features that are required for a positive identification. In many cases a single tooth can be used for identification if it contains sufficient unique features. Equally, a full-mouth series of radiographs may not reveal sufficient detail to render a positive conclusion. The discretion of identification lies with the odontologist who must be prepared to justify the conclusions in court, surely the ultimate in peer-review.

Reconstructive Postmortem: Dental Profiling

When circumstantial evidences required to establish a presumptive identification are not available; it is necessary to assess personal features such as:

a. Age at death—prenatal/young/adult,
b. Sex, and
c. Race/ethnicity, along with opinion from forensic anthropologists and associated findings.

These conclusions can be used to estimate who the decedent most likely is—It narrows down the search, likely antemortem records are obtained.

Age

Pathologic age; related to various conditions and disease process that results in deterioration of many tissues over time. Dental experts can estimate this by

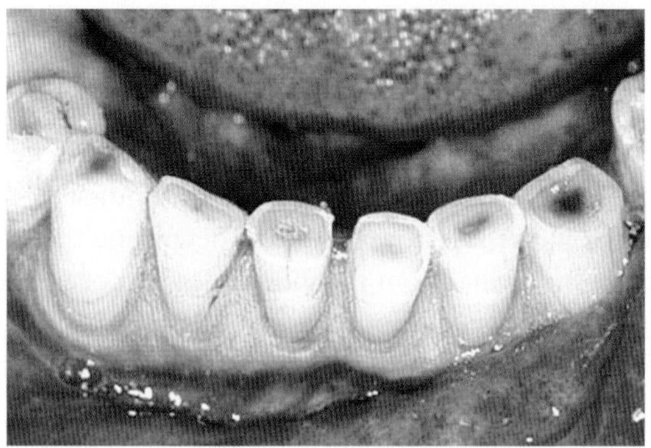

Fig. 2.7: Attrition reflecting an aging phenomenon

examining for arthritic changes in TMJ, attritional wear **(Fig. 2.7)** of teeth, root dentine transparency.

Physiologic age; determined by natural/ expected changes that occur through growth and development. Examination of development of roots (apical closure) **(Figs 2.8A and B)** and comparison with tables that record the amount of development vs age.

Chronologic age (the time from birth to death) age that investigators are most interested in. The detailed descriptions of various methods for age estimation in different age groups are provided in another chapter of this title, "age estimation". Readers are advised to please refer to the same for all details and procedures.

Sex (Fig. 2.9)

Forensic odontology tells us a lot about determination of age from various methods. In addition to determination of age, sex can also be determined from the teeth. Various features of teeth, like morphology, crown size, root lengths etc. are characteristic for male and female sexes. There are also differences in the skull patterns. These will help a forensic odontologist to identify the sex. New developments like PCR amplification etc. will assist in accurately determining the sex of the remains.

Also, it has been pointed out that skeletal development maturation in females is accelerated over that of males after the third or fourth year of life. However, differentiation of sexes by skeletal radiology is unreliable until after puberty. It is then that the sexual characteristics discernible by radiography begin to appear. In general, the male skeleton is more robust and heavier, with more prominent attachment for muscles and tendons.

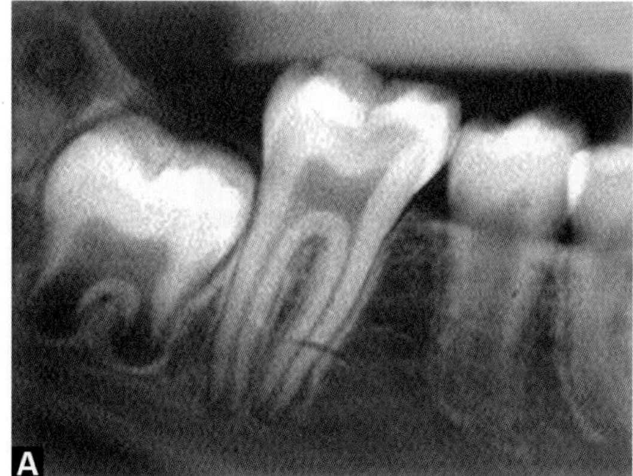

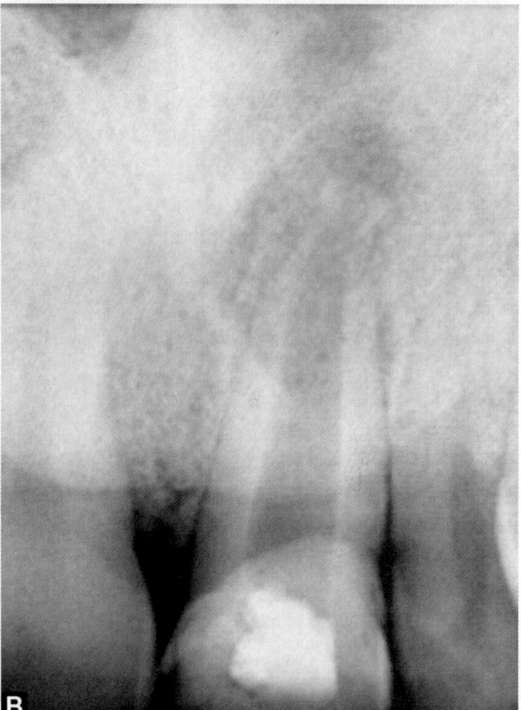

Figs 2.8A and B: (A) An IOPA showing the open apices of 1st and 2nd permanent molars, (B) Another IOPA showing the open apices of maxillary incisor

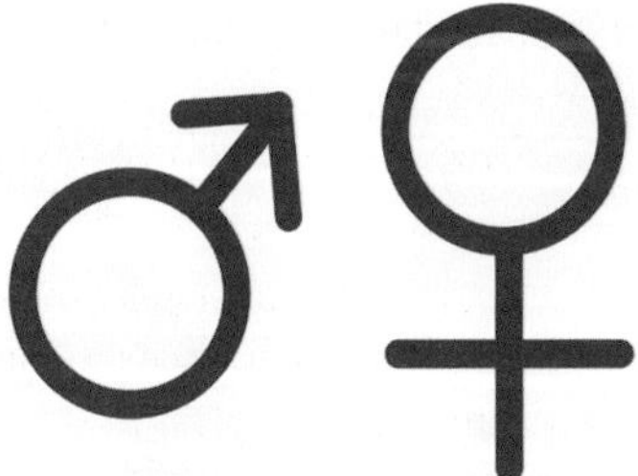

Fig. 2.9: Male and female logos

With aging, there is a tendency for more degenerative and hyperostotic changes in the male skeleton. Male long bones are about 110% the length of female long bones. The male femoral head is larger in all dimensions. All of these general findings are helpful but not definitive in establishing the sex of unidentified human remains. There are certain skeletal components, and both skeletal and extra-skeletal findings, which are more useful in determining sex.

Role of Skull and Mandible (Figs 2.10A and B)

Bony characteristics of the skull and mandible may be useful in assigning sexual identification to unknown remains. The male skull tends to range from mesocephalic to dolichocephalic; the female skull is more likely to be mesocephalic to brachycephalic. The male has a larger brow or supraorbital ridge and a more sloping forehead. The male zygomatic arch is wider and heavier. The male inion or nuchal crest is prominent. The male mastoid process is larger and heavier. The male mandible is larger and more rugged with a wide ascending ramus. Male orbits tend to be larger and higher. The inferior nasal spine is longer in the male. Hyperostosis interna frontalis is an overgrowth of the inner table of the frontal bone, often florid, found almost exclusively in middle-aged or older females and is a valuable characteristic for sex determination. Parietal thinning is a condition of postmenopausal females in which profound osteoporosis causes symmetrical resorption and virtual disappearance of the outer table and diploë of the parietal bones.

Forensic odontology plays an important role in establishing the sex of victims with bodies mutilated beyond recognition due to major mass disasters.

However it is not possible to determine the sex of an individual from the morphologic appearance of teeth alone. Although previously assumed that larger teeth are male characteristics have been disapproved.

Sex differences in dentition are based largely on tooth size and shape. Male teeth are usually larger, whereas female canines are more pointed and a narrower buccolingual width **(Fig. 2.11)**. There

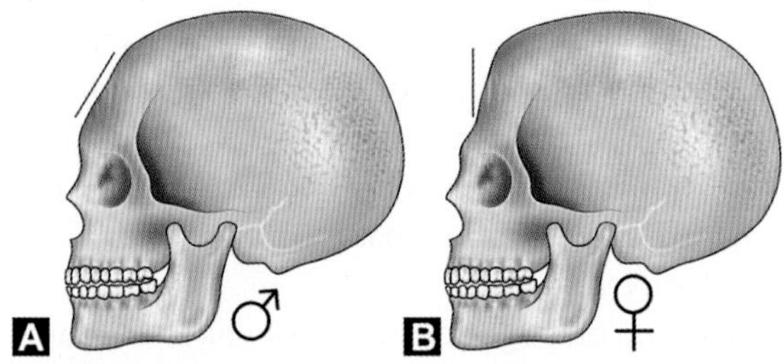

Figs 2.10A and B: Graphical representation showing the characteristic differences between male and female skull. The differences are highlighted by darker and solid lines

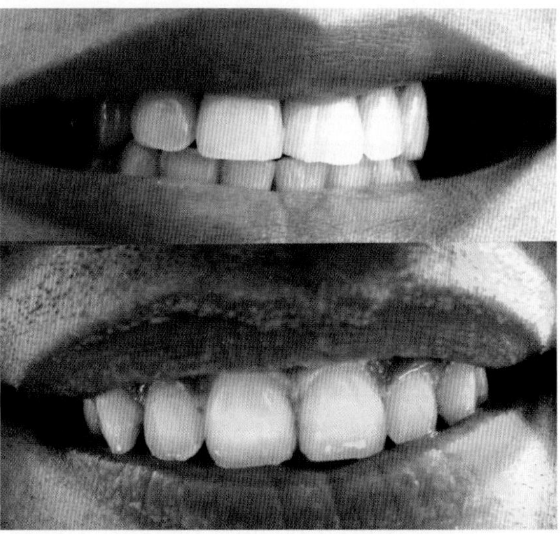

Fig. 2.11: Smile close-up photographs of female (upper) and male (lower) patients

also appear to be greater differences in size between maxillary central and lateral incisors in females as compared to males. Seno and Ishizu reported in 1973 on the use of the Y chromosome in dental pulp to determine sex differences. Success in sexing unknown remains based on this technique have resulted in several published accounts. In 1984, Mudd reported on the use of the Y chromosome in hair specimens. Sundick in 1985 reported on sex determination by Y chromosome detection in unidentified remains at the annual meeting of the American Academy of Forensic Sciences in Las Vegas. Each of these studies involved the detection of the Y chromosome using quinacrine and fluorescent microscopy. This microscopic approach to sexing would appear more reliable to the forensic odontologist than metrics, at least on difficult, incomplete remains. More recently, there have been a number of articles in the forensic literature reporting the successful isolation of sex-specific banding patterns in DNA profiles of the X and Y chromosomes developed from fresh and degraded specimens. All reports indicate the need for high molecular weight genomic DNA.

Classification of Methods

1. Visual method or clinical method.
2. Microscopic methods.
3. Advanced methods.

1. Visual/Clinical Methods

(A) *Sex differences in tooth size:* Teeth may be used for differentiating sex by measuring their mesiodistal and buccolingual dimensions. This is of special importance in young individuals where skeletal secondary sexual characters have not yet developed. Studies show significant differences between male and female permanent and deciduous tooth crown dimension. One is reminded that tooth size, or odontometrics, is under considerable influence of the environment. Such measurements are, therefore, population specific, and do not apply to the world at large.

Amongst teeth, mandibular canines show greatest dimensional difference with larger teeth in males than in females. Premolars, first and second molars as well as maxillary incisors are also known to have significant differences.

(B) *Sex determination using canine dimorphism:* In the field of forensic odontology, permanent canine teeth and their arch width (distance between the canine tips) contribute to sex identification through dimorphism. The study of permanent mandibular and maxillary canine teeth offers certain advantages in that they are the least extracted teeth, are less affected by periodontal disease and the last teeth to be extracted in respect of age (Bossert and Marks, 1956; Krogh, 1968).

The dimensions of canine teeth have been studied by several methods, including Fourier analysis (Minzuno, 1990), Moire topography (Suzuki et al, 1984) and the measurement of linear dimensions such as mesiodistal width, bucco-lingual width and inciso-cervical height (Garn et al, 1967; Anderson and Thompson, 1973; Rao et al, 1988). The use of Fourier analysis and Moire topography were limited to small samples whereas measurement of the linear dimensions of canine teeth was used in large populations because it is simple, reliable, inexpensive and easy to perform.

A study by Anderson and Thompson (1973) showed that mandibular canine width and inter-canine distance was greater in males than in females and permitted a 74.3 percent correct classification of sex.

Garn et al (1973) studied sexual dimorphism by measuring the mesiodistal width of canine teeth in different ethnic groups. They concluded that the magnitude of canine teeth sexual dimorphism varies among different ethnic groups. Furthermore, the mandibular canine showed a greater degree of sexual dimorphism than the maxillary canine.

Sherfudhin H et al (1996) investigated the occurrence of canine tooth dimorphism in Indian subjects and compared the use of two statistical methods of evaluation. These were the methods of NG Rao and co-workers published in 1988 and quadratic discriminant analysis for correct classification of sex. Parameters considered were: (i) the mesiodistal width of maxillary and mandibular canines, (ii) the maxillary canine arch width (intercanine distance) and (iii) the mandibular canine arch width.

The results indicated significant dimorphism of the maxillary and mandibular canine teeth. When the results of the arch widths were subjected to the two statistical methods, differing results were obtained in the accuracy of sex classification. The percentage of correct classifications of sex was higher when using quadratic discriminant analysis. In another study, Iscan Kedici (2003) could accurately establish sex in 77 percent of the cases using maxillary and mandibular canines, and mandibular second molar.

The role of the maxillary canine arch width in establishing sex identity has not been reported in the literature.

The sexual dimorphism specific to canines has been explained by Eimerl and DeVore on the basis of their function which, from an evolutionary point of view, is different from other teeth. During the evolution of primates, there was a transfer of aggressive function from the canines in apes to the fingers in man. Until this transfer was complete, survival of the species was dependant on the canines, especially those of males. Of late, researchers are trying to determine the influence of the X- and Y-chromosomes on tooth morphology. While the role of sex chromosomes in dental development has been proved, Scott considers that there is little dimorphism apparent at a phenotypic level.

(C) *Root length and crown diameter:* Using optical scanner and radiogrammetric measurements on mandibular permanent teeth sex determination can be done with 80 percent accuracy by measuring root length and crown diameters.

(D) *Dental index:* In addition to absolute tooth size, tooth proportions have been suggested for differentiating the sexes. Aitchison presented the 'incisor index' (Ii), which is calculated by the formula Ii = [MDI2/MDI1] × 100, where MDI2 is the maximum mesiodistal diameter of the maxillary lateral incisor and MDI1 is the maximum mesiodistal diameter of the central incisor. This index is higher in males, confirming the suggestion of Schrantz and Bartha that the lateral incisor is distinctly smaller than the central incisor in females. Another index, the 'mandibular canine index' proposed by Rao and associates has given an accurate indication of sex in an Indian population. Using the mesiodistal (m-d) dimension of the mandibular canines, these researchers obtained the formula:

[(Mean m-d canine dimension + (Mean m-d canine dimension in female + SD) in males – SD)]/2

The value obtained using this formula was 7.1, i.e. 7.1 mm is the maximum possible mesiodistal dimension of mandibular canines in females. The same dimension is greater in males. The success rate of determining sex using the above formula was close to 89 percent. However, relative to the near 100 percent accuracy using pelvis and skull, sexing by odontometrics is relatively poor.

(E) *Odontometric differences:* The odontometric difference between males and females is generally explained as a result of greater genetic expression in males. Following is the table showing the odontometric difference between males and females (see **Table 2.3**).

Iscan and Kedici caution that an overlap exists between male and female tooth dimensions, and this makes accurate diagnosis of sex challenging, even for experienced dentists. They emphasize that success is greater when all available teeth are used.

Table 2.3: Showing the odontometric difference between males and females

Tooth No.	Mesiodistal Buccolingual			
	Male	Female	Male	Female
11	8.9	8.5	7.1	7.0
12	7.0	6.65	6.5	6.2
13	8.3	7.6	8.4	7.9
14	6.9	6.8	9.3	8.9
15	6.7	6.65	9.8	9.3
16	11.0	10.6	11.0	10.9
17	10.4	9.9	11.0	10.7
41	5.5	5.3	6.2	6.1
42	6.1	5.9	6.5	6.5
43	7.2	6.6	7.55	7.4
44	7.1	7.0	7.9	7.6
45	7.4	6.9	8.6	8.2
46	11.1	10.8	10.4	10.2
47	10.5	10.2	10.3	9.9

Source: M Hemanth et al. Sex determination using dental tissue. Medico-Legal update Vol 8, No. 2(2008-07_2008-12)

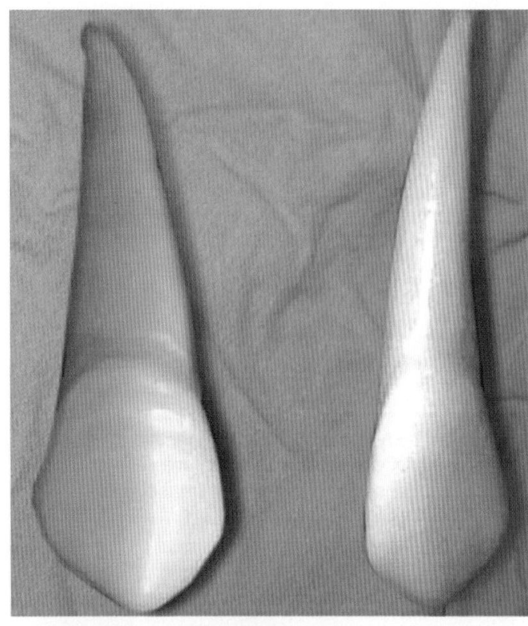

Fig. 2.12: Picture showing the sexual dimorphism in human canines

(F) *Tooth morphology and sexing:* In addition to the canines being the most sexually dimorphic teeth in terms of size, Scott and Turner II highlight that the 'Distal Accessory Ridge', a non-metric feature on the canine" is the most **(Fig. 2.12)** sexually dimorphic crown trait in the human dentition, with males showing significantly higher frequencies and more pronounced expression than females". Rao and Rao have reported greater incidence of four-cusps (absence of the distobuccal cusp or distal cusp) on the mandibular first molar in females (40.6 percent) compared to males (16.2 percent) in a south Indian population. They cite Anderson and Thomas who opine that the reduction in the number of cusps is a reflection of an evolutionary trend towards overall reduction in the size of the lower face, with male apparently resisting this trend.

2. Microscopic Methods

Sex determination using barr bodies.

Sex can also be determined by the study of X and Y chromosomes in the cells which are not undergoing active division. Presence or absence of X chromosome can be studied from buccal smears, skin biopsy, blood, cartilage, hair root sheath, and tooth pulp. After death it persists for variable periods depending upon the humidity and temperature in which tissue has remained. X chromatin and intra-nuclear structure is also known as Barr body **(Figs 2.13A and B)** as it was first discovered by Barr and Bertam (1949). It is present as a mass usually lying against the nuclear membrane in the females.

It was found that in cases after fires, high impact crashes and explosions fragmentation and thermal trauma renders other methods impossible to determine sex of the remains except the above said method from pulp. Pulp tissue cells become embedded firmly into the dried fibrosis matrix. Duffy et al have shown that Barr bodies and F bodies of Y chromosomes are preserved in dehydrated pulp tissues upto one year and pulp tissues retain sex diagnostic characteristics when heated upto 100°C for 1 hour.

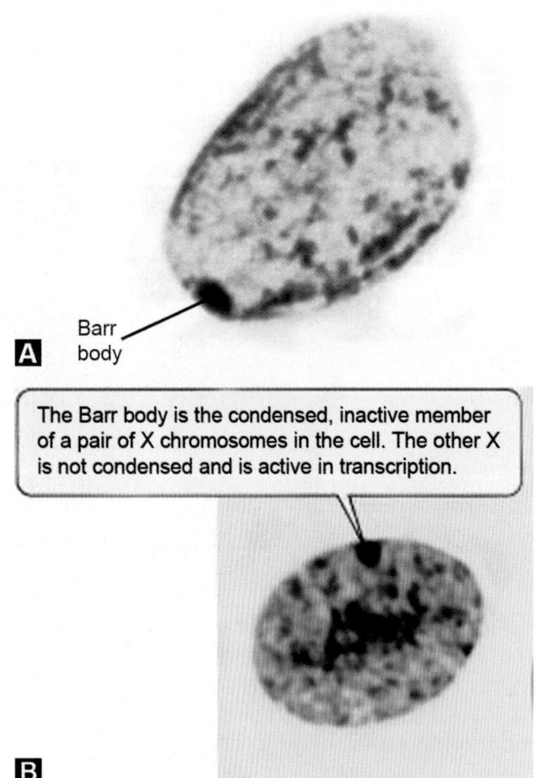

Barr body
A
The Barr body is the condensed, inactive member of a pair of X chromosomes in the cell. The other X is not condensed and is active in transcription.
B

Figs 2.13A and B: Microscopic appearance of Barr bodies in the squamous epithelial cells obtained from the buccal mucosa

3. Advanced Methods

(A) *Sex determination using PCR:* Polymerase chain reaction (PCR) is a method of amplifying small quantities of relatively short target sequences of DNA using sequence-specific oligonucleotide primers and thermostable Taq DNA polymerase.

The teeth can withstand high temperature and are used for personal identification in forensic medicine. In the case of few teeth or missing dental records, there is not enough information to identify the person. The dental pulp enclosed by the hard tissue is not influenced by temperature, unlike the buccal mucous membrane, saliva and calculus.

A procedure utilizing Chelex 100, chelating resin, was adapted to extract DNA from dental pulp. The procedure was simple and rapid, involved no organic solvents, and did not require multiple tube transfers. The extraction of DNA from dental pulp using this method was as efficient, or more so, than using proteinase K and phenol-chloroform extraction. In a study by Tsuchimochi T et al (2002), they used Chelex method to extract DNA from the dental pulp and amplified it with PCR and typing at Y-chromosomal loci to determine the effects of temperature on the sex determination of the teeth.

Hanaoka et al (1996) conducted a study to determine sex from blood and teeth by PCR amplification of the alphoid satellite family using amplification of X (131 bp) and Y (172 bp) specific sequences in males and Y specific sequences in females. It was showed to be a useful method in determining the sex of an individual.

Sivagami and coworkers (2000) prepared DNA from teeth by ultrasonication, and subsequent PCR amplification, they obtained 100 percent success in determining the sex of the individual.

(B) *Sex determination from the enamel protein:* Amelogenin or AMEL is a major matrix proteins found in the human enamel. It has a different signature (or size and pattern of the nucleotide sequence) in male and female enamel.

The AMEL gene that encodes for female amelogenin is located on the X chromosome and AMEL gene that encodes for male amelogenin is located on the Y chromosome. The female has two identical AMEL genes or alleles, whereas the male has two different AMEL genes. This can be used to determine the sex of the remains with very small samples of DNA.

Race

The world has traditionally been divided into six prominent geographic races **(Figs 2.14A and B)**: White, Black, East Asian, Melanesian/Australian, Native American and Polynesian.

However, now a days this is not a qualitative nature because many more hybrid conditions exist

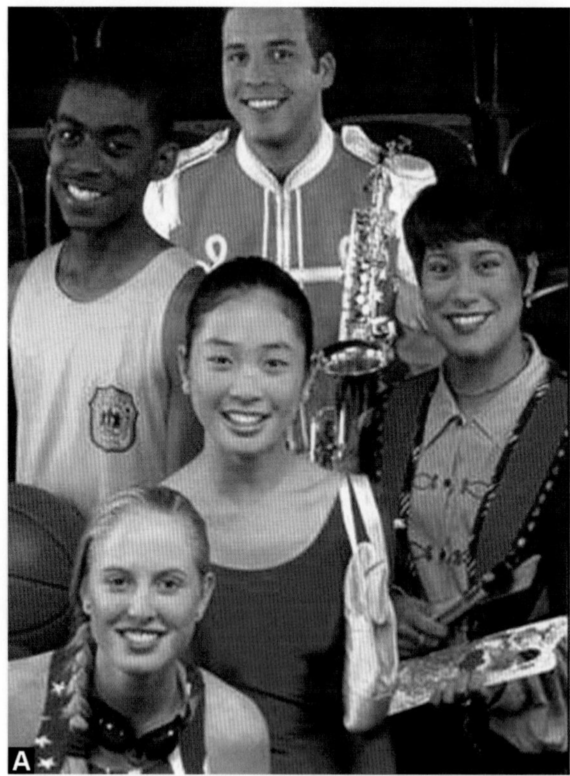

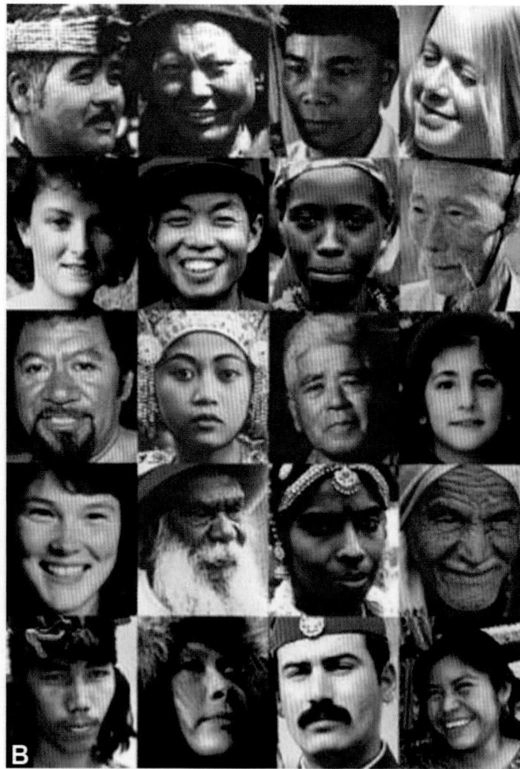

Figs 2.14A and B: Composite pictures showing the various races of the world. Note that many of the differences lie within the facial middle third area

than are described above. No single or combination of trait can be considered completely diagnostic. Assessment of skeletal aspects of corpse by physical anthropologists can be helpful. Generally speaking, assessment of certain anatomic landmarks is done and compared with published standards

Many of the best traits are found in mid face skeleton including the following:

- Area of nose, mouth and cheek bones
- Shape of cranium, lateral projection of zygomatic arches
- Shape, contour of orbits and nasal aperture
- Shape of dental arches
- Facial profiles

Certain dental traits as— shovel shaped incisors, multiple cusps on lower premolar, cusp of carabelli.

Race determination in skeletal remains traditionally focuses on craniofacial characteristics such as the proportions of the orbital and nasal areas, nasal aperture characteristics, lower nasal border features, lower facial prognathism, palate form, cheekbone contours and incisor shoveling.

St Hoyme and Iscan in 1989 reviewed the determinants of sex and race relative to accuracy and assumptions in reconstructions of life from the skeleton. For each of the osteological clues, they pointed out the need to consider:

1. Its basic etiology: Whether it is primarily biochemical, hormonal, or activity-related in order to predict its variation pattern,
2. Its range of variation by sex in various racial/ ethnic groups,

3. Its manifestation by age: The age at which it appears and its pattern of change from childhood to old age,
4. How it is influenced by health, nutrition, occupation, or other circumstances of an individual's life,
5. Whether there are secular changes in its expression, and
6. Whether the characteristics are real, but temporary.

From a dental perspective, both the mandible and dentition reflect racial characteristics. Projecting chins **(Fig. 2.15)** are found in Europeans and some Asiatics. Rounded, almost receding, chins are found in Australian aborigines and in some South Pacific Islanders. Most African and Afro-American chins are intermediate. General jaw shape corresponds with general skull shape. Prognathous palates are associated with long, narrow mandibles with low rami; whereas large bizygomatic widths with wide mandibles have deep rami and significant gonial flare. The greatest eversion is found in Eskimos and Amerindians.

Rocker jaws seem associated with Hawaiian crania. These general characteristics reflect relative ethnic dental markers. According to these authors, the most useful racial clue in dentition is "shovel-shaped" incisors found in most Asiatic Mongoloids and Amerindians and in less than 10 percent of whites and blacks. Tooth size and shape including shovel tooth incisors, Carabelli's cusp **(Figs 2.16A and B)** or tubercle, enamel pearls, and dental pulp shape (taurodontism vs cynodontism) **(Fig. 2.17)** have been listed as racial determinants.

Carabelli's tubercle or cusp is an anomalous cuspule on the mesiolingual surface of maxillary incisors appearing in 50 percent of American whites, 34 percent of Afro-Americans, and 5 to 20 percent of Amerindians. Taurodontism or "bull toothness", especially in maxillary molars, enamel pearls on premolars, and the frequent congenital lack of upper third molars, are commonly noted features in Mongoloids.

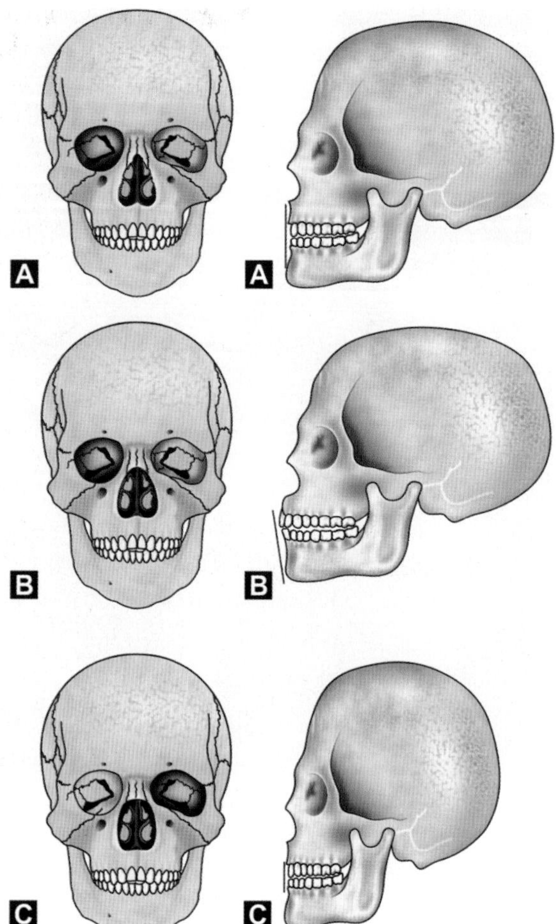

Fig. 2.15: Graphical picture emphasizing characteristic differences in the skull between humans of diverse population ancestry in frontal and lateral views. AA: Caucasoid; BB: Negroid; CC: Mongoloid

The form of the palate and the shape of the dental arches are subject to considerable variation. Stewart in 1946 described these forms as ovoid, "U" shaped, and horseshoe-shaped. Martin and Saller in 1956 described these forms as semicircular, half ellipse, paraboloid, and broken angular line. The proportions of the palate and the associated dental arches are indicated by the palatal index, the ratio of the width to the length of the palate (width/length × 100). The resulting decimal

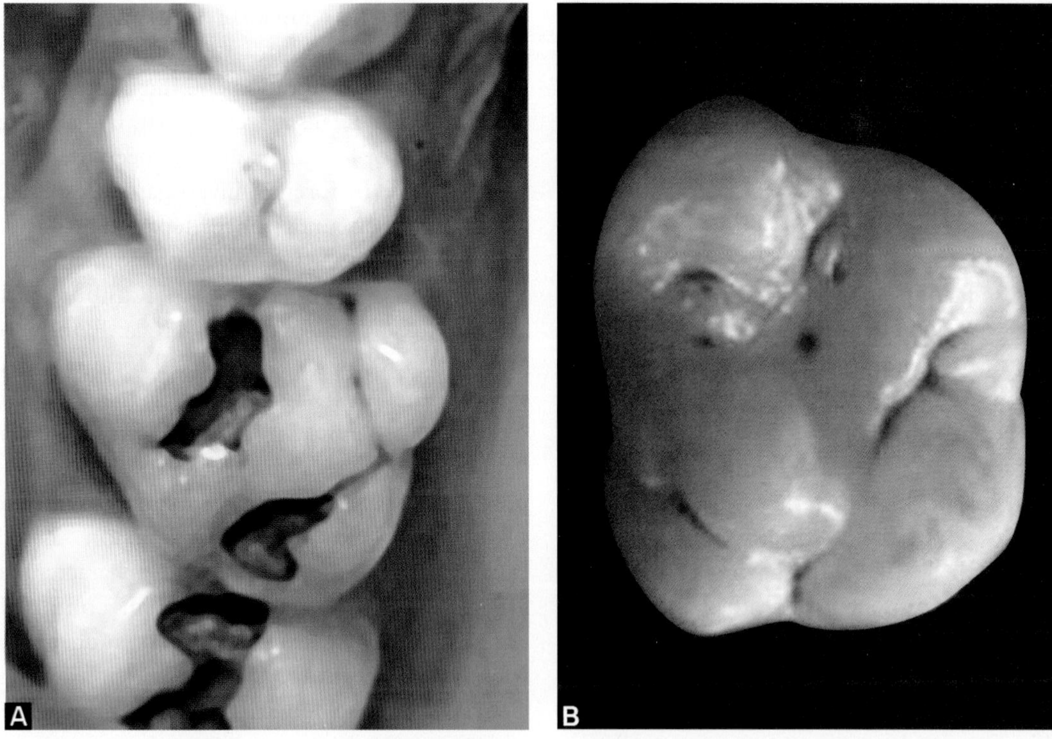

Figs 2.16A and B: Cusp of carabelli, located on the mesioplatal aspect of permanent maxillary molars

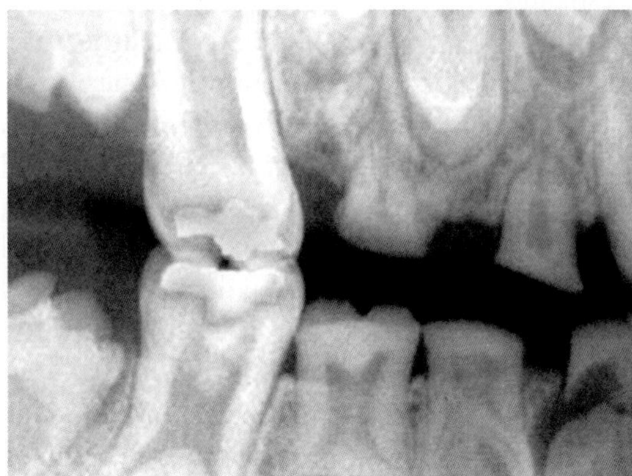

Fig. 2.17: Taurodontism or bull-shaped tooth, an atavistic feature as shown by enlarged pulp space and root canals in the bitewing radiograph

fraction approaches 100.0 as the palate becomes wider and shorter. The anthropometric divisions of this index are:

a. Below 80,
b. 80 to 85, and
c. Above 85.

An index of less than 80 indicates an elongated narrow palate typical of aboriginal Australians, Kaffirs and Zulus. Most Europeans and Amerindians have middle to high indices whereas numerous Orientals and some Pacific islanders have high palatal indices, indicating a short, rounded palate. In general, there are large-toothed and small-toothed races. Aboriginal Australians, the Melanesians, and the American Indians including the Eskimos tend to be large-toothed, with wide crowns. The Lapps and Bushmen are small people with small teeth. American blacks tend to have large crowns. Skull measurements have been used by many examiners as a basis for racial determination. In South America, the Bonwill triangle, an equilateral mandibular triangle connecting the apex of the mesial contact areas of the two central mandibular central incisors with the two mandibular condyles, has been used on the assumption that the studied population groups are not mixed and retain consistent hereditary characteristics.

According to Stewart, metric means of cranial race determination usually follow the discriminant analyses of Howells and Giles-Elliot. Dental decay and occlusal wear, often attributed to advancing technology and increased carbohydrate consumption, are not confirmed when a number of groups are studied such as prehistoric Amerindians, or Southeastern Asians, and ancient Hawaiians. However, cultural usages are often helpful such as black stains from betel nut consumption in Indonesia and other southeastern Asian regions or teeth with excessive slanted wear resulting from pulling fibrous, siliceous fern fronds in native peoples from South Pacific areas. Removal, modification, or decoration of anterior teeth can be useful indicators of sex or race. These cultural characteristics often reflect geographic ethnic patterns.

These craniofacial and dental issues take on some relevance when efforts are made to reconstruct likely visages based on skeletal craniofacial characteristics. Caldwell described four current methods of facial reconstruction:

1. Modeling in clay directly on the skull (three-dimensional),
2. Construction of artists' drawings (two dimensional),
3. Restoration of disrupted or damaged tissues, and
4. Photographic or portrait superimpositions.

Webster et al. reported on the identification of human remains using photographic reconstructions in two methods, comparative and superimpositions. This report used photographs, portraits, and dental studies to confirm the identifications. It is noteworthy not only for its success but also because it utilized several complementary methods of identification. The process of facial restoration and the importance of physiognomic details is well known, largely based on the work of Krogman, and has been used since by a number of forensic investigators, especially anthropologists and police departments, with reasonable success. Caldwell also compared the facial reconstruction studies of Rathbun et al, Lenorovitz and Sussman, and Zavala. Rathbun et al emphasized the eyes, lips, nasal form, and hair style as the most significant facial features in recognition. Lenorovitz and Sussman listed skin, hair, skin color, ears, face shape, eyebrows, eyes, nose, lips, eye color, chin age, and cheeks in order of importance to visual recognition. Zavala expanded that list twice-fold. These characteristics are also the same features which composite computer or overlay techniques such as the Identikit utilize in facial reconstructions. These efforts have also led to further computerized techniques such as computer age progression studies which have proven to be a valuable identification technique in missing persons investigations. Fierro discussed this technique in a comprehensive review of human identification problems in unknown decedents and the variety of techniques used to resolve these problems. Computer age progression has been actively used by the FBI and by the National Center for Missing and Exploited Children. In contrast, computerized regression studies, that is taking a visage and scientifically relating it to earlier ages of the individual are not currently available.

Scott and Turner II suggested unique dental features that have evolved over time as a result of genetic and environmental influences in different population groups.

Dental features used to describe these differences are broadly categorized as:

- Metric (size), not much important
- Non metric (shape/features)

More than 30 non-metric features of both crown and root have been analyzed—Scott and Turner II.

Crown

Shovelling/double shoveling, Carrabelle's feature, Lower molar groove pattern (+, Y, X), Odontome, Lateral incisor variants, Premolar lingual cusp, Parastyle, Protostylid, Premolar lingual cusp.

Root

Two rooted upper premolar/molar, Two rooted lower canine, Tomes root, Single rooted lower molar.

Based on above features, various races in the world have been found to possess following features unique to them as exemplified below:

European/West and South Asians—4 cusped lower 2nd molars, two rooted lower canine, Carrabelle's feature, 3 cusped upper 2nd molar

East Asians — Shovelling, odontome, 3 rooted lower 1st molars, 3 cusped upper 2nd molars, single rooted lower 2nd molars.

Opinion from Forensic Anthropologists

For a number of practical reasons, many forensic odontologists have resisted pressures to characterize an unknown dentition by age, race, or sex except in general terms. Lasker and Lee and Aitchison, often referenced, both described racial traits in the human dentition. Even aging methodologies appear equally shared among forensic odontologists, anthropologists, pathologists, and often radiologists. Both anthropologists and radiologists rely heavily on radiographic evidence of aging, dental eruption patterns, and changes in the facial structures with age such as the angle of the mandible, zygomatic arches, and lateral pterygoid plates.

Harris and McKee in 1990, studied tooth mineralization characteristics in blacks and whites from the southern US in individuals ranging in age from 3.5 to 13 years. They found that females develop more rapidly than males, and that blacks are nearly twice as sexually dimorphic (7.2 percent) as whites (3.7 percent). Within each sex, blacks achieved mineralization stages significantly earlier, by approximately 5 percent, than whites. Anthropologists also appear more eager to use a variety of observations to assist them in obtaining a dental age with a skeletal age for comparison. Sexing parameters generally in use involve classical anthropometric measurements. Rogers in the *"Testimony of Teeth: Forensic aspects of human dentition"*, reviewed the efforts of many authors to use the human dentition for determinations of age, sex, race, and individualization. He focused on several useful categories:

1. Heredity—Size and genetic peculiarities,
2. Wear characteristics,
3. Pathology—Caries and periodontitis, and
4. Restorations—Dental fillings and prostheses, such as crowns, bridges and dentures.

This approach represents a composite analysis of general features and is useful for presumptive sorting of unknown remains. In 1976, Burns and Maples reported on three parameters of dental aging: formative, degenerative, and histological. The formative parameter includes tooth mineralization, crown completion, eruption of the crown, and complementary roots. Degenerative measurements include tooth wear, tooth color, and periodontal attachments. Histological assessments include the degree of secondary dentin deposition, cementum apposition, root resorption, and root transparency. The histological measurements and grading follow Gustafson's efforts. In 1978, Taylor published a text on variation in tooth morphology relative to anthropologic and forensic aspects which emphasized the structural qualitative rather than quantitative differences of teeth and dentition.

Taylor, in studying variations in dental patterns, suggested six parameters for evaluation:

1. Type of tooth structure—Family characteristics,
2. Personal characteristics found throughout a dentition—Crowns, occlusal ridges, cusps, and root robusticity, as well as branching patterns, furcation, and fusion,
3. Imposed characteristics based on the anatomical relationships of the crowns and roots,
4. Complexity factors such as tubercles, pits, additional ridges, grooves and fissures,
5. Acquired characteristics resulting from differences during tooth formation such as hypoplasia, pathology, trauma, function, personal habits, and restorations, and finally
6. Ethnic considerations.

Rogers and Taylor, both anthropologists, rely heavily on general dental structural characteristics and their relationship to the environment and cultural modifications.

Shown below are the various established cranial anatomical landmarks associated with the race and sexual dimorphism **(Tables 2.4, 2.5 and 2.6)**.

Other Methods of Dental Identification

The two processes described above, comparative identification and postmortem profiling, represent the most common methods of dental identification. However, in some instances more novel and innovative techniques have been applied. There have been a number of requests from individuals and dental organizations over the years to insist that dental prostheses are labelled with the patient's name or a unique number. Labeled dentures **(Fig. 2.18)** can be of great assistance in the identification of individuals.

Unlabeled dentures have been recovered from patients and then fitted to casts retained by the treating dentist or laboratory, and this has been an accepted method of identification. Other dental appliances, such as removable orthodontic braces have also been used for identification purposes. Whittaker describes a case where a removable orthodontic appliance was used to identify a victim of a house fire. Authors have also described the use of palatal rugae patterns rendered on dental

Table 2.4: Showing skeletal anthropologic variations associated with sexual characteristics of the skull

Parameter	*Male*	*Female*
Size	Large	Small
Glabellar ridges	Pronounced	Not developed
Mastoid process	Large	Small
Occipital area	Pronounced muscle lines	Minimal muscle lines
Mandible	Larger, broader ramus	Smaller
Forehead	Steeper/slopes vertically	Rounded/more vertical

Table 2.5: Showing skeletal anthropologic variations associated with racial characteristics of the skull

Parameter	*White*	*Black*	*Asian/Native American*
Width	Narrow	Narrow	Broad
Height	High	Low	Intermediate
Profile	Straight	Prognathic	Intermediate
Orbit	Triangular/teardrop	Square	Circular
Nasal opening	Tapered	Wide	Rounded
Palate	narrow	wide	Intermediate

Table 2.6: Showing the morphological features for racial assessment of the skull and mandible

Feature	*Caucasoid*	*Negroid*	*Mongoloid*
General configuration	Mesocephalic	Dolichocephalic	Brachycephalic
Saggital contour	Round	Coronal flat or notching	Arched
Parietal bossing	+–++	0	+++
Bite	Slight overbite	Prognathic	Even
Face	Long, narrow	Prognathic	Flat
Orbits	Rectangular	Oval	Rounded
Intraorbital distance	Inermediate	Wide	Wide
Nasal aperture	Narrow, oval	Round	Wide with inferior gully
Inferior nasal spine	Sharp	Short or troughed	Dull
Nasal bones	Intermediate	Short, depressed	Prominent
Zygomatic arches or malar prominence	Slight, retreating	Slight retreating	Prominent, inferior projection
Mandibular angle	Slightly obtuse	Obtuse	Nearly right angle
Chin, mental process	++	–	+

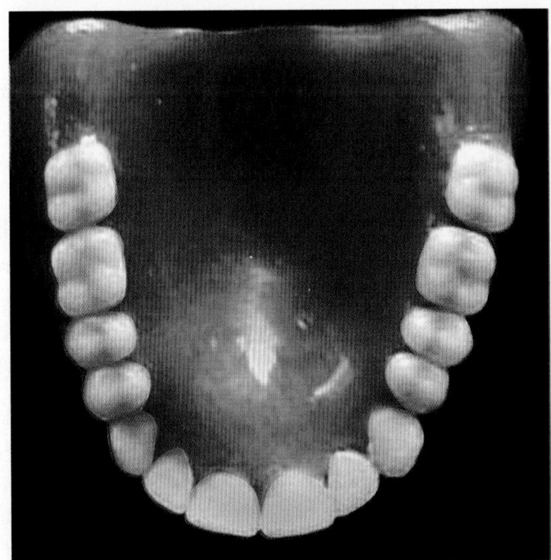

Fig. 2.18: Labeled denture, showing the name of the wearer and the unique identification number. Such incorporated features may be of immense value in case of unfortunate events for the purpose of identification

casts to compare with found remains. Positive identifications have resulted from this technique.

Dental materials have provided clues to assist identification. One of the authors has used SEM-EDX to identify the composition of a glass-ionomer restoration and then traced this back to a prison where the filling was placed. Dental records secured the identification of the individual. In another case, it was possible to identify Kevlar fibers that had been placed within a lower denture to reinforce it. This rare procedure enabled an identification of the wearer who was a victim of homicide.

Role of DNA Molecule in Identification

Except for identical twins, everyone's DNA is different. The application of DNA analysis to individualize biologic evidence is quite similar to specific point of references on the human body that are accepted broadly as being visually distinctive(height, hair, color). The molecular biologists targets specific point of reference on the human genome that are accepted broadly as being biochemically distinctive. The variation in sequence of four nucleotides provides the basis for its unique role in identification.

When conventional dental identification methods fail, this biological material can provide the necessary link to prove identity. With the advent of the polymerase chain reaction (PCR), a technique that allows amplification of DNA at pre-selected, specific sites, this source of evidence is becoming increasingly popular with investigators. Comparison of DNA preserved in and extracted from the teeth of an unidentified individual can be made to a known antemortem sample (stored blood, hairbrush, clothing, cervical smear, biopsy, etc) or to a parent or sibling.

Forensic identification is based on finding differences: Polymorphisms between different individuals. These differences can take many forms, such as differences in facial appearance, differences in ear lobe conformation, differences in retinal arterial structure, differences in hair color, differences in height, etc. Some variations are unique and some are not. Indeed, individual variation is a tenet of biology. Fingerprint friction ridge patterns and dentition are useful for identification precisely because they are different in each individual. Polymorphisms can either be acquired or inherited. A surgical scar is an obvious example of an acquired identifier. The friction ridge patterns of fingerprints have an obvious genetic component, but are predominantly established from local perturbations during fetal development, hence identical twins have different dermatoglyphics. Most acquired features used for identification may change with time, for example dental features can change over time. The polymorphisms within the DNA molecule are the basis for all inherited polymorphisms and they do not change over the lifetime of an individual.

Although dental identification is an excellent and convenient means of positive identification, there are limitations to its use. Dental identification requires the availability of a good quality, reasonably up-to-date dental radiograph. The dentist or orthodontist who has the radiograph in his file must be found. Due to the water fluoridation programs in many of the countries, there are now fewer dental restorations in younger people. Restorations have provided the basis for most dental identifications. Massive head trauma or decapitation may render dental identification impossible. Consequently, not all remains can be identified through dental comparison techniques.

Dental identification takes advantage of the polymorphic nature of the hardest structures in the body—precisely those structures which are most likely to remain available for identification purposes. Although dental structures are more likely to survive traumatic and decompositional changes than other traditional means of identification such as fingerprints, scars, facial appearance, etc. DNA has a still greater likelihood of survival. Any tissue or bone fragment can be used for DNA testing, with the possible exception of those which have undergone severe incineration or prolonged water (particularly saltwater) immersion. Perhaps most significantly, body fragments, unless of a hand with fingerprints, a portion of a jaw with teeth, or an articulable limb, will not ordinarily be identified except by laboratory tissue identification techniques.

A common obstacle to fingerprint and dental identification is the lack of antemortem data for comparison. The common availability of families as sources of reference material for comparison purposes is a particularly important aspect of DNA identification. Furthermore, dental and fingerprint identification are relatively slow and tedious in a large mass disaster. Future DNA testing technologies will permit high-volume, low-cost testing. In significant mass disasters, the speed of batch laboratory testing may prove critical. For many years, tissue identifications could only be accomplished by traditional serologic markers, particularly ABO blood group typing. DNA testing is far superior to those other tissue-typing techniques for a variety of reasons. DNA is the basis for all blood group types, red cell antigens, and protein isoenzymes. Due to the degeneracy of the genetic code, there will always be more polymorphisms in DNA than in the resultant phenotypes. The discriminatory power of DNA is far greater than any set of traditional markers, including HLA typing. Traditional markers typically yield values of one in thousands, whereas DNA tests often yield values of one in millions. DNA testing can be performed on any tissue or fluid. DNA tests, particularly PCR-based DNA tests, are more sensitive than traditional serologic markers. DNA tests can be performed on specimens which are far older than is the case with traditional markers and DNA is less susceptible to environmental insults.

Forensic DNA profiling methods such as PCR technique to amplify small amounts of recovered DNA at specific genetic loci are sensitive enough to discriminate one individual from all others with a high level of confidence by starting with only 1 ng or less of target DNA.

Ultraviolet light, extreme pH, severe heat, microbial contamination and certain environmental conditions (high humidity) can damage molecular arrangement and make DNA unsuitable for analysis. Most collection and preservation protocols for DNA evidence focus on providing a cool, dark, dry environment, secure from sources of chemical/ biological contamination.

Human DNA: This is found in two main cellular organelles that is nucleus and mitochondria, providing an unique opportunity to forensic odontologists for DNA profiling of the deceased. Each of these have unique properties as summarized herein.

The DNA Molecule

Basic Structure (Figs 2.19A and B)

The basis for all inheritance is found within the DNA genome of cells. This information is coded

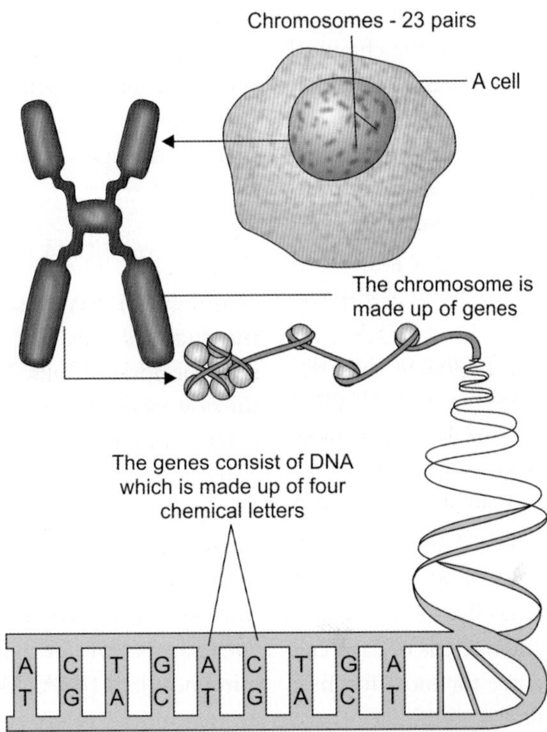

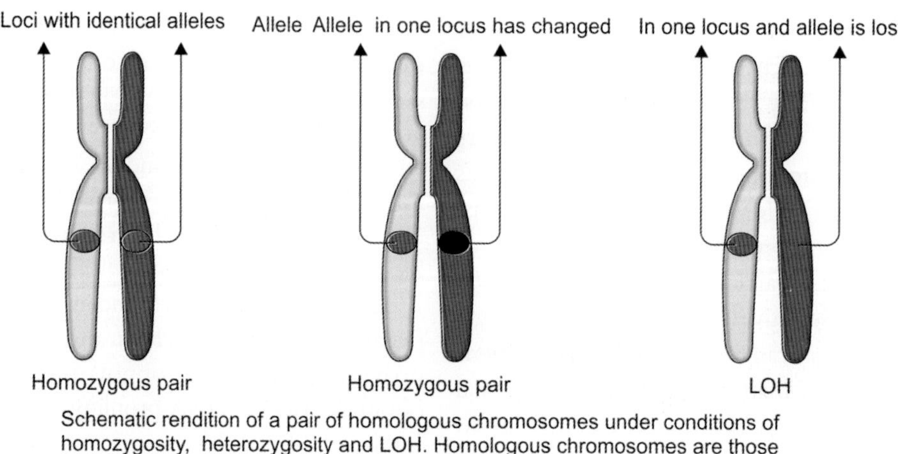
Loci with identical alleles
Allele Allele in one locus has changed
In one locus and allele is lost
Homozygous pair
Homozygous pair
LOH
Schematic rendition of a pair of homologous chromosomes under conditions of homozygosity, heterozygosity and LOH. Homologous chromosomes are those pair during mitosis, have the same morphology, and contain genes governing the same characteristics. Note that one of the chromosomes, say the blue one, came from the father, and the other, the red, from the mother.
B

Figs 2.19A and B: The basic genomic structure showing the DNA and chromosomes

within the chemical structure of the DNA molecule or, more accurately, the set of DNA molecules known as the genome. Nucleotide bases are arranged in specific sequences within the chemical structural scaffolding. Only four bases (adenine, cytosine, guanine, and thymine) make up the genetic alphabet that produces the words, sentences, paragraphs, and chapters which are eventually read into proteins that comprise biological organisms. These bases are present in pairs in a complementary fashion to form base pairs, such that every A is paired with a T, every C with a G, and vice versa. The consequence of this base pairing is that half of the molecule can be stripped away from the other half and the base sequence of one strand can be used to determine the sequence of the opposite strand, or to create a specific DNA hybridization probe.

Genomic DNA

Genomic DNA is found in the nucleus of each cell and represents the DNA source for most forensic applications, (there are no nuclei, and hence there is no DNA, in red blood cells.) When body tissues have decomposed, the structures of the enamel, dentine and pulp complex persist. It is necessary to extract the DNA from the calcified tissues. Teeth represent an excellent source of genomic DNA. Indeed, many authors have found that even root-filled teeth supply sufficient biological material for PCR analysis

Mitochondrial DNA (Mt DNA) (Fig. 2.20)

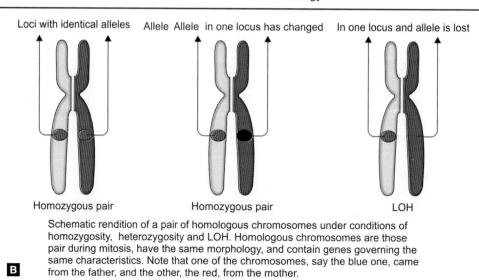

Not only is DNA present within chromosomes in the nuclei of cells, but DNA is also present in the mitochondria of cells. Mitochondria are known as the powerhouses of the cells as they are the primary machinery for accomplishing oxidative metabolism. Tens, hundreds, or even thousands of mitochondria are present within a single cell and each mitochondrion may contain several mitochondrial "DNA particles". Consequently, a cell contains only one copy of nuclear DNA, but literally thousands of copies of the 16,000 bp mitochondrial DNA (MtDNA) sequence; hence a mitochondrial DNA type can be obtained when

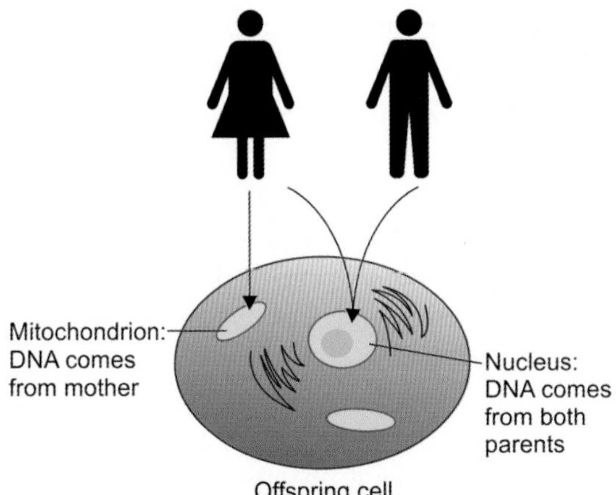

Fig. 2.20: The mitochondrial DNA, which is only inheritable from the mother

the nuclear DNA type cannot be. Since no significant regions of repetitive DNA exist in MtDNA, only sequence polymorphisms are typed. The region of MtDNA which is analyzed for human identification is the noncoding region known as the displacement loop (D-loop) or control region. The degree of polymorphism in the D-loop is so great that direct sequencing may be the most efficient method of typing MtDNA, although a commercial dot/blot system is in development. Another unique feature of MtDNA is its mode of inheritance—one half of nuclear DNA is from the mother and one half from the father. Mitochondria are inherited in a strictly mother-to-child manner; there is no paternal contribution. Because there is no recombination and because only a single (unpaired) copy is present in the cell, an exact sequence match is anticipated. Accordingly, MtDNA can be traced through a family via maternal lineages for many generations. Mitochondrial DNA sequencing has great application to severely decomposed and skeletonized remains. However, the discriminatory power is limited; discriminatory powers are often of the order of one in a hundred. Very few laboratories are performing this kind of testing at this point in time.

Stability of DNA

DNA is a robust molecule which can tolerate a remarkable range of temperature, pH, salt, and other factors that destroy classical serologic markers. Validation testing in forensic science laboratories has shown that DNA mixed with detergents, oil, gasoline, and other adulterants did not alter its typing characteristics. Indeed, it is this ruggedness which allows DNA longevity and has permitted DNA typing of Egyptian mummies and 30-million-year-old insects preserved in amber. Bone or tissues that have been in soil environments for extended lengths of time often yield no DNA typing results by traditional means, especially when the soil is moist. However, even relatively ancient skeletal remains may yield an informative mitochondrial DNA sequence.

DNA Polymorphisms

DNA polymorphisms can be length-based or sequence-based. Length-based polymorphisms are a characteristic of repetitive DNA that generally does not code for any protein (so-called "junk" DNA). DNA fragments vary in size between individuals due to the presence of variable numbers of tandem repeats (VNTRs); i.e. a core of 7 bases may be repeated 3 times in one individual or 12 times in the next individual. Traditional restriction fragment length polymorphism (RFLP) analysis, as is commonly associated with the DNA testing in crime labs, involves cut fragments (restriction fragments) which include internal VNTR regions (loci) and thus vary in fragment length. VNTR fragments can also be amplified instead of cut, hence, amplified fragment length polymorphisms (AmpFLPs). DNA identity information is found not only in fragment length variation, but also within the DNA sequence of similarly sized DNA fragments.

Sequence polymorphisms consist of difference, changes in one or more bases in a DNA sequence at a particular location in the genome. Sequence variations can manifest as regions of alternative alleles or base substitutions additions, or deletions. Most sequence polymorphisms are mere point mutations. They may be found in coding or noncoding DNA. Sequence polymorphisms can be detected by DNA probes or by direct sequencing.

DNA Typing Methods

RFLP Methods: The DNA typing method that was first described, and most commonly employed by crime labs initially, is known as restriction fragment length polymorphism (RFLP) analysis. The six steps in RFLP testing include:

1. Extraction of DNA from a biologic source
2. Cutting the DNA into relatively small fragments at specific sites with "restriction enzymes"
3. Separating the fragments by size using agarose gel electrophoresis
4. Transferring and immobilizing the separated DNA fragments onto a nylon membrane
5. Denaturation of the DNA into single strands and hybridization to radioisotopically-labeled probes (small fragments of single-stranded DNA)
6. Autoradiography, in which an X-ray film is placed over the membrane for several days, resulting in exposure of the film at the point of the probe.

The RFLP testing is often called "Southern blotting" because the DNA transfer technique was first described by Professor Southern. Typically, RFLP testing will take several weeks to perform. For every probing, the membrane is stripped of the previous probe and rehybridized and autoradiography performed anew. However, alternatives to radioisotopic labels now exist, particularly chemiluminescent and fluorescent probe labels, which permit much faster testing.

Unfortunately, RFLP is not useful where the DNA is degraded, because random fragmentation thwarts detection of a specific large uncut fragment population. Since DNA rapidly breaks down after death, RFLP testing is of limited value in testing cadaveric tissue for identification of human remains, unless the remains are fresh.

PCR Methods

The polymerase chain reaction (PCR) is a method of copying or "amplifying" a particular segment of DNA. A few strands or even a single strand of DNA can be used to reproduce millions of copies of target DNA fragments. Kary Mullis **(Fig. 2.21)** was awarded the Nobel Prize in 1993 for the discovery of the PCR process, which has led to a revolution in the life sciences. PCR amplification **(Figs 2.22A and B)** is a sample preparation technique which enables further testing to detect various polymorphisms. Non-amplified DNA becomes undetectable against the amplified background target sequence. PCR testing is not only very sensitive, but it is quicker, less labor intensive, and less tedious than RFLP testing. Most significantly for remains identification, it is often successful even though the tissue specimen is

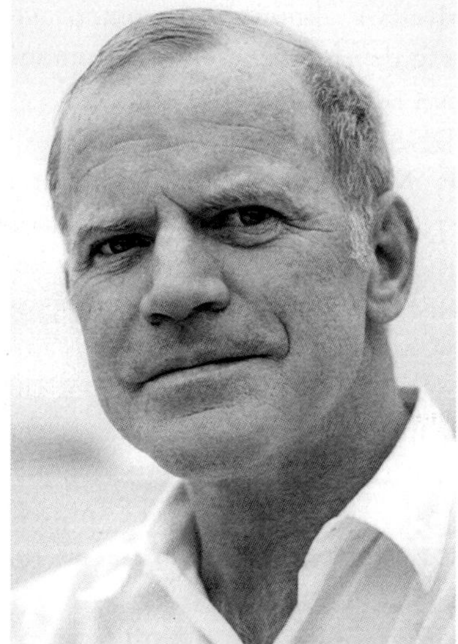

Fig. 2.21: The most notable contributor to the field of medicine and biology, Karry Mullis, the author behind the invention of PCR technique

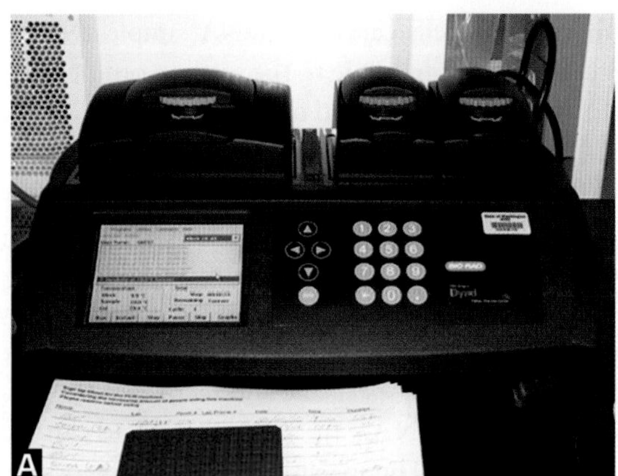

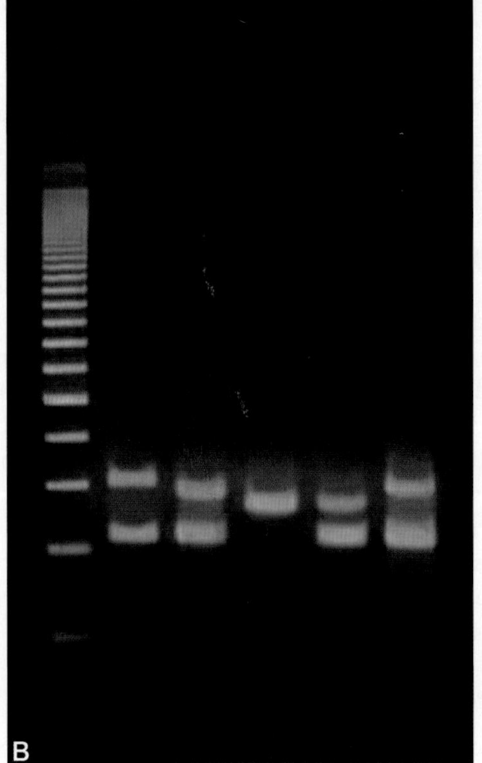

Figs 2.22A and B: (A) The PCR machine, (B) The pattern obtained after PCR and Fluorescent labeling technique showing the specific banding at specific levels

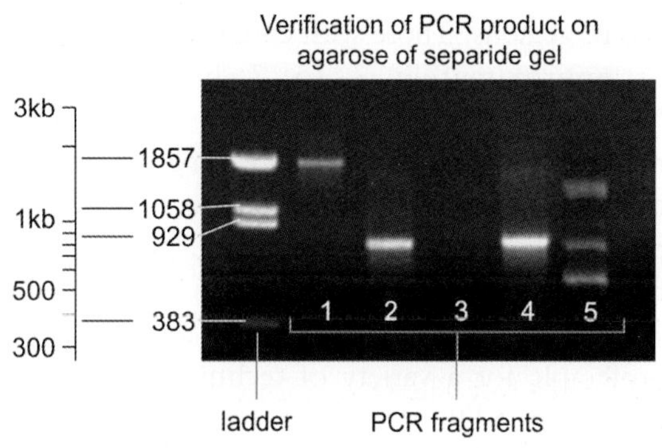

Fig. 2.23: Results obtained after PCR on a agarose gel

degraded because only a few copies of relatively short segments need to remain intact. However, PCR testing is susceptible to inhibition and the potential for cross contamination.

Dot/Blots (Fig. 2.23)

Sequence information can be obtained through the use of DNA probes. A DNA probe is a small piece of single-stranded DNA (oligonucleotide) which will bind to another single-stranded DNA with the complementary sequence. A sequence-specific oligonucleotide (SSO) probe, also known as an allele specific oligonucleotide (ASO) probe, is a single-stranded DNA fragment sufficiently long to confer specificity, but short enough to bind only to the exact sequence complement. Commercial kits, i.e. DQ-alpha and Poly-Marker systems, are based on a dot/blot format for SSO typing and are currently in use by many crime labs. The resultant dot/blot strip has a series of spots that turn blue if the reaction is positive and in this way give a series of yes/no results. These dot/blot tests are quite rapid and work reasonably well despite sample degradation, but do not harbor the same discriminatory power as RFLP tests.

AmpFLPs and STRs

VNTR polymorphisms can be typed by both RFLP and by PCR methods. Since smaller loci are desired for amplification, generally the VNTR loci typed by PCR methods are different from those that are typed using RFLP methods. Regions with core repeat sequences greater than 7 base-pairs (bp) have been called "minisatellite" or "long tandem repeat"

(LTR) regions. Those with core repeat sequences of approximately 3 to 7 bp are called "microsatellite" or "short tandem repeat" (STR) regions. Dinucleotide repeats are not generally used in forensic science laboratories due to the artifactual production of so-called "shadow" and "stutter" bands.

The shorter STR fragments are generally preferable for a variety of technical reasons. A number of STR systems are available for use in identification, and commercial kits are available. These STR systems work well despite significant degradation and are quite amenable to automation. Sufficient numbers of STR systems can be performed to achieve discriminatory powers similar to current RFLP testing. The British and Canadian crime labs are moving towards using STR systems exclusively.

Specimen Selection, Collection, and Preservation

DNA can be isolated and tested from virtually any postmortem tissue, although after death it will undergo progressive fragmentation. DNA is generally broken down (degraded) into fragments through autolytic and bacterial enzymes, specifically DNases. Nevertheless, the sequence information is still present within the DNA fragments and therefore the information is not completely lost despite the fairly extensive fragmentation which occurs from decomposition. However, not all DNA testing is appropriate or possible when the DNA is degraded. Traditional RFLP testing will require non-degraded high molecular weight DNA, whereas PCR-based analysis can be performed on degraded samples and mitochondrial DNA can be obtained from skeletal remains when nuclear DNA cannot. In relatively fresh cadavers, unclotted blood (EDTA anti-coagulated in a purple-top tube) is the preferable source of DNA. Although heme is an inhibitor of PCR, laboratories are accustomed to blood as a DNA specimen and although only white blood cells carry the DNA, ample DNA is present for testing. Due to the settling out of white blood cells, clotted blood may not be a good source of DNA.

Blood is a good culture medium and bacterial growth may render blood samples useless. Virtually any tissue can be used successfully for DNA typing purposes. Brain tissue is said to be a particularly good source in intermediate post-mortem time periods. Hard tissues (bone and teeth) are the best source of DNA in cases of advanced decomposition. The specimens should be kept cold or preferably frozen (although repeated freezing and thawing is not good). Desiccation, even simple air drying, may be an adequate method of storage of some DNA specimens, e.g. bloodstains and bone. Tissues in formalin are not optimal, but can often be used for PCR-based DNA testing. No tissues or biologic fluids should be discarded as inadequate without first attempting DNA testing. Due to the degree of sensitivity of PCR-based technologies, great care should be taken to prevent contamination of one specimen by other sources of DNA. Specimens should be collected with gloves and pristine instruments. Fresh tissues should be collected by an incisional biopsy technique, where possible. Similarly, laboratory testing should be carried out with particular precautions against the possibility of contamination, including separating the pre-PCR sample preparation area from the post-PCR analysis area.

Dental DNA Evidences

Teeth themselves can be excellent sources of DNA. In fact, the same reasons that permit the survival of teeth for dental identification similarly protect the DNA within teeth. Accordingly, teeth are a better source of DNA than skeletal bones, which are better than soft tissues in cases of much decomposed remains. DNA is present in the vascular pulp of the tooth, but it is also found throughout the tooth in varying levels, particularly in the odontoblastic processes, accessory canals, and cellular cementum. Most information necessary for traditional dental identification is present in the crown (enamel and dentin) of the tooth.

Two important conclusions can be withdrawn from this DNA profiling methods:

1. In a reconstructive profile —Sex of the decedent through analysis of Amelogenin sex linked gene.
2. Direct/indirect reference sample—Through comparisons of DNA from the found body.

Obtaining the Dental DNA

A. *Conservative approach:* Sectioning of teeth and opening the crown to extirpate the pulp. Consequently, a tooth can be sectioned horizontally through the cervical root subjacent to the cemento-enamel junction, preserving most restorations for traditional dental comparison purposes. Although somewhat greater amounts of DNA are obtained by crushing the entire tooth, this conservative method of sampling DNA from teeth has been found to be quite adequate and also it is crucial in cases where preservation of sampled tooth is important as in mass fatality incidents.

B. *Cryogenic grinding:* Requires following instruments and equipments **(Fig. 2.24)**

- Freezer mill (2 to 4 minutes)
- Liquid nitrogen
- Lysis buffers
- PCR.

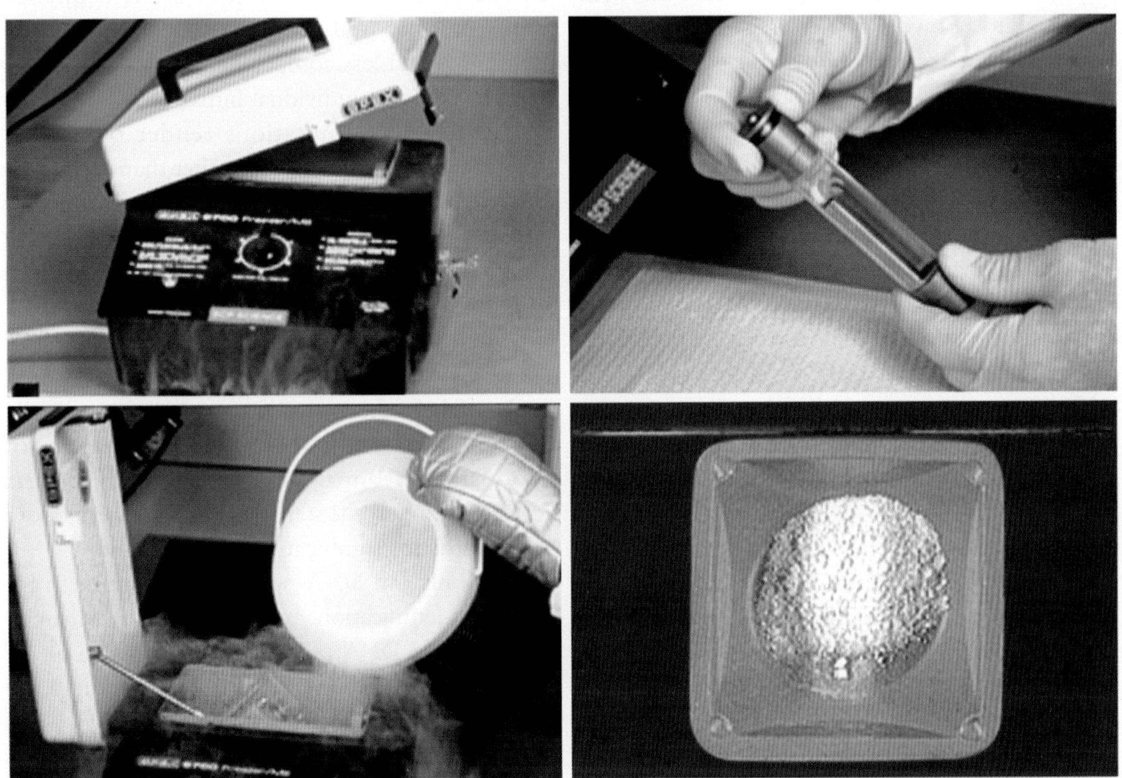

Fig. 2.24: The process of cryogenic grinding, showing the apparatus, freezer mill, an oscillator and the powder obtained after such procedure

DNA profiling: Multiplexing-analyze many genetic loci simultaneously, requires smaller sample, faster than previous methods such as restriction fragment length polymorphism.

Cryogenic grinding is used to extract DNA from calcified tissues such as teeth. The first step in extraction of DNA from bone or teeth is to break up the tissue to expose the DNA to the extraction medium. Early techniques involved the fracturing of bone by freezing it in liquid nitrogen, but subsequent protocols specify breaking the tissue with a mortar and pestle and then grinding the tissue into a coarse powder in a grinding mill. In a freezer mill a ferromagnetic plunger is oscillated back-and-forth in alternating electric current. Liquid nitrogen is used to cool the sample, which results in making it extremely brittle and also protects DNA from heat degradation. The tooth is reduced to a powder to increase surface area and expose trapped cells to biochemical agents that release DNA into solution. Protocols have differed in requiring or not requiring a decalcification step. But many authors have found that decalcification is not only unnecessary, but approximately half of the DNA is lost through the dilution and imperfect recovery involved. The next step in most protocols is incubation in a proteinase-K solution to enzymatically digest proteins and release the DNA. After incubation in a buffer solution, standard DNA extraction procedures may then be performed.

Reference Samples/Databases

The lack of an antemortem dental X-ray or fingerprint record is the most common reason for the inability to obtain identification by traditional identification methods, whereas reference specimens for DNA testing are generally available from family members. Specimens from the spouse and children will permit "reverse paternity" testing using nuclear DNA probes. Parental specimens, and possibly those from siblings, will permit identification, particularly in closed populations. Reconstruction from scattered relatives is often possible, but the statistical inference is substantially diminished. Mitochondrial DNA analysis must be performed on maternal kindred (mothers, siblings, children only in the case of a female), but unlike nuclear DNA identification, it can be performed even in distant relatives (maternal aunts and uncles, children of sisters). It is not always possible or desirable to use families for reference specimens. Sometimes family members are no longer alive. Sometimes the family members are not known or their whereabouts cannot be determined. Some individuals are adopted into their families and therefore the family is not appropriate as reference specimens. Often it is awkward to approach families on the mere possibility of an identification. Except in the case of mitochondrial DNA sequence comparisons, pedigree analysis permits only inferential and less compelling conclusions than a sample from the individual himself.

Furthermore, mutations render occasional identifications problematic. Rather than secondary reference samples from family members, primary DNA specimens of the individual may be available from toothbrushes, biopsies or tissue slides archived in a hospital's pathology department, from stored blood donations, from licked envelopes and stamps, or in the case of mitochondrial DNA from locks of baby hair or clippings from an electric shaver. All states in US require the taking of bloodstains from infants for phenylketonuria (PKU) testing; some state health departments store these cards for significant periods of time.

Not only can DNA be obtained from teeth for primary identification, but it can also be obtained for reference DNA purposes. Numerous cases are there in which teeth have been identified, and the DNA from the tooth used as a reference DNA source to identify other tissue fragments. The majority of states now have legislation creating DNA databases of convicted sex and violent offenders;

other states will likely enact such legislation. These state DNA databanks will be linked by the FBI's National DNA Identification Index (also known as the Combined DNA Index System or CODIS) and will include a file for unidentified and missing persons. This computer system is separate and apart from the NCIC. Due to the tremendous utility of DNA identification, the military established the DOD DNA Registry for the purpose of human remains identification. The DNA Registry is comprised of the Armed Forces DNA Identification Laboratory and the DOD DNA Specimen Repository. By the year 2001 in USA, all active duty military members had their buccal swabs and dried bloodstain DNA specimen cards on their file. The DNA Registry has already proven itself to be of great benefit. With the establishment of the DNA Registry, the military's duplicate panograph program will be phased out. DNA identification represents a significant new adjunct to traditional methods of identification.

Problems Applying DNA Test Results

Irrespective of the analytical approach general acceptance or relevancy courts, legal commentators, and the treatise writers generally agree DNA profiling, as a novel scientific procedure, has received broad support and has been admitted into evidence. Professor Imwinkelried, concludes that courts have been receptive to the technology and most have found DNA typing a trustworthy technique. If there are shortcomings in which technicians conduct DNA tests, such shortcomings do not affect the admissibility of the test results, only the weight a judge or jury should accord it. Hence, a judge or jury might give little or no weight at all to the expert's testimony.

The success of the application of DNA profiling in the identification of defendants, by its very nature, depends largely on a case-by-case analysis. This approach is in keeping with Judge Cox's classification that some novel scientific evidence can neither be accepted nor rejected outright. However, the most frequent challenges that opponents to DNA profiling raise are (1) adequacy of genetic interpretations; (2) quality assurance of testing procedures; and (3) the inference of unfairness to defendants.

Adequacy of Genetic Interpretations

After a proponent has successfully proffered evidence establishing the DNA technique and that sound laboratory procedures were followed, there must be a scientifically reliable method of determining the probabilities or frequency of a matching profile. The purpose of frequency estimates is to give meaning to the match by showing the likelihood that an unrelated person in the reference population would be a chance match. As the NRC noted, it is meaningless "to say that two patterns match, without providing any scientifically valid estimate (or, at least, an upper bound) of the frequency with which such matches might occur by chance".

To develop their frequency estimates, forensic laboratories establish databases of analyzed blood specimens (usually several hundred) of different ethnic groups from different parts of the US. By using its RFLP radioactive probes on the samples, the laboratory creates band patterns or images on the autoradiograph. Each band represents one particular match allele. The bands are then grouped by the size of DNA fragments and then placed into "bins" for purposes of comparing the percentage of the public that has that band. The percentage of bands falling into a particular bin is established as the percentage of the population possessing that particular allele. The percentages for each allele, reflected in each "probe" in the "series" performed for a particular DNA analysis, are multiplied together. That result is then multiplied by, reflecting the composition of an individual's DNA from the combination of each parent's DNA. The result of this final multiplication is the statistical probability of that particular DNA being repeated in the general population.

Bibliography

1. Adams BJ. Establishing personal identification based on specific patterns of missing, filled, and unrestored teeth, J Forensic Sci. 2003; 48:487-96.
2. American Board of Forensic Odontology. Body identification guidelines. J Am Dent Assoc 1994; 125:1244-54.
3. Andersen L, Juhl M, Solheim T, Borrman H. Odontological identification of fire victims potentialities and limitations. Int J Legal Med 1995; 107:229-34.
4. Burris BG, Harris EF. Identification of race and sex from palate dimensions. J Forensic Sci 1998; 43:959-63.
5. Clark DH. An analysis of the value of forensic odontology in ten mass disasters. Int Dent J 1994; 44:241-50.
6. Hemath M, Vidya M, Nanda prasad. Bhavana VK. Sex determination using dental tissue. Medico-Legal update. Vol. 8, No. 2 (2008-07_2008-12).
7. Hutchison CA, Newbold JE, Potter SS, Edgell MH. Maternal inheritance of mammalian mitochondrial DNA. Nature 1980;251:536-8.
8. MacLean D, Kogon S, Stitt S. Validation of dental radiographs for human ID, Int. Dent. J. 1994;39: 1195-1200.
9. Marella GL, Rossi P. An approach to identification by means of dental prostheses in a burnt corpse. J Forensic Odontostomatol 1999;17:16-9.
10. Steyn M, Iscan MY. Sexual dimorphism in the crania and mandibles of South African whites. Forensic Sci Int 1998;98:9-16.
11. Sweet D, Hildebrand D. Recovery of DNA from human teeth by cryogenic grinding, Journal of Forensic Sciences 1998 Nov;43(6):1199-1202.

Chapter 3

Dental Records and Forensic Photography

Nitul Jain, Gaurav Atreja

Chapter Overview

- Long-term storage of dental records
- Forensic photography

The production, retention and release of clear and accurate patient records are essential part of the dentist's professional responsibility. Success in this task will assist the dentist's medicolegal claim and can assist the police and coroners in the correct identification of individuals. Dental professionals are compelled by law and duty of care to produce and maintain adequate patient records. With the increasing awareness amongst the general public of legal issues surrounding health care, and with the worrying rise in malpractice cases, a thorough knowledge of dental record issues is essential for any practitioner—especially those who are just beginning their careers.

INTRODUCTION

The ability of clinical practitioners to produce and maintain good dental records is essential to good quality patient care as well as being a legal obligation. Unfortunately dental records are often unsatisfactory. A study performed by two Regional Dental officers in the UK identified charting as inaccurate in 38 percent of examined records and absent in 14 percent, less than half (48 percent were considered satisfactory).

In another observational study on the quality of dental records, Swedish researchers found a large discrepancy in the quality of examined records. In the study they examined ten years worth of patient records which had been submitted for the purposes of forensic identification. A startling statistic is that ten percent of the patients were identified incorrectly on their records! Other areas of concern included signatures in only five percent of records and the documentation of a treatment plan in only eight percent. These simple mistakes can lead to errors of treatment, confusion when transferring records and opens the practitioner to criticism should a medicolegal claim be made against them.

What is a Patient Record?

In brief, the patient's record is the complete story of the history, physical examination, diagnosis, treatment and care of a patient. The record may consist of several different elements; common ones include written notes, radiographs, study models, referral letters, consultants' reports, clinical photographs, results of special investigations, drug prescriptions, laboratory prescriptions, patient identification information and comprehensive medical history (**Figs 3.1A to C**). Clearly this is a large amount of information and it is essential that a practitioner maintains this in an easily accessible manner.

Within the written notes the established minimum information is:

A. Identification data—Name, date of birth, phone numbers and emergency contact information.

B. Medical history—Thorough investigation to include a minimum of:
   - Name and phone number of physician
   - Dentists' own evaluation of patient's general health and appearance
   - List of systemic disease—Diabetes, rheumatic fever, hepatitis etc.
   - Any ongoing medical treatment
   - Any bleeding disorders, drug allergies,
   - Smoking and alcohol history
   - Any cardiac disorders.

C. Relevant family medical history.

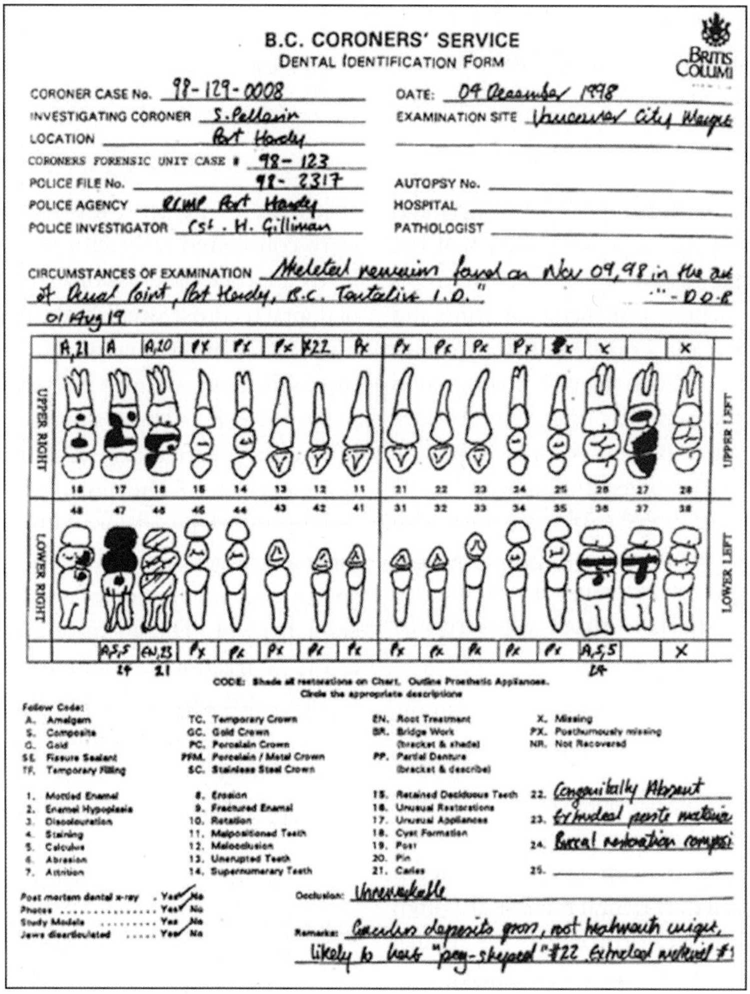

B.C. CORONERS' SERVICE
DENTAL IDENTIFICATION FORM

CORONER CASE No. 98-129-0008 DATE: 04 December 1998
INVESTIGATING CORONER S. Pellasin EXAMINATION SITE Vancouver City Morgue
LOCATION Port Hardy
CORONERS FORENSIC UNIT CASE # 98-123
POLICE FILE No. 98-2317 AUTOPSY No.
POLICE AGENCY RCMP Port Hardy HOSPITAL
POLICE INVESTIGATOR Cst. H. Gilliman PATHOLOGIST

CIRCUMSTANCES OF EXAMINATION Skeletal remains found on Nov 09, 98 in the area of Dual Point, Port Hardy, B.C. Tentative I.D. "..." - D.O.B. 01 Aug 19

UPPER RIGHT: 18 17 16 15 14 13 12 11 — UPPER LEFT: 21 22 23 24 25 26 27 28

LOWER RIGHT: 48 47 46 45 44 43 42 41 — LOWER LEFT: 31 32 33 34 35 36 37 38

CODE: Shade all restorations on Chart. Outline Prosthetic Appliances.
Circle the appropriate descriptions

Follow Code:

A. Amalgam	TC. Temporary Crown	EN. Root Treatment	X. Missing
S. Composite	GC. Gold Crown	BR. Bridge Work (bracket & shade)	PX. Posthumously missing
G. Gold	PC. Porcelain Crown		NR. Not Recovered
SE. Fissure Sealant	PFM. Porcelain / Metal Crown	PP. Partial Denture (bracket & describe)	
TF. Temporary Filling	SC. Stainless Steel Crown		
1. Mottled Enamel	8. Erosion	15. Retained Deciduous Teeth	22. Congenitally Absent
2. Enamel Hypoplasia	9. Fractured Enamel	16. Unusual Restorations	23. Extruded paste material
3. Discolouration	10. Rotation	17. Unusual Appliances	
4. Staining	11. Malpositioned Teeth	18. Cyst Formation	24. Buccal restoration composite
5. Calculus	12. Malocclusion	19. Post	
6. Abrasion	13. Unerupted Teeth	20. Pin	
7. Attrition	14. Supernumerary Teeth	21. Caries	25.

Post mortem dental x-ray ..... Yes No
Photos ..... Yes No
Study Models ..... Yes No
Jaws disarticulated ..... Yes No

Occlusion: Unremarkable

Remarks: Calculus deposits gross, not mouthwash unique, likely to have "peg-shaped" #22 Extruded material #1

Fig. 3.1A: A typical case history performa

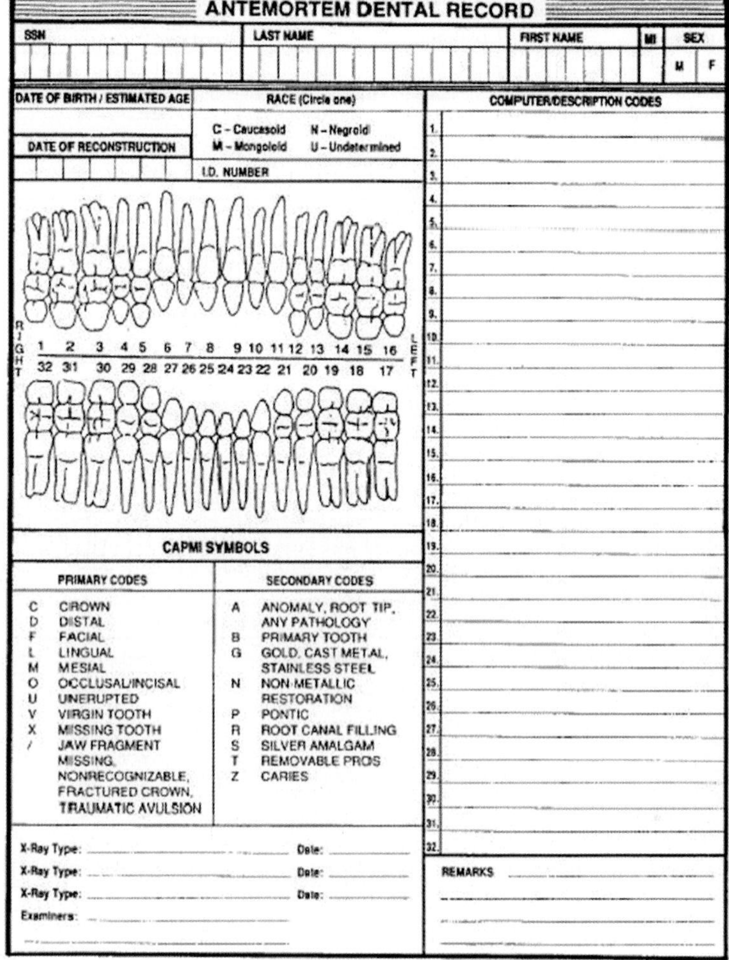

ANTEMORTEM DENTAL RECORD

SSN | LAST NAME | FIRST NAME | MI | SEX: M F

DATE OF BIRTH / ESTIMATED AGE

RACE (Circle one)

C - Caucasoid N - Negroid
M - Mongoloid U - Undetermined

DATE OF RECONSTRUCTION

I.D. NUMBER

COMPUTER/DESCRIPTION CODES

1. 2. 3. 4. 5. 6. 7. 8. 9. 10. 11. 12. 13. 14. 15. 16. 17. 18. 19. 20. 21. 22. 23. 24. 25. 26. 27. 28. 29. 30. 31. 32.

RIGHT 1 2 3 4 5 6 7 8 9 10 11 12 13 14 15 16 LEFT
32 31 30 29 28 27 26 25 24 23 22 21 20 19 18 17

CAPMI SYMBOLS

PRIMARY CODES		SECONDARY CODES	
C	CROWN	A	ANOMALY, ROOT TIP, ANY PATHOLOGY
D	DISTAL	B	PRIMARY TOOTH
F	FACIAL	G	GOLD, CAST METAL, STAINLESS STEEL
L	LINGUAL	N	NON-METALLIC RESTORATION
M	MESIAL	P	PONTIC
O	OCCLUSAL/INCISAL	R	ROOT CANAL FILLING
U	UNERUPTED	S	SILVER AMALGAM
V	VIRGIN TOOTH	T	REMOVABLE PROS
X	MISSING TOOTH	Z	CARIES
/	JAW FRAGMENT MISSING, NONRECOGNIZABLE, FRACTURED CROWN, TRAUMATIC AVULSION		

X-Ray Type: ______ Date: ______
X-Ray Type: ______ Date: ______
X-Ray Type: ______ Date: ______
Examiners: ______

REMARKS ______

Fig. 3.1B: Antemortem dental record performa

D. Pregnancy history in case of female patients.
E. Dental history.
F. Clinical examination to include an accurate charting:
   - Diagnosis
   - Treatment plan
   - Documentation of informed consent.

Creation and Maintenance of a Patient Record

Lawney describes a simple ten step procedure to ensure that your records are adequate. A modified and expanded version, appropriate to the dentists, is given below:

1. Use a consistent style for entries—The appearance of the record is enhanced by using the same color and type of pen, use the same abbreviations and notations etc.
2. Date and explain any corrections—It may be a fatal error in a malpractice case if records appear doctored in any way. These unexplained corrections can undermine the credibility of the entire record and of the treating dentist.

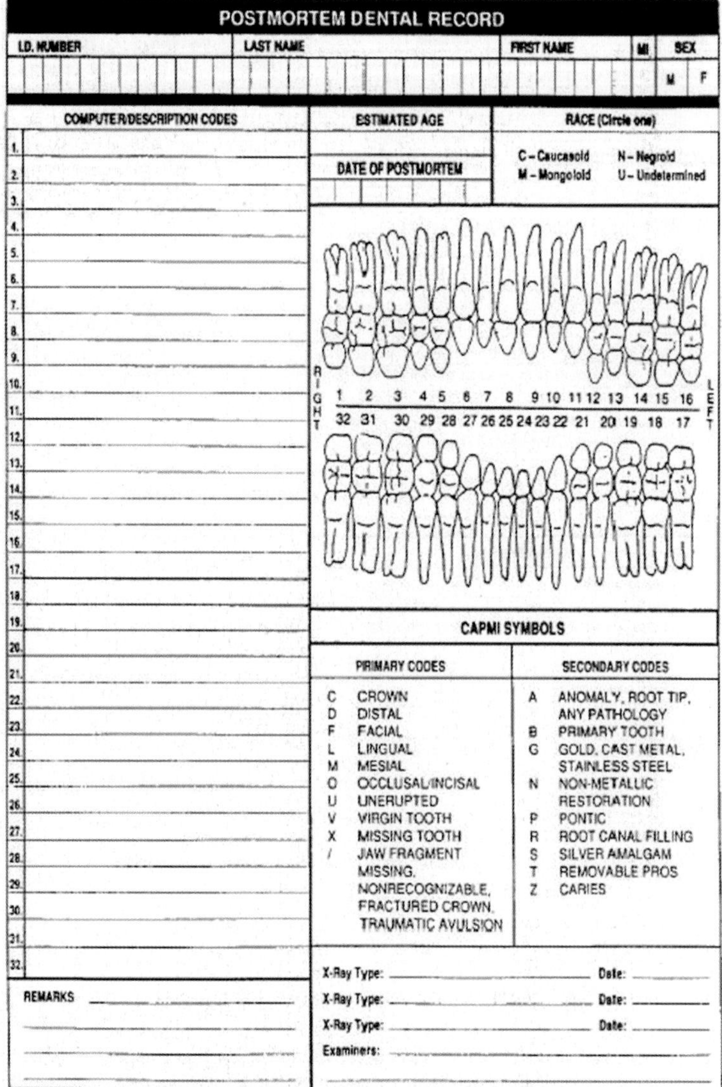

POSTMORTEM DENTAL RECORD

I.D. NUMBER	LAST NAME	FIRST NAME	MI	SEX
				M F

COMPUTER/DESCRIPTION CODES	ESTIMATED AGE	RACE (Circle one)
1.	DATE OF POSTMORTEM	C – Caucasoid N – Negroid M – Mongoloid U – Undetermined

1. through 32.

RIGHT — 1 2 3 4 5 6 7 8 9 10 11 12 13 14 15 16 — LEFT

32 31 30 29 28 27 26 25 24 23 22 21 20 19 18 17

CAPMI SYMBOLS

PRIMARY CODES	SECONDARY CODES
C CROWN D DISTAL F FACIAL L LINGUAL M MESIAL O OCCLUSAL/INCISAL U UNERUPTED V VIRGIN TOOTH X MISSING TOOTH / JAW FRAGMENT MISSING, NONRECOGNIZABLE, FRACTURED CROWN, TRAUMATIC AVULSION	A ANOMALY, ROOT TIP, ANY PATHOLOGY B PRIMARY TOOTH G GOLD, CAST METAL, STAINLESS STEEL N NON-METALLIC RESTORATION P PONTIC R ROOT CANAL FILLING S SILVER AMALGAM T REMOVABLE PROS Z CARIES

REMARKS

X-Ray Type: Date:

X-Ray Type: Date:

X-Ray Type: Date:

Examiners:

Fig. 3.1C: Postmortem dental record performa

3. Use single-line crossout—This preserves the integrity of the record and shows that you have nothing to hide.
4. Do not use correction fluids—Not only is this messy, but it is conspicuous and may indicate that there has been an attempt to hide information.
5. Use ink—Pencil can fade and opens up the question of whether or not the records have been altered.
6. Write legibly—An illegible record may be as bad as no record at all. Difficult to read entries can lead to guesswork by others and this may not be favorable to you.

7. Express concerns about patient needs—By doing this you are documenting that you have listened, empathized, understood and acted upon the wishes of your patient. It also enables an explanation to be given should a patients' wishes be unobtainable or unrealistic and can help instantly diffuse a malpractice case. Use quotations to indicate patient comments as distinct from your own.
8. Never write derogatory remarks in the record—Superfluous entries only serve to convey a feeling of unprofessionalism and may give doubts to the overall credibility of the remainder of the record. Negative views about patients, such as their failure to follow your advice or attend appointments, should be recorded in a dispassionate and objective manner.
9. Document fully—There is no need to be sparse with notes, a detailed explanation is always better than one lacking information. It is important to note, however, that each entry should pertain directly to patient care.
10. Only use accepted abbreviations for treatments—This is helpful both in a malpractice situation and also when transferring records to a different dentist for referral, prior approval or a change in dentist of record.
11. Collate documents—Insurance details and other materials from third parties should be separate from those items which pertain directly to patient care.
12. Maintain a chronological order—The use of a hole punch and metal retainer clips in the top of the record may be helpful to keep loose sheets organized.

By following these steps the production of accurate and defensible records is possible.

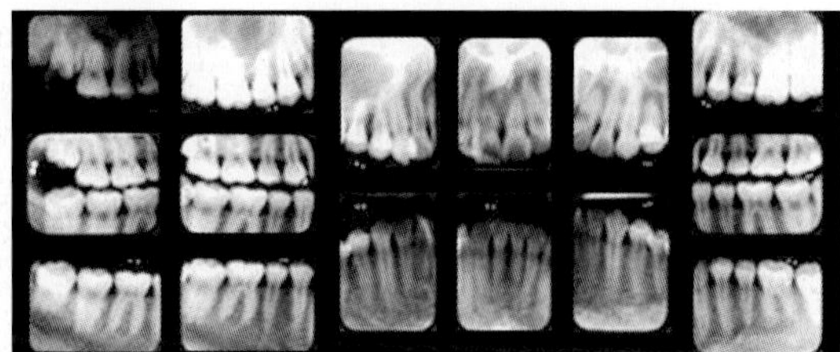

Fig. 3. 2A: An example of complete radiograph records

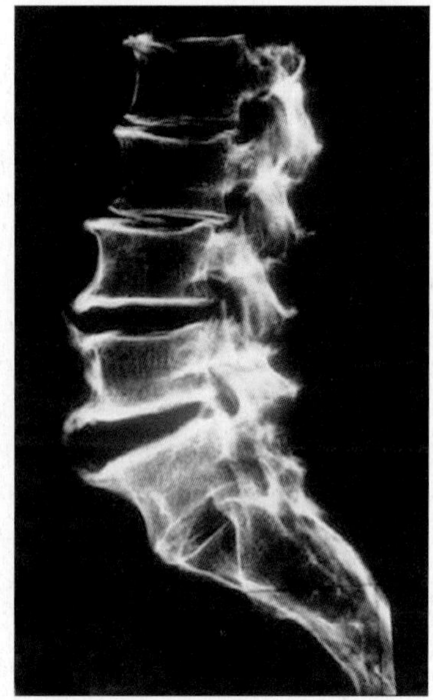

Fig. 3.2B: A spine radiograph obtained from patient's previous physician

Radiographs Keeping (Figs 3.2A and B)

The production, storage and documentation of radiographs is highly variable. In the Swedish study only 40 percent of the radiographs were identifiable to the patient. In the NHS system (UK) the most common technique for radiograph storage is in a small envelope with the patient's details, type of radiograph and date listed on the front. The patient's record can quickly become filled with these envelopes and establishing a time line can be difficult and confusing, especially when endodontic films become co-mingled with diagnostic films. A mounting method can be a more effective solution to radiograph storage. This mount will easily fit within the patient's record sleeve.

A common problem experienced when viewing a patient's radiographic history is that of degradation of the films. This is usually due to processing errors, especially a failure to properly fix and rinse the films. This is most frequently found on those films used for endodontic procedures as the developing is often hurried and commonly self-developing films are used.

As well as the need for accurate, well-stored and documented radiographs, the frequency of radiographic examination is also important. A patient's record that is lacking up-to-date radiographs may jeopardize a malpractice case and is against the patient's best interest. There are established guidelines for the frequency of radiographic examination. These guidelines should be modified for the individual patient's requirements, based on caries risk and presence or absence of periodontal disease and other pathologies.

Like all parts of the dental record, radiographs should be stored for 11 years or up to the age of 25, in the case of children, for protection against the 1987 Consumer Protection Act (UK).

Retention of Patient Records

The NHS Terms of Service state that dental records should be kept for a period of two years. The Regulations state that treatment records, radiographs, photographs and study models should be retained after the completion of any course of treatment and care under a continuing care or capitation arrangement for this period. However, a patient has the right to raise an action for damages based on accusations of negligence or breach of contract. There are strict time limits applied to such actions.

It is therefore possible that a claim for negligence could happen many years after the event, and that retention of records for the minimum two years is inadequate. The defense organizations suggest that records be kept permanently. This is often impossible due to space constraints and so the advice given by defense organization (UK) is as follows:

A. Treatment records, X-rays, study models **(Figs 3.3A and B)** and correspondence retained for 11 years after the completion of treatment
B. For children, retention of records until the patient is 25 years old
C. *Orthodontic models-* **(Fig. 3.4)** retain the original pre and postoperative models permanently, discard any intermediates after a period of 5 years.

The storage area of these records should be secure and access strictly controlled. By following these guidelines, the dental records of a patient will be available for you should a claim ever be made.

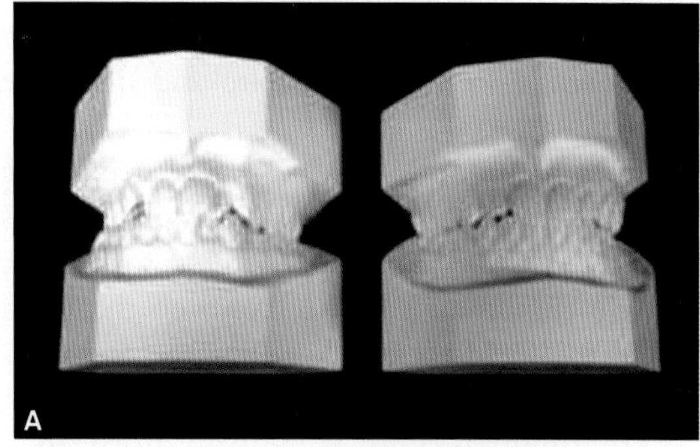

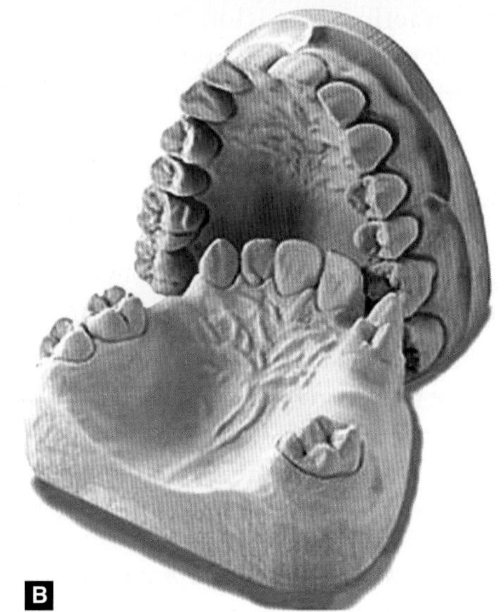

Figs 3.3A and B: Well-mounted and articulated casts

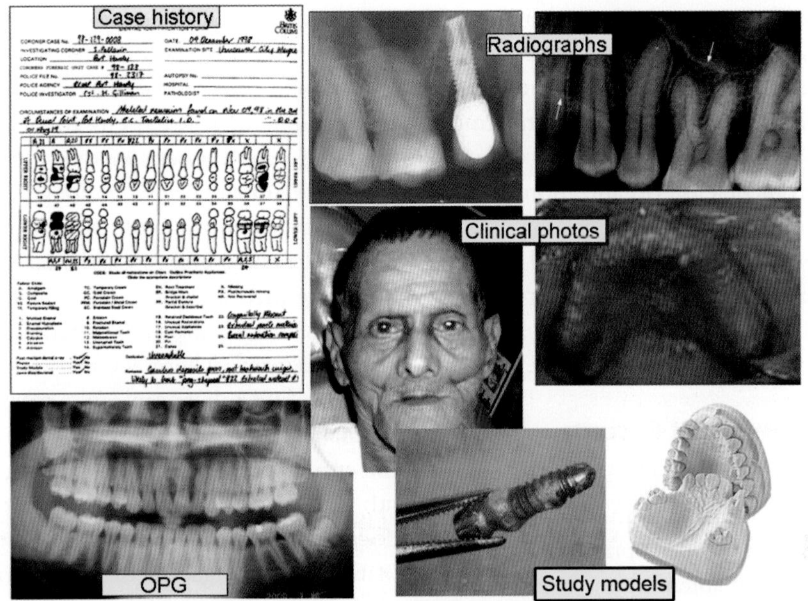

Fig. 3.4: Composite diagram showing various types of dental records that may be useful in the case need arises for the identification

Long-term Storage of Dental Records

For records which are dormant, and yet need to be retained, computer technology provides an economical solution. The use of high density, removable storage media, such as Iomega Zip disks, allows large quantites of data to be stored easily and economically. Paper records and radiographs can simply be scanned into a personal computer using a desktop scanner. This data is then compressed using technologies such as JPEG, enabling many records to be stored on a single disk. Commonly used programs such as Adobe Photoshop contain the JPEG compression system. Should the record ever be needed again then the files can simply be printed to a high quality laser printer. By using these techniques the dentist can protect themselves from malpractice claims without using valuble storage space. The removal of inactive files streamlines the filing system leading to an improvement in record system efficiency.

Access to Patient Records

Patients, their legal representatives and police officers may gain access to dental records. The Access to Health Records Act 1990 (UK) provides the following legislation:

Personal inspection—A patient can request to see their notes and be guided by the dentist through the contents with explanations of terminology and technical language.

Photocopies—A dentist can provide a photocopy of the notes if the patient requests so in writing. The record photocopy must be provided within 21 days of the request or within 40 days if no treatment has been carried out in the past 40 days. Only details of the record from 1st November 1991 can be provided under this Act, however, it may be necessary to provide earlier entries to explain subsequent treatment.

The dentist may charge reasonable photocopy and postal charges. When asked by a patient for access to records, a caring attitude and prompt delivery may well help prevent any future claim. If the request for disclosure of notes comes from a solicitor then this may indicate that the patient intends to take legal action. Not all of the treatment record is relevant to the matter in question and so always consult your defense organization prior to releasing any documents in this situation. As an additional note it must be remembered that the Data Protection Act 1984 allows patients to view any information about themselves held on computer, following a written request.

Forensic Uses of Patient Records

Forensic dentistry is the overlap of the dental and legal professions. The most common element of forensic dentistry that a general practitioner is likely to encounter is supply antemortem (before death) records to aid in human identification. Forensic dentists are frequently called upon to identify the remains of individuals who cannot be identified visually. This encompasses a large number of situations such as burnt, grossly decomposed or mutilated remains. The identification is normally carried out by the comparison of antemortem (before death) and postmortem (after death) records.

The identification of deceased individual is an essential element in the process of death certification and is a crucial component in the investigation of homicides or other sudden deaths. It is vital to have expeditious and accurate identification both for police officers and relatives. Until identification can be confirmed, estates cannot be settled, death benefits cannot be paid and surviving spouses are unable to remarry. Perhaps of most importance is that the identification of the dead is an essential component of the grieving process and is a necessary part of human dignity in a civilized society.

The police officers in charge of the case will normally call upon the dentist to provide details of dental records. It must be remembered that police officers have no statutory rights to inspect or remove a patient's records without their consent. However, the law allows for special circumstances and it is reasonable to hand over an individual's record if it enables them to be identified or excluded. The consent of the nearest relative or estate executor may also be sought if required.

The availability of contemporaneous and clear notes is essential in forensic dental identification If notes are incorrect or dated, this can complicate and even negate a positive identification. It is in such situations where the errors highlighted by Borrman and others can cause crucial mistakes to be made. When a request for records is received the entire record is useful, including such items as lab prescriptions and study models. Many documented cases have used the unique pattern of the palatal rugae recorded on an orthodontic study model to identify a young individuals with no dental restorations.

The police may require access to an individual's record for another criminal matter. They may, for example, want to see an appointment book to establish an alibi or time line. In these circumstances a warrant is required, if the patient has not agreed to the release, as it can be argued that the release of notes in this instance is not in the patient's best interest.

Confidentiality of Records

Dentists are in a privileged position to learn much about patients and this knowledge is acquired under the assumption that it is confidential. Confidentiality encourages open and honest communication, enhancing the dentist-patient. relationship, and encourages respect for patient autonomy and privacy. Confidentiality is taken very seriously by professional bodies and an alleged breach of this trust would be investigated by the Professional Conduct Committee of the General Dental Council (UK).

There are circumstances in which information can be disclosed, and they include:

1. Sharing of relevant information with other health care professionals involved in a patient's treatment.
2. Information may be passed to a third part if the patient or legal adviser gives written consent, e.g. an insurance company.
3. Where information is requested about a deceased patient and consent of the estate or relative is sought and the investigation of sudden, suspicious or unexplained deaths.
4. Information required in the preparation of legal reports containing only relevant dental treatments.
5. Investigation of sudden, suspicious or unexplained deaths.
6. Access to dental records by the police. Search and seizure warrants may not include dental records, and therefore should be carefully checked.
7. Clinical research protocols and peer review procedures. The name of the patient must be kept confidential. If information is to be used for teaching purposes then the patient's consent must be obtained.

The area of confidentiality of children's dental information can be confusing. Those individuals of 16 years and older should be considered adults, however for those 16 and under, the dentist still has a duty of care and therefore confidentiality to the child. This duty is combined with a duty to the parents, especially in the area of consent to treatment. Children who are victims of abuse require special management and the dentist may have an overriding responsibility to break confidentiality and report their findings to the appropriate authorities. Special guidelines exist for AIDS/HIV and sexually transmitted diseases. Strict confidentiality must be maintained when dealing with these individuals. Disclosure of such information could lead to a complaint of serious professional misconduct.

Indian Scenario and Lacunae in the System

As published in the journal of Indian Dentist Research and Review, issue 2, September 2007, the total number of dental colleges in world is approximately 960. Out of these 960 dental colleges, around 260 dental colleges, that is a staggering 26 percent of the total are alone present in India. Also, India has got a population which is supposed to be one fifth of the world. Unfortunately our country also happens to be one of the countries in the world where there are maximum number of causalities arising out of terrorist attacks, fire disasters, horrific bombing incidents and lastly the curse of Mother Nature in terms of earthquake, floods and landslides.

Given the above considerations, it is clear that many of the causalities arising because of the above situations, do not get their identity and hence their grieved families never get any thing that can console them of the loss they suffered.

We have so many numbers of dental clinics and dental colleges and hospitals in India, still it does not help us out to resolve the identity crisis in such happenings. Because scenario in India is not the same as it is in the western countries. So the tremendous vast potentiality of dental records in the identification protocol does not help out to come to any conclusion in case of such events. So the question arises where are we lagging behind. Answers to all the above questions become clear as because of the reasons mentioned below:

1. Not many people in India visit dentist even once in their life.
2. Records are not kept and even if kept, are not maintained for a long time.
3. Inability to locate the dentist in case of any causality and subsequently obtain AM records.
4. Poor quality of AM records/non availability.
5. Patients treated on emergency basis may have few records.

6. There is no law and rule in India, which reinforces the dental record keeping mandatory.
7. Lack of funding to sustain and maintain the records.
8. Also, at present no specialization in the field of forensic odontology.

With above considerations, it is clear that a dentist can be an important source for providing valuable data to answer questions that arise during a death investigation. As a tooth can withstand insults where all other tissues may not survive to be recognized, the importance of such tooth can be of interest in identification of persons, provided good ante mortem records are available.

There are fewer AM records available particularly in our set-ups, we need to keep an accurate and ordered dental records of all the patients which may be of immense value in unfortunate events, thus making us to serve people even better with more responsibility and care.

Thus, when nothing remains out of a body, except for a fragment of tooth, identifying the person to whom it does belongs to, may at least make something at last to be returned to the grieved families **(Fig. 3.5)**.

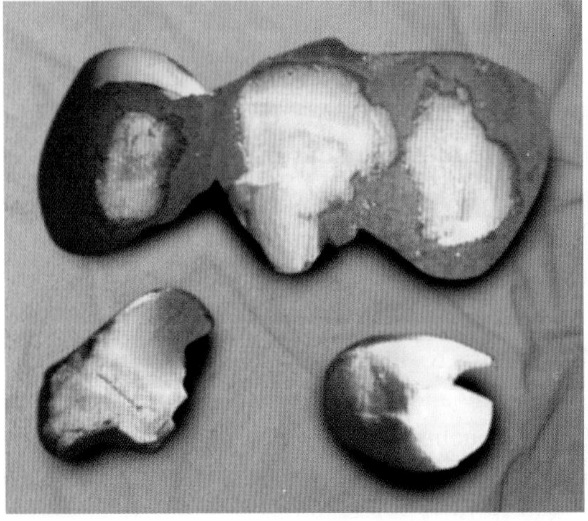

Fig. 3.5: A recovered bridge from the remains of a victim of a disaster, making the identification easier

Forensic Photography

Need for the Photography

Accurate photography is crucial to forensic investigation as a means of documenting evidence. The need to photographically record injury patterns as they appear on skin is paramount to the odontologist and pathologist. Since vast amounts of time often elapse between the commission of a crime and the trial of the perpetrator, photographs frequently are the only permanent record of the injuries to the victims. Therefore, it is imperative that the forensic investigator be able to properly photograph injury patterns as a means of preserving such evidence.

Photography is one of the most important applied protocols of forensic dentistry. The demands on the photographer can be great, especially in situations where an injury is the only evidence tying a suspect to the crime. Time, patience, and preparation in forensic photography are requirements for successful pattern injury documentation. While often frustrating and time consuming, when done properly the results yield good evidence, bringing with it a sense of accomplishment and satisfaction that the forensic dentist has made a significant contribution to the case. Developing the skills necessary to competently document these injuries with visible and nonvisible light is one of the great challenges in forensic dentistry.

The Technical Considerations

The process of photographically recording images on film, videotape, or other media occurs through the capture of electromagnetic radiation (light) of specific wavelengths. These wavelengths, measured in millionths of millimeters, are referred to as nanometers and abbreviated as (nm). Photographic images are recorded on photographic films which are sensitive to light wavelengths in the range of 250 to 900 nm. Visible light, which comprises the range of **(Fig. 3.6)** electromagnetic radiation seen by the naked human eye, is from 400 to 760 nm in range. Most modern camera equipment and film is specifically designed to record images seen in the visible range of light. In the visible spectrum, the image is recorded on the film as it is seen by the eye through the lens when the lens is focused on the image. It is also possible to record images specifically illuminated in the shorter ultraviolet range (210 to 400 nm), and longer infrared range (750 to 900 nm) wavelengths.

Because ultraviolet and infrared light are outside the visible range of electromagnetic radiation, they are commonly referred to as "non-visible light". Photography using non visible light requires special techniques to record the injury. It may also require some minor focusing adjustments, called "focus shifts", to correct for the optical properties of lenses which were designed for visible light photography.

The Basic Optics of Photographic Process

When light strikes skin, four basic events occur. The first of these is reflection, which occurs when some of the electromagnetic radiation hits the skin and bounces back from it. It is this reflection of visible light that accounts for the colors seen by the human eye. Not all light energy on an object is reflected. Some of the light can be absorbed.

The second of these is the absorption of light by an object that makes it appear black. The action of the absorption of light associated with the injury being photographed is significant in nonvisible light photography.

A third reaction of light striking skin is the transmission and scattering of the energy associated with the light through successive layers of cells until the energy of the light has dissipated. The final reaction that occurs when light energy strikes an object is a molecular excitation called fluorescence. Excitation at the molecular level causes the emission of a faint glow that lasts only as long as the excitation energy is applied to the object. Once the excitation energy is spent, the fluorescent glow ceases. Fluorescence is not readily seen because of the short duration of the emittance, lasting only about 100 ns and because the reflected light energy

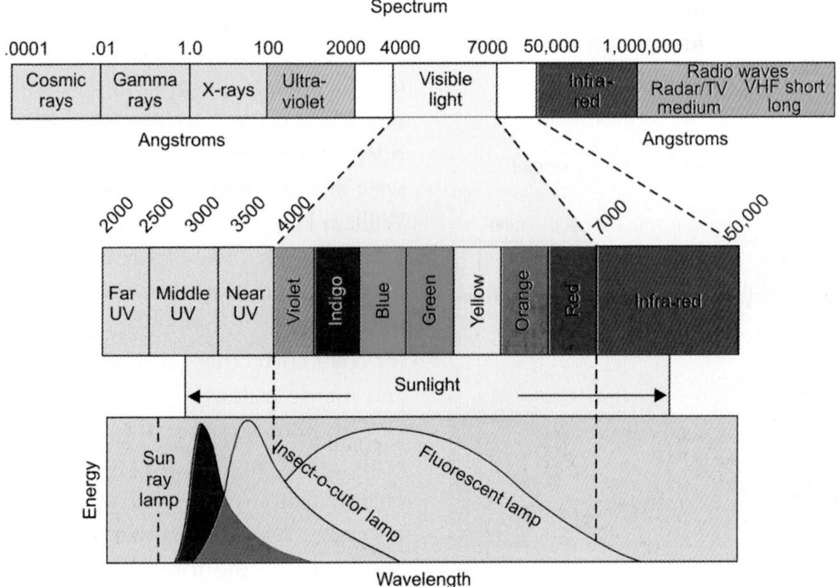

Fig. 3. 6: Light spectrum

is so much greater that it overwhelms any fluorescent light detectable by the naked eye. When light strikes human skin, all four of the previously mentioned events occur simultaneously. Depending on the wavelength of the source of the incident light and the configuration of the camera, it is possible to record, individually, any of the four reactions of skin to light energy. Ultraviolet light only penetrates a few microns (thousandths of millimeters) into skin whereas infrared light can penetrate skin to a depth of up to 3 mm **(Fig. 3.7)**.

What is usually seen when visible light strikes the skin is reflected light energy. What is not seen, however, is the light energy that is absorbed by the skin. By varying the wavelength of incident light used for illumination and setting up the appropriate configuration of the camera, lens, filters, and film, it is possible to photograph any of the four events which occur. This ability creates an opportunity for interesting pictures, especially when looking at bruises and other injuries to skin. Sharp surface details can be seen with ultraviolet light, while images well below the surface of the skin can be seen using infrared light. The techniques and photographic protocol for documenting injuries to human skin in visible and nonvisible light will be described.

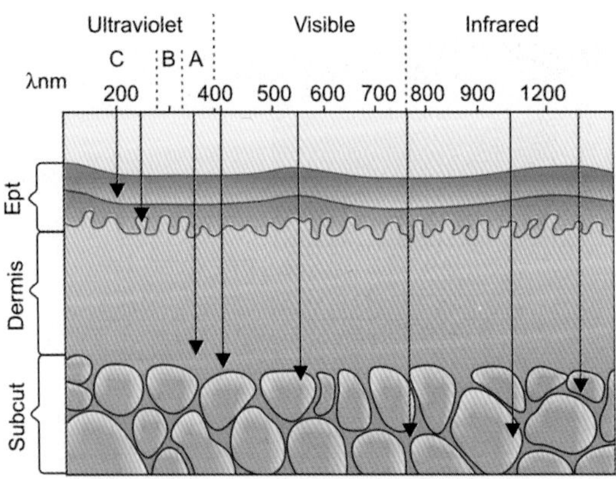

Fig. 3.7: A graphical representation illustrating the penetration of various types of wavelengths of light into the skin

Types and Techniques

When presented with an injury, the forensic dentist or investigator must decide

a. What information the injury may contain?
b. The extent of the injury, and
c. How best to photographically record it?

As previously mentioned, preserving the detail of the injury with photographs may involve a combination of color and black and white visible light photographs as well as the use of the non-visible ultraviolet and infrared photographs.

The Standard Technique

The photographer should develop a standard technique which includes orientation photographs showing where the injury occurred on the body. Additionally, this protocol should include close-up photographs for detail, **(Figs 3.8A to C)** and photographs, placing the lighting source (flash and light guide) at different angles in relation to the injury. Photographs should be taken with and without a scale. The use of a scale serves as a reference to record the relative size of the injuries in the photographs. While there are a number of acceptable scales, including coins, when unavailability of appropriate scales occurs, many forensic investigators use the ABFO No. 2 **(Fig. 3.9)** scale in their photographs. This right-angled scale was developed by a photogrammetrist (Mr William Hyzer) and a forensic dentist (Dr Thomas Krauss) for the purpose of minimizing photographic distortion and assuring accuracy in measurement. It has a black, white, and gray scale for color correctness, as well as three perfect circles and metric scales.

The photographer should retain the original scale used in the photograph in the event enlargement to life-sized reproductions becomes necessary. It is essential that the standard technique developed by the forensic photographer includes exposing many photographs for each case. One

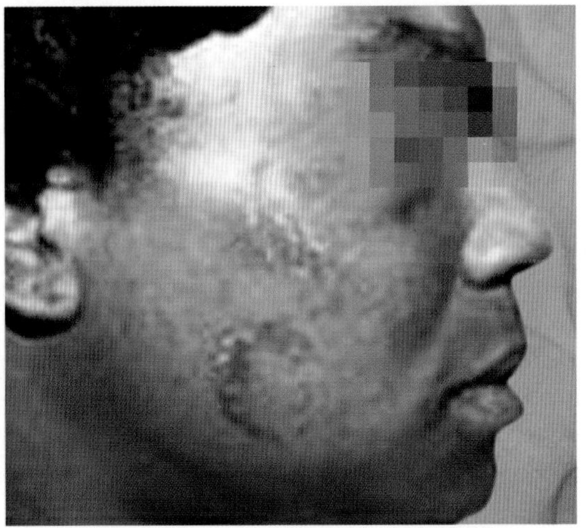

Fig. 3.8A: A color orientation picture of patient highlighting the site of injury and its overall relationship to the surrounding tissues

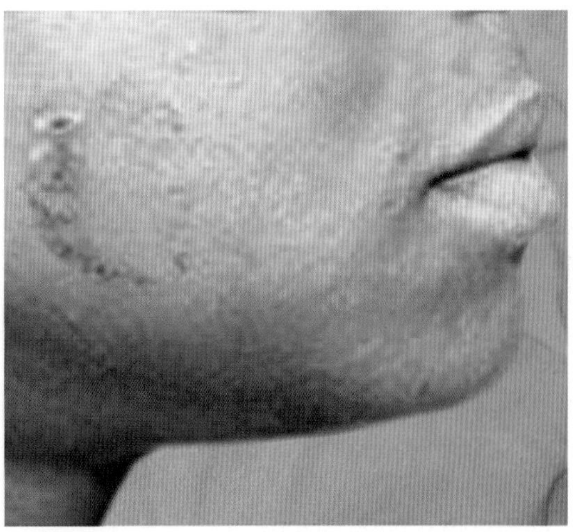

Fig. 3.8C: A B/W picture, taken in order to see the details of injury which may be masked in the color picture

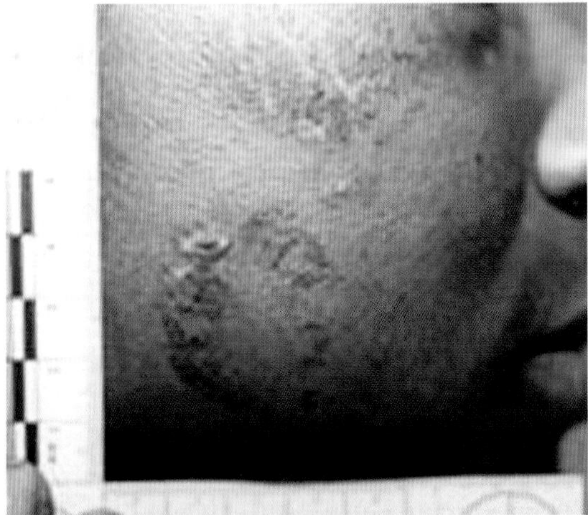

Fig. 3.8B: A close-up picture of the same patient to illustrate the injury in more detail

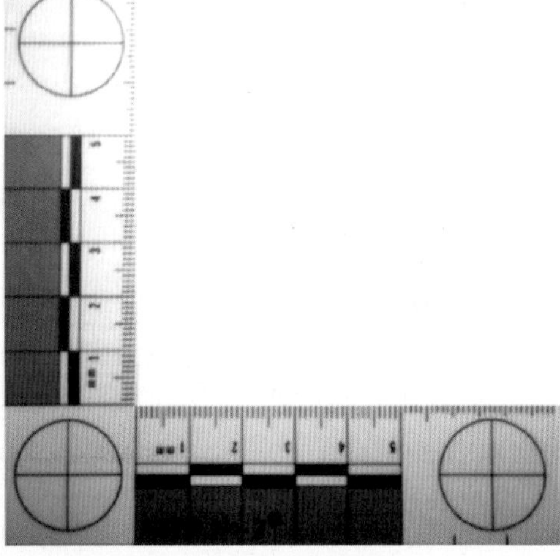

Fig. 3.9: ABFO Scale No. 2 "(ABFO: American Board of Forensic Odontology)

should not be hesitant about using several rolls of film for a photo shoot.

Types of Technique

Various types of photographic technique are available today in order to cater the different need arising out of different situations. Some of these technique are used routinely, easier to perform and a mere more standardized adaptation to what we use in our day to day life, while others are more complex, requiring a thorough knowledge of optics and its principles, along with the advanced knowledge of various kind of camera systems, lens properties, and the processing techniques. In this part of the chapter, described first will be the simpler technique followed by the more complex other techniques. Following is the list of various techniques that are used in forensic photography.

1. Visible light photography
   a. Digital photography
   b. Visible light color photography
   c. Visible light black and white photography
2. Alternate light imaging (ALI) and fluorescent techniques
3. Non-visible light photography
   a. Reflective long-wavelength ultraviolet (UVA) photography
   b. Infrared photography

Visible Light Photography

By far, the most common type of photography utilized today is photography using visible light, both in color and black and white. Manufacturers of photographic equipment and films develop and market equipment and supplies that are specifically designed to have an optimal performance in the 400 to 760 nm range of the electromagnetic spectrum. For the photographer wishing to take pictures in this range of light energy, there is relatively little practice required to ensure highly detailed and sharply focused photographs.

Many 35 mm SLR cameras available today are considered "automatic" point-and-shoot cameras. By definition, the object to be photographed is viewed through the lens and the camera automatically adjusts the focus and exposure variables before exposing the film. However, depending on the type of film used and the spectrum of electromagnetic radiation to which the film has sensitivity, it can become possible to "fog" (alter or distort) a visible light exposure with ultraviolet and infrared light. With visible light photographic techniques, ultraviolet light may cause color shifts toward an undesirable bluish tint in the photographs, while infrared light may create more red tints than desired. To prevent ultraviolet and infrared wave energy from fogging visible light photographs, modern day manufacturers produce coated lenses and filtered flash units, allowing only visible light to reach the film. Most 35 mm cameras have serious size limitations when it comes to recording life-size images. The limitation comes from the small area of film (24 mm × 35 mm rectangle) which records the image. Since there are very few objects which will fit into that small area, considerable enlargement of the photographs may be necessary to see the injuries life-sized. Since evaluations and comparisons of the injuries to the teeth, weapons, or tools which created them are often done in direct relation to the life-sized object, it is necessary to have photographs that can be enlarged to life-size without loss of the detail necessary for the comparison.

Film manufacturers have designed photographic films that record light wavelengths from 250 to 700 nm. Special infrared films are available that can record photographs taken in light from 250 to 900 nm. Choosing the proper film is critical for successfully recording the detail of an injury. The film must be sensitive to the wavelength of light being used to photograph the injury or no image will appear when the film is developed. There are many quality photographic negative films manufactured, both in color and black and white.

In addition to the photosensitivity range of the film, the correct film speed must also be determined. Films come with a rating, referred to as the ASA/ISO number, which serves as an indicator of the amount of light energy necessary to properly expose the film. The higher the ASA/ISO number, the faster the film; in other words, less light is needed to expose an image. Films with high-speed ratings (ASA 1600 or 3200) require very little light energy exposure, but caution must be exercised. The higher the ASA/ISO number, the lower the grain density on the film where the image is recorded, which translates into less versatility during enlarging. Large-grain fast films tend to produce prints which appear to lose focal sharpness and detail as they are enlarged toward their normal limits, i.e. life-sized or 1:1. Just as there are good and bad attributes for high-speed films, slower speed films can also have limitations. Using a film speed that is too slow for the amount of available light will result in an underexposed picture that may also lack clarity and detail. There are some situations where the photographer does need to underexpose for better detail, particularly during fluorescent photography. The basic recommendation is to use the slowest film speed which will have the most grain density for the lighting present. Problems caused by having the wrong film or improper lighting may be minimized by bracketing the exposures over a wide range of camera settings (bracketing means to expose individual photographs in a range of f-stops and shutter speeds).

a. Digital Photography (**Figs 3.10A and B**): This technique utilizes a special computer hard disk in the camera that stores the images as digital information. These images can be later written to CD-ROM for storage. The advantage of digital photography is that the image can then be immediately viewed on a computer monitor or printed on a color printer. The image could also be transferred to traditional photographic films. This technology works superbly for color and black and white visible light photographs, but requires special computer chips for non-visible light photographs.

Before approaching any photographic subject for close-up documentation of either a injury pattern or tool mark, remember to take an orientation shot. For example, in photographing a bite mark, typically a few preliminary photos would be taken at a distance which includes the location and orientation of the bite mark relative to its position on the body. This is to communicate to subsequent observers exactly where the injury occurred and its positional orientation. After the orientation photos, numerous close-up photographs using a macro lens should be taken, both with and without a scale in place. If the camera has a macro lens and is used for close-ups, be certain the scale is in the same focal plane of the object being photographed before exposing the film.

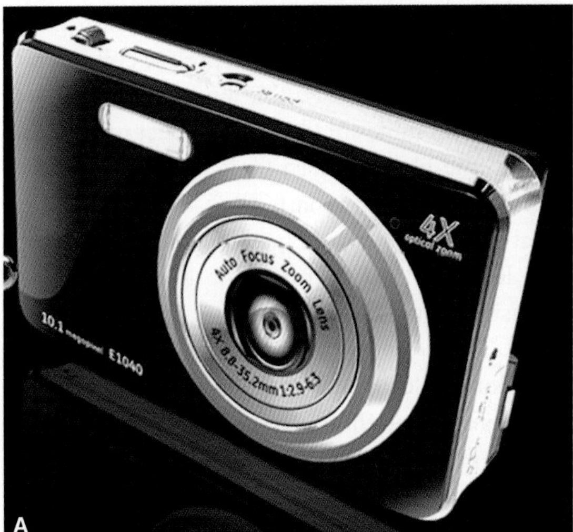

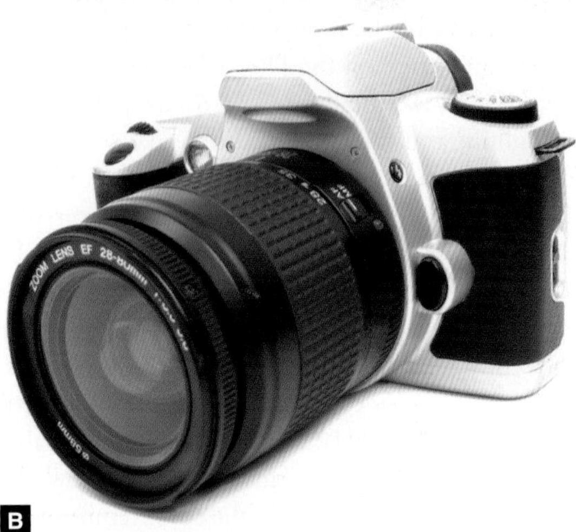

Figs 3.10 A and B: Types of digital and SLR cameras available in the markets

b. Visible Light Color Photography: Advancements in design and manufacture of modern 35 mm cameras have greatly simplified color photography.

These cameras have the capability to photograph objects with great accuracy and precise color detail. As discussed previously, the lenses have coatings and the flash units are filtered to direct only visible light to the film. Modern films record the images in brilliant colors and sharp detail. The most critical variables to consider when taking still photographs in color are (1) the type of the film and (2) the intensity of the light present when the film is exposed.

Color visible light photography is by far the most common type of photography used today. Modern cameras readily available today are manufactured and configured to take photographs using **(Fig. 3.11)** visible light. There are generally no special requirements or equipment needs assuming there is enough visible light energy available to properly record the image on the film. When choosing the type of film, use the lowest speed film possible for the lighting available and proceed to take orientation exposures, gradually moving to the specific site of the injury. With routine color slide or print film illuminated by flash, a film of ASA 100 is generally adequate for close-up photography. To insure color accuracy, it would be helpful to include a color correction guide in one or more of the exposures. One popular color correction guide is the Macbeth Color Chart **(Figs 3.12A and B)**, which is available in camera shops. Use of this guide will allow the film processing lab to correct the color temperature of the negative to the real color composition of the image before printing the photograph.

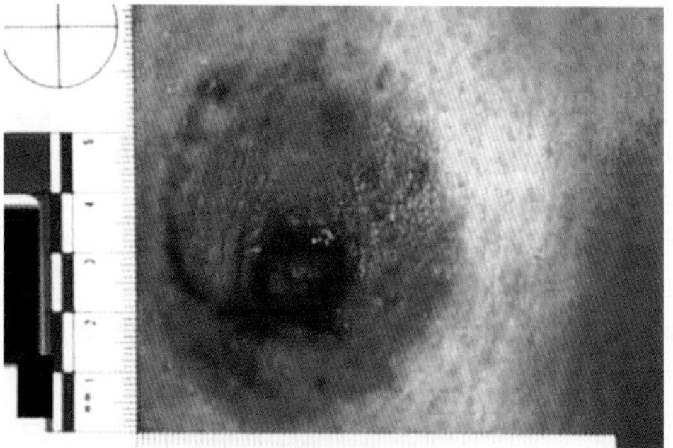

Fig. 3.11: A normal close-up color picture of the bite mark with correct placement of ABFO Scale No. 2

106 81 67	182 149 130	103 122 154	95 108 69	129 128 174	133 189 170
194 121 48	79 91 162	170 85 97	84 62 105	167 186 73	213 162 57
54 62 149	101 148 76	152 48 58	228 199 55	164 83 144	63 134 163
242 241 236	200 200 199	159 160 159	122 121 120	84 84 84	53 53 53

A

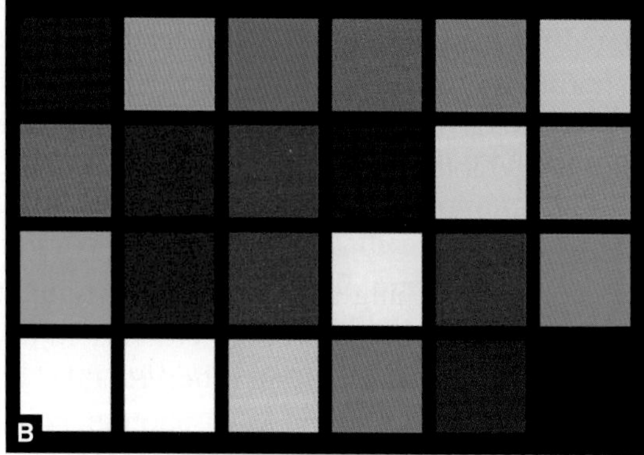

Figs 3.12A and B: Macbeth color charts used for color correction purposes

c. Visible Light Black and White Photography: Changing from color film to black and white film, the forensic photographer proceeds to re-photograph the injury. Use the same orientation and standard technique that was used when the color photographs were taken. In order to simplify this process, many photographers maintain two complete camera systems, with interchangeable bodies; one loaded with color film, the other with black and white. It may seem redundant to re-record the injury with black and white photographs when color photographs of the same injury were just taken—or is it?

This is because of the fact that the human eye is very adapt at seeing images in color. Because of the color information processed optically by the retina, other important details of the injury may be overlooked. When the injury is photographed in black and white, the eye is not distracted by the color composition of the injury and the normal surrounding areas. Consequently, this absence of color allows the viewer to see more detail in the injury. When exposing film for black and white photographs, the same criteria for exposing color photographs are followed. In many situations there may only be one chance for photographs. If that is the case, take a minimum of three or four rolls of black and white and color photographs, bracketed widely, and illuminated from different angles.

Alternate Light Imaging (ALI) and Fluorescent Techniques

The field of forensic investigation has seen a tremendous growth in the utilization of alternate light imaging for both locating and photographing latent evidence. Fingerprints, serological fluids left behind at a crime scene (blood, semen, saliva), types of ink used to counterfeit or falsify documents, and bruises or other pattern injuries left on human skin that were sustained during violent crimes can now be more easily detected and also transformed into exciting and important exhibits with the utilization of fluorescence. The application of this new technique has numerous titles. For simplicity, here it will be referred to as alternate light imaging (ALI). The technique of photographing evidence with alternate light is called fluorescent photography.

Fluorescence: It is the stimulation and emission of radiation from a subject by the impact of higher energy radiation upon it.

Luminescence: It is a general term for the emission of radiation that incorporates both fluorescence and phosphorescence, as well as other electrochemical phenomena like bioluminescence.

The technique requires an alternate light source which is capable of producing the monochromatic beam. The particular wavelength one tunes to depends upon what trace evidence the forensic investigator is seeking. There are optimal wavelengths for different applications; therefore the color (frequency) of the light and blocking filters will vary. Research and investigation of pattern injuries on human skin has shown that peak fluorescence of the epidermis occurs at 430 to 460 nm, and is blue in coloration. Most of what strikes the surface of the skin is reflected. Of the rest, about 30 percent penetrates below the surface. Some of it gets scattered, some is absorbed, and some is remitted as fluorescent light. The natural light-absorbing organic components of tissue are called chromophores. Examples of chromophores are hemoglobin, bilirubin and melanin.

Since the fluorescent light is always less bright than the incident light, one must observe the fluorescence of an object with filters which allow only the fluorescent light through to the eye and block the more powerful reflected source light.

Principles and techniques previously described are used in fluorescent photography. Light returning to the film must be filtered to allow only the fluorescent image to be captured on the film emulsion. In documenting injury patterns, this filtration is accomplished with a yellow filter such as the Kodak gelatin 15 filter which blocks light transmission in the 400 to 500 nm range. Fluorescent photography is best accomplished successfully in complete darkness, where all other sources of light are eliminated. One can imagine the difficulty in setting up and capturing this kind of photo, especially when the exposure times can range up to 2 to 4 seconds in length and the subject is alive and moving. Use of a tripod-mounted camera is mandatory.

It has been shown that slightly underexposing the film will produce better results than the actual metered exposure. This is true because during longer exposures even the fluorescent light coming back to the film is still bright enough to wash out some of the fine detail in the injury at the so-called "correct" exposure factor. Several variables can influence the photographic protocol and parameters of exposure. Skin color (amount of melanin), skin thickness, wound healing response, light intensity, film speed, and location of the injury are but a few factors which affect the exposure times. Thick skin as found on the palm of the hand and sole of the foot fluoresces more than the thin skin covering the face. Darkly pigmented skin will require longer exposure times than lighter skin because more light is absorbed by the melanin pigmentation of the **(Fig. 3.13A)** darker skin. Persons who bruise easily, such as the elderly, will produce injuries which may require shorter exposure times due to the thinness of the skin; but one can also expect longer exposures when greater hemorrhaging occurs beneath the skin since the blood absorbs light.

Advantages of using ALI:

1. The primary advantage which alternate light imaging (ALI) imparts to the forensic investigator is improved detail and visibility of the subject matter.
2. Fibers which are not easily located under normal light can become like beacons as they fluoresce under alternate light.
3. Gunshot residue on a dark background can be made to stand out as though it were photographed against a white background with the employment of ALI
4. Illegal narcotic drugs such as rock cocaine or a latent fingerprint which may have otherwise gone undetected, can not only be located but may become crucial evidence by using ALI
5. For documenting injuries to victims of violent and sexual crimes or human abuse, fluorescent photography using ALI will frequently provide more information about the actual pattern injury than one would observe under normal flash photography.

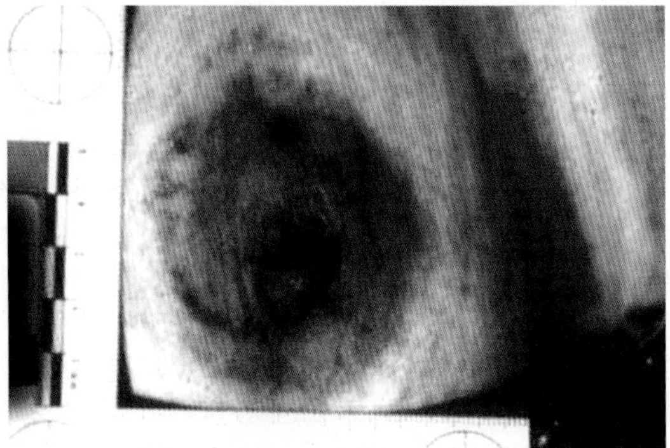

Fig. 3. 13A: Special photograph of the same bite mark case as shown in the picture 3.11 with an alternate source of fluorescent light

Non-visible Light Photography

The photographic requirements for recording injuries on film using non-visible light become somewhat more complex. The appearance of the injury using nonvisible light illumination cannot be seen by the naked eye. Therefore, special techniques must be employed to record the injury on film and then print the image on photographic paper for viewing in visible light. Just as in ALI, these techniques require that band-pass filters be used. They are placed between the injury and the film, usually in front of the lens of the camera. The filters allow only the selected wavelengths of light to pass to the film. It is important that several factors be considered when attempting to photograph injuries in non-visible light:

First, one must consider the type of film being used. The film's photo emulsion must be sensitive to the light wavelength the filter is allowing it to "see". Additionally, the light source must be strong enough to expose the film. The camera's exposure settings (f -stop and shutter speeds) must be set to properly bracket for the type of light being used. The camera's ASA/ISO value must be correctly set for the film being used, and the lens must be focused correctly for the type of nonvisible radiation being used.

There are two major problems encountered with nonvisible light photography. First, it is difficult to acquire a predictable light source that emits enough of the desired wavelength to adequately illuminate the injury being photographed. Second, the exact amount of focal shift to produce a sharp photograph must be determined. Developing confidence and getting predictable results in nonvisible light photography will require some trial and error experimentation. Available and predictable sources of nonvisible lighting are listed below for both ultraviolet and infrared photography.

Ultraviolet (UV) Light Sources

1. *Sunlight:* A good source of long UV light but not practical for situations requiring indoor or night-time exposures.
2. *Fluorescent tubes:* Routinely used for indoor lighting; some useful UV emission. The best of these types of lights is known as a "black light", which emits good UV radiation; the brighter the better.
3. *Mercury vapor lights:* Particularly useful in lighting small areas with intense UV light. Problems include long warm-up time for the light and limited availability.
4. *Flash units:* Many older units provide adequate UV light emission. Some newer units emit a measurable amount of UV but will require experimentation to determine the correct output.
5. *Combination fluorescent/black light:* This light combines the emission of the two light sources in one light fixture; commonly known as a Wood's lamp.

Infrared (IR) Light Sources

1. *Flash units:* Most commercial flash units emit sufficient IR light to be adequate, but require experimentation to determine their acceptability in infrared photography
2. *Tungsten lamps:* Used routinely in forensic investigations. The brighter the Kelvin value, generally the more IR output.
3. *Quartz-halogen lamps:* Good source of IR radiation if unfiltered; more readily available and easy to use.

Focus Shift

After securing a source of predictable nonvisible light illumination, the problem of focus shift must be addressed. By definition, focus shift is "the distance between the visible focus and either the infrared or ultraviolet focus". Focus shift is necessary because nonvisible wavelengths do not behave in the same way as visible light as they pass through a compound lens. The focal length of a lens is specific to a given wavelength of light. Most lenses are chromatically corrected to work within the 400 to 700 nm wavelengths (visible light). When the light energy falls outside of the visible spectrum, the optimal visual focus is no longer the optimally focused point for the nonvisible light energy used to expose the film.

While some manufacturers have developed achromatic lenses which act to bring two different wavelengths to a single coincident focus, many readily available chromatic lenses may require a focus shift for nonvisible light wavelengths. Kodak has suggested the easiest method, and the one recommended to be tried first. It is their opinion that the focus shift required for ultraviolet photographs may be accounted for by simply increasing the depth of field. The recommendation is to decrease the lens aperture at least two stops if shooting from wide open. Since the construction of compound lenses used in 35-mm photography can be so different, Kodak suggests that test exposures at various aperture settings be performed to determine the exact change for an individual lens. The downside to this modification is that it may significantly alter exposure times, lighting, and film speed. Other authors have suggested small focus shifts by turning the focusing ring slightly from the visible focus position. The majority of modern high-quality achromatic compound lenses have a focus color correction to achieve sharp photos.

a. Reflective Long-Wavelength Ultraviolet (UVA) Photography

Ultraviolet photography is used by the forensic photographer primarily for two reasons: The first is to increase the observed detail of the surface of the injury. The second reason is to recapture an injury on film after the injury has "healed" and is no longer visible to the human eye. This second use occurs because ultraviolet light is strongly absorbed by pigment in the skin. Any area of the injury having excess pigmentation when compared to the surrounding normal tissue will be recorded with excellent results using reflective ultraviolet photography. It is also possible to photograph a healed injury up to several months after the injury.

Ultraviolet light does not appreciably penetrate the surface of skin, so photographs are taken using lower numbered f-stops that do not have too much depth of field at the focused distance. Bracketing exposures sequentially from f-4.5 to f-11, at shutter speeds of 1/125 to 2 seconds for each f-stop with the Kodak Wratten 18A band-pass filter in front of the lens should be included in the standard technique. The resultant photographs will contain detail "seen" by ultraviolet light. It is mandatory that the camera be mounted on a tripod before taking ultraviolet photographs due to the long exposure times. The UV exposed film records the unseen information contained in the affected area of the injured skin which later becomes visible to the human eye on the photographic print, assuming that proper UV photographic techniques were applied to the injury. Changing the position (angle) of the UV light source relative to the injury, while keeping the camera perpendicular to the injury, will frequently allow surface details to be enhanced.

b. Infrared Photography

Just as in reflective UV photography, infrared photography also requires special techniques. The infrared band of light is at the opposite end of the light spectrum from the ultraviolet band. Ultraviolet light is about one half of the wave length of infrared light. Because infrared is longer it penetrates up to 3 mm below the surface of the skin. Since the depth of the injury recorded with the infrared technique is below the surface, the infrared focus point will not be the same as the visible focus point **(Fig. 3.13B)**. Just as in UV photography, some allowance must be made for the differences in these focus points. After obtaining a through-the-lens focus, the lens must be moved slightly away from the injury. In other words, the lens-to-object distance must be increased (moved back) from the visible focus point, thereby making the correction. By using an aperture setting of f-11 or smaller to increase the depth of field, the discrepancy in focus points will be minimized. Fortunately, many lenses are marked with a small dot (usually red) on the lens that indicates the infrared focus shift point. The photographer simply observes reference lines on the focusing ring of the lens which indicate the normal focus position, and moves the red dot to that location to acquire the correction.

Exposing infrared photographs requires several special considerations over conventional visible

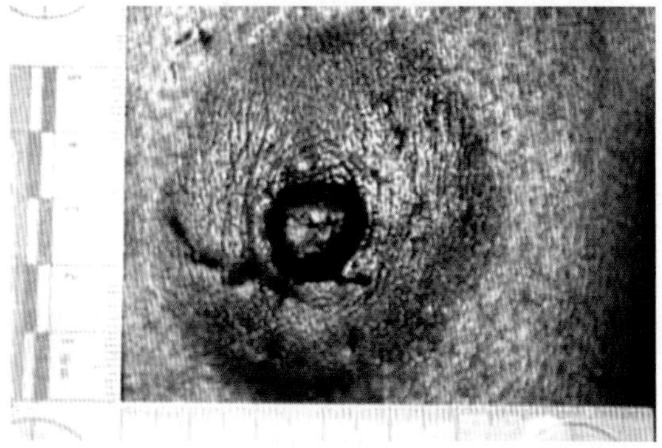

Fig. 3.13B: Same picture taken with the infrared cameras.

light photographs. The first is the camera setup. Unlike most films commercially available, Kodak high-speed infrared film does not come with a preset ASA/ISO speed rating. Each photographer's camera equipment should be tested in trial sessions to determine the optimum speed setting for the technique. Many cameras work best in the ASA/ ISO range of 25 to 64. Whatever speed found best should be noted and marked on the surface of the canister containing the film so that it is processed correctly for developing and printing. Kodak suggests that the infrared film "can advantageously be developed for a 30 percent increase over the average time. The additional fog is negligible and the resultant pattern is strengthened".

Just as in the UV technique, infrared illuminated photography records the part of the injury "seen" with non-visible light on a film emulsion, that when developed, will be viewable in the photographic prints. Because of that fact, the injury documented with infrared technique will not appear the same as photographs taken using visible light.

The majority of biological infrared images are formed from details not on the outside of the subject. This accounts for the misty appearance of many infrared reflection records. Successful infrared photography is a trial and error process, particularly when dealing with injury patterns. Since there is no way to know what injury detail is being recorded using this nonvisible light technique, wide bracketing and many exposures are highly recommended. If the injury did not cause sufficient damage to the deeper skin tissues, i.e. no bleeding below the surface of the injured skin, or if the surface of the injured skin is too thick for the infrared light to penetrate to find the site of the bleeding, there may be no infrared detail recorded in the photographs. No image appearing on the developed film and subsequent photographic prints should not be interpreted as a failure of the technique. Expectations of 100 percent success with the technique are not realistic. One should not be discouraged as a result of a non-productive photo session. Nor should the lack of an image be interpreted incorrectly as though nothing was present. Additional sessions may be required to re-photograph the injury to successfully capture it on film.

Handling of Photographic Evidence

The photographs documenting a victim's injuries may become part of the legal system and, as such, are subject to chain of evidence rules. This requires an accountability as to what individuals had possession of the evidence from the time it was collected until it is marked and introduced into the legal system. As part of the standard technique, the forensic photographer should routinely mark each photograph with a categorizing system, usually consisting of numbers or letters which include the case number, as well as an identifying mark of the forensic photographer. This can be his or her initials or a signature, so that the photographs can be identified as originals and the chain of evidence maintained.

It is strongly suggested that the forensic photographer should not part with the original negatives. Under no circumstances should both the negatives and prints be out of the possession of the photographer. If through carelessness they became "lost", there could potentially be no photographic evidence of the injuries and no way to recover from the mistake.

Bibliography

1. Arheart KL, Pretty IA. Results of the 4th ABFO Bitemark Workshop, 1999, For Sci. Int. 2001;124: 104-11.
2. Golden G. Use of alternative light source illumination in bite mark photography. J. Forensic Sci. 1994;39(3).
3. Guidelines for bitemark analysis, American Board of Forensic Odontology. J Am Dent Assoc. 1986;112:383-6.
4. Robbins SL, Angell M, Kuman V. Inflammation and repair. Basic Pathology, 3rd ed.; WB Saunders, Philadelphia 1981;28.

Chapter 4

Oral and Maxillofacial Radiology: An Approach to Forensic Aspects

Vishal Saxena

Chapter Overview

- Radiology and Forensic Sciences
- Scope of Forensic Radiology
- Limitations of Dental Radiography

Radiology and Forensic Sciences

By its very nature, the science of radiology solves mysteries as it reveals deep within the body hidden secrets that are otherwise inaccessible to exposure. This potential was obvious from the first few images Röntgen produced in those first fateful 50 days in Würzburg. The discovery of "a new kind of ray" while working alone in the laboratory on an autumn afternoon firmly established the place of Wilhelm Conrad Röntgen **(Fig. 4.1A)** among the great investigative scientists of all time. Working with his screens and plates, Röntgen made all of the fundamental observations that were the basis for his first two papers on the "X" rays: so named because "X" was the symbol for the unknown. It is no wonder then, that on January 23, 1896 a large crowd of representative scientists and members of the Society, university faculty and students, city officials, and representatives from the army filled the auditorium of the Physical Institute for Röntgen's first and only lecture on the X-ray **(Fig. 4.1B)**. How ever some credit Professor A W Wright of Yale University with being the first American to produce an X-ray image.

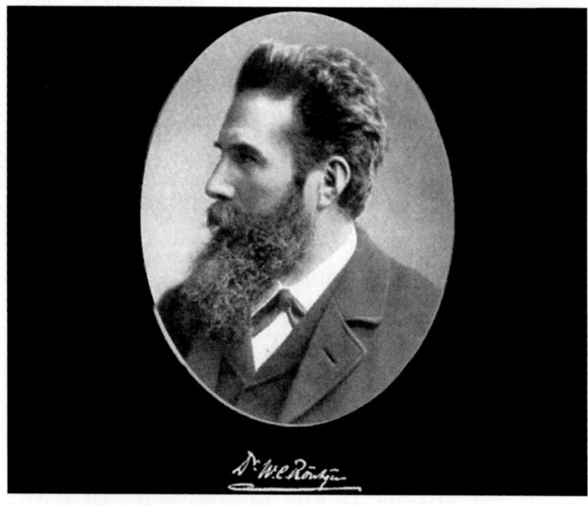

Fig. 4.1A: Sir Wilhelm Roentgen, the person behind the invention of X- rays

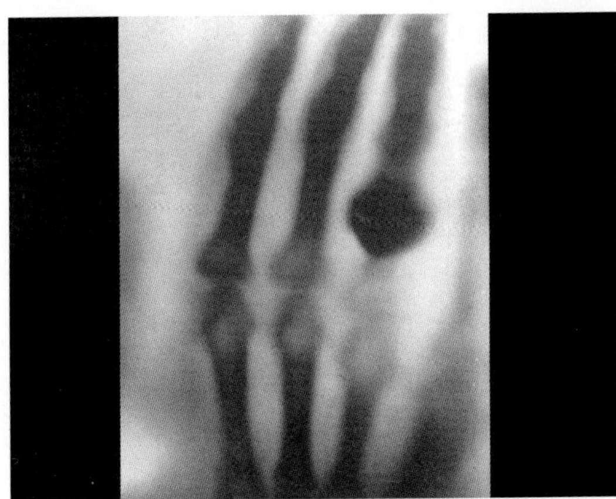

Fig. 4.1B: The first radiograph taken by sir W Roentgen. The radiograph shown is of wife of Roentgen. Note the image of the ring worn by the lady

Historical Perspectives

Actually, the first court case involving the X-rays in North America commenced on Christmas Eve, 1895 (three days before Röntgen submitted his first communication to the Physical-Medicine Society of Würzburg).

In Montreal, Mr George Holder shattered the peace of that wintry evening by shooting in the leg of Mr Tolson Cunning. Attempts to locate the bullet by probing failed; the wound healed but remained symptomatic. A professor of physics at McGill University, John Cox, was requested by Cunning's surgeon Dr RC Kirkpatrick, to make an X-ray photograph of the wounded extremity. In the physics lecture theater appropriate equipment was assembled and, with a 45 minute exposure, a plate was obtained which showed the flattened bullet lying between the tibia and fibula. Dr Kirkpatrick removed the bullet, and Mr Cunning was discharged 10 days later. The X-ray plate was submitted to the court during the trial, with the subsequent conviction of Mr Holder for attempted murder. He was sentenced to 14 years in the penitentiary.

The first instance, in which a Roentgenogram was brought to court in England was a personal injury case tried by Mr Justice Hawkins and a special jury in Nottingham.

The first civil case in which X-ray evidence was accepted into a US court took place in Denver.

The first criminal case in the US involving X-rays was the October, 1897 Haynes murder trial in Watertown, New York. The victim was shot in the jaw with a .32 caliber bullet. Another foreign object was discovered lodged in the back of the head. Was this a second bullet or a fragment from the first? Dr Gilbert Cannon gave testimony on the findings of the roentgenogram (not a second bullet) which subsequently was accepted as evidence by Judge Wright.

In February, 1896 W Koenig was taking intraoral films of the teeth, leading the way for the science of Forensic Odontology which has flourished only since the 1940s. The case of Adolph Hitler dates from that decade. Hitler had many residual physical symptoms and disabilities. Persistent headaches finally forced him to follow the advice of his otolaryngologist, Dr Paul Giesler. On September 19th he was driven to an army field hospital at Rastenburg where three roentgenograms of his skull were obtained. Those films survived the war; Hitler **(Fig. 4.2)**, of course, did not – although speculation and rumors abounded that he had somehow escaped. The dental work displayed on Hitler's roentgenograms **(Figs 4.3A to C)** was quite distinctive, however, and the Russians were able to make comparison with the burned remains found in the ruins of the chancellery garden. Although positive identification was made by this dental comparison, the Russians kept secret this information for more than two decades.

Dental Radiology and Forensic Sciences

In 1923, the first practical X-ray machine for dental use was introduced. Film for intraoral radiographs

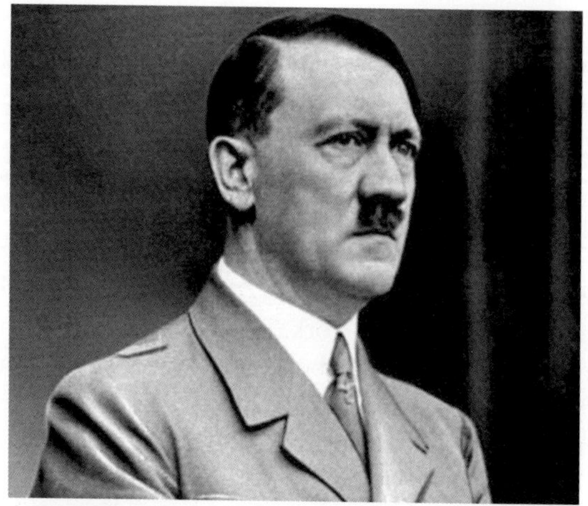

Fig. 4.2: Adolf Hitler during his last days

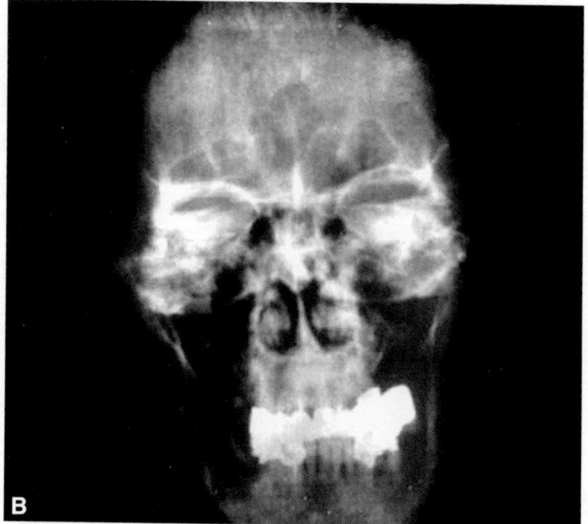

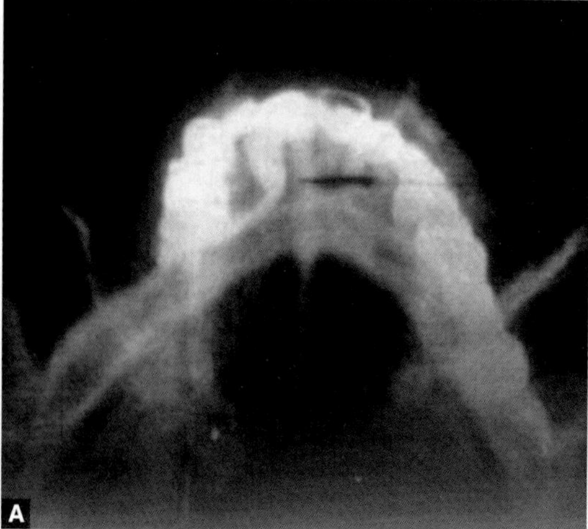

Fig. 4.3A: Postmortem radiograph of the lower jaw remains obtained form Hitler's corpse. Note the telephonic bridge fabricated within his mandibular arch

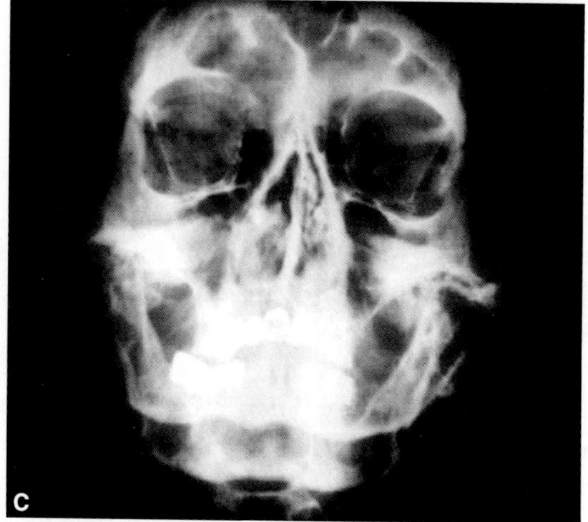

Figs 4.3B and C: The Antemortem radiographs of the skull of Hitler. Note the well placed restorations within both of the arches

was developed 10 years earlier by Kodak. Each film had to be hand wrapped. The earliest case of an identification on an unknown decedent made through comparison of sinuses in skull radiographs was published in 1926. The first reported use of dental radiography in a forensic identification occurred in 1943. Dental radiology was used to help identify 72 of the 119 victims who perished in the 1949 fire on board the steamship Noronic which burned in Toronto.

Today, radiographs are routinely used to identify unknown decedents, individually and in mass disasters, and have confirmed identifications in such notable cases as Adolf Hitler, Josef Mengele, and Lee Harvey Oswald.

Radiology has been used extensively in conventional dental identification, anatomically based identification and identification using maxillofacial skeletal landmarks such as the frontal sinus (**Figs 4.4A and B**). Examples of these are well documented in the literature.

This chapter is devoted to revisit the methods where radiographic methods may be used to determine identity using the teeth, the root structures and the frontal sinuses. Additionally suggestions are offered for management of radiography in mass disasters and cases where age determination is required. Computer assisted tomography can be used in the assessment of the degree of fit of a weapon to a wound in cases of blunt force skull injury and plane films can assist in depicting the pattern of postmortem skull fractures. Microcomputed tomography has been used in matching weapons to wounds in sharp force injury cases. There are gaps in the science where radiological methods are used.

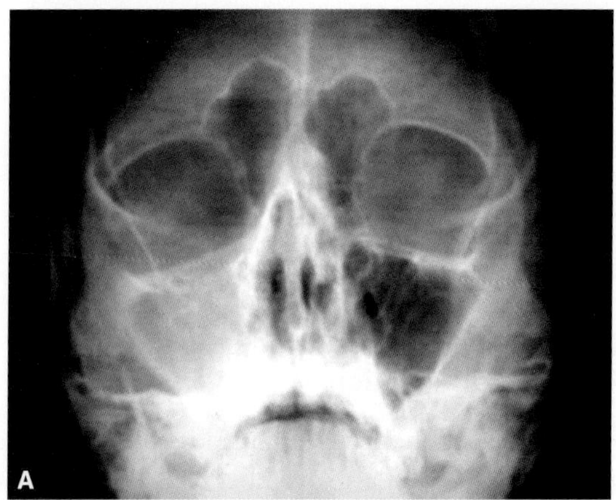

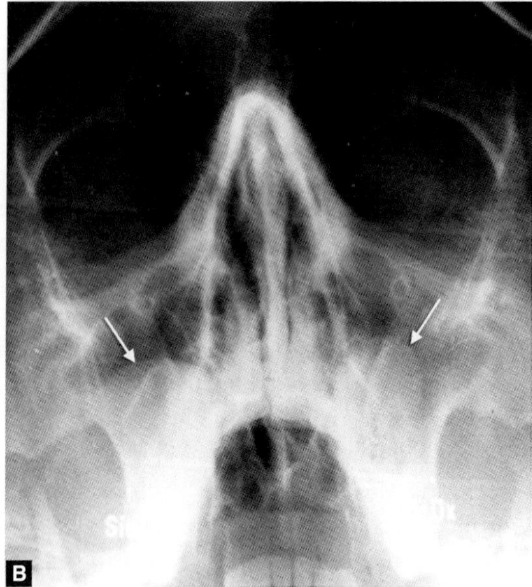

Figs 4.4A and B: Water's view of the skull for the visualization of the sinuses

Scope of Forensic Radiology

Forensic radiology, as do all other academic and scientific disciplines, rests on the sometimes unsteady four-legged stool of service, education, research, and administration. The scope of forensic applications of diagnostic medical radiology as currently understood and practiced is summarized in the following table. As the field of diagnostic radiology has undergone rapid expansion in technology and utilization in the past quarter-century, so may the range of forensic applications burgeon in the near future. The following fields are the main areas of interests harboring tremendous scope in forensic radiology.

I. Service

A. Determination of identity
B. Evaluation of injury and death
   1. Accidental
   2. Non-accidental
      a. Osseous injury
      b. Missiles and foreign bodies
      c. Other trauma
      d. Other causes
C. Criminal litigation
   1. Fatal
   2. Nonfatal

D. Civil litigation
   1. Fatal
   2. Nonfatal
E. Administrative proceedings

II. Education

III. Research

IV. Administration

Oral and Maxillofacial Radiology in Person Identification

Dental identification was used prior to Roentgen's discovery of X-rays on November 8, 1895. The first recorded use of radiographic techniques in identification was by Schuller in 1921. Radiographically assisted dental identification may be comparative or reconstructive in type. The former "compares" radiographs exposed prior to death to those exposed after death. Reconstructive identification may use radiographs as an aid in the generation of a biological profile of a person for whom the putative identity remains unknown. Comparative identification utilizing dental radiographs is now common in the evaluation of human remains. When the identity is suspected, and comparative means of identification are contemplated, the basic algorithm for dental radiographic identification is:

a. Examine the antemortem radiographs for quality, type and time of examination;
b. Examine the postmortem specimen and expose radiographs that will duplicate the areas of interest seen in the antemortem films using similar image geometry, suitable exposure factors and archival processing;
c. Use a system of marking or mounting the films so that their identity as postmortem or ante mortem films is known;
d. Visually analyze the radiographs, taking into account ancillary information such as dental chart notations, dental models and photographs;
e. Tabulate the points of concordance and explain, if possible, discordant points between the ante mortem and postmortem radiographic examinations;
f. Make a decision as to whether the materials provided allow the observer to make a positive identification, a possible identification or a negative assessment (no identification).

In the absence of dental radiographs, dental charts may be used. The issue in using dental charts is their veracity. There are numerous incidents of dental fraud reported in the lay press. Clearly, written records may be falsified outright. Alternately there can be honest errors in written records and in recorded treatments. Radiographic records provide objective evidence of the anatomical conditions and the dental treatment provided up to the point in time. Most cases of comparative identification use radiographic evidence of dental intervention (restorations, root fillings, crowns, and extractions) **(Figs 4.5A and B)** as common points of identification.

Less commonly anatomical features are used as concordant points. Dental interventions, especially restorative ones, in many cases provide unique identifiers that are common in antemortem and postmortem examinations.

Objectives in Radiographic Comparisons

The objective of using radiographs in identification is to compare and evaluate similarities between antemortem and postmortem films. The tasks for the forensic investigator include six steps:

i. Securing antemortem radiographs
ii. Making postmortem radiographs
iii. Comparing meaningful features (those which are stable and distinctive)
iv. Accounting for discrepancies
v. Assessing uniqueness
vi. Verbalizing the degree of confidence in the identification.

Radiographic Anatomic Landmarks of the Jaws (Fig. 4.6A)

Fixed anatomic features are present in all individuals. These landmarks are relatively similar

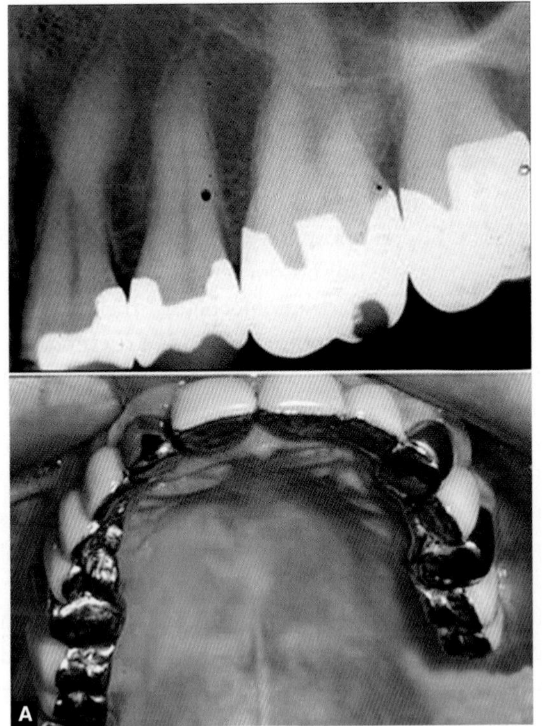

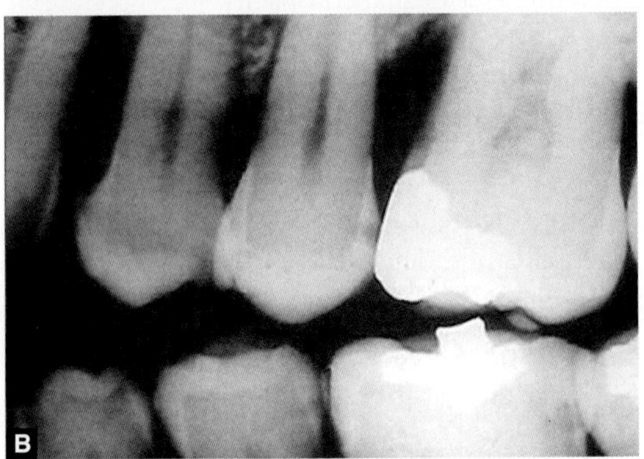

Figs 4.5A and B: Picture and radiograph of the patient showing crown, bridge and the restorations

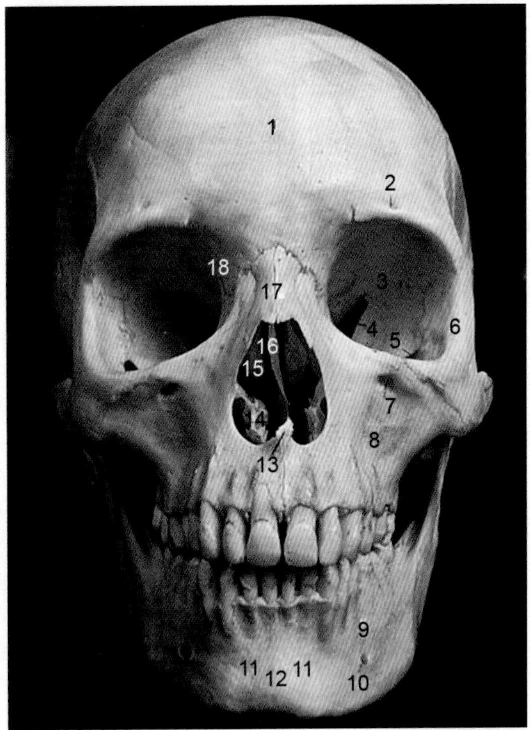

Fig. 4.6A: Skull showing the various anatomical landmarks

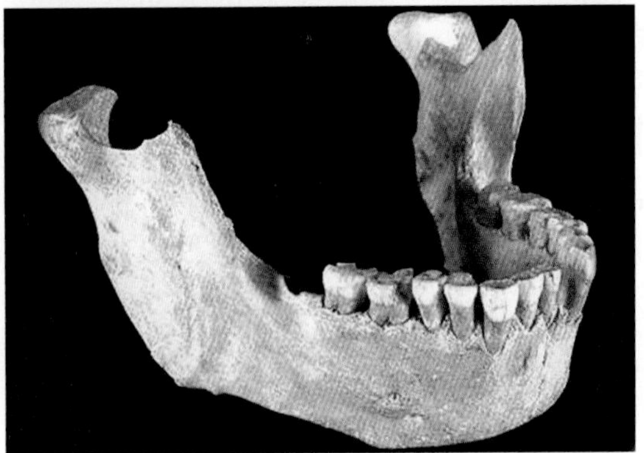

Fig. 4.6B: Mandible bone

in most people and, unless showing distinctive variation, should not be considered as individual identifiers. These landmarks are not always visible in radiographs due to technical and anatomic variations.

Mandibular Landmarks (Fig. 4.6B)

The mandibular canal is a tubular canal running centrally within the body of each hemimandible and appearing as a linear radiolucency outlined both superiorly and inferiorly by a thin opaque border. It begins at the mandibular foramen located in the middle of the ramus, running below the teeth and terminating as the mental foramen, a circular lucency near the apex of the second premolar. The mandibular nerve and vessels are the contents of this canal. The genial tubercles are the bony attachments for several muscles. They appear as an oval radiopacity sometimes showing a central radiolucency (lingual foramen) below the roots of the central incisors in the mandibular midline. The internal and external oblique ridges are opaque bony ridges in the superior part of the posterior body extending diagonally toward the anterior ramus. The external ridge is buccal and more superior than the lingual internal ridge, which is at the level of molar root apices. The coronoid process is a flat triangular protrusion of bone extending superiorly from the anterior ramus. It is the area of attachment of the temporalis muscle. Extending superiorly from the posterior ramus is the condylar neck to which is attached the mushroom-shaped condylar head. The "valley" in-between the two "hills" formed by the coronoid process and condylar neck is the sigmoid notch. The condyle fits into the glenoid fossa of the temporal bone to form the temporomandibular joint.

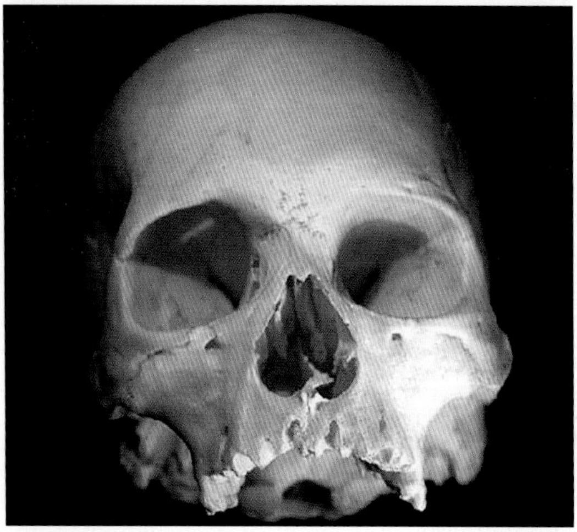

Fig. 4.6C: Skull with mandible removed highlighting the maxillary bone

Maxillary Landmarks (Fig. 4.6C)

The incisive foramen is a circular opening in the palatal midline between the apices of the central incisors. Superimposition of the radiopaque nasal spine on its superior border renders a heart-shaped rather than circular radiolucency to the foramen. There is variability in the size of this structure. The floor of the nasal cavity and the maxillary sinuses are visible in dental radiographs. From the maxillary midline above the incisor roots, the floor of the nasal cavity slopes superiorly as it extends distally toward the long canine root. The maxillary sinus presents as a radiolucency extending from the distal aspect of the canine root to the second molar. Its lower border is scalloped and dental roots often project into the sinus floor. The malar bone and inferior border of the zygomatic arch may be projected over the sinus in the molar region, appearing as a U-shaped opacity.

Radiological Anatomical Features and the Spatial Relationship of the Teeth (Fig. 4.6D)

In the Western world, water fluoridation and improved dental care have resulted in a decrease in dental caries. This decrease is associated with a concomitant decrease in the number of restorative

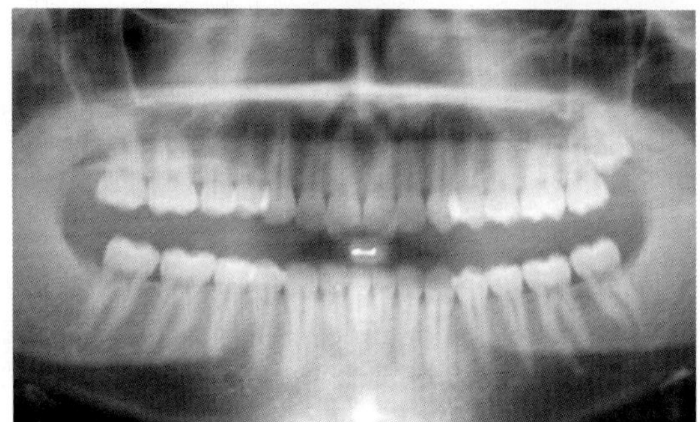

Fig. 4.6D: An OPG showing various normal anatomic landmarks

interventions. If there is no evidence of dental intervention then the forensic odontologist must rely on anatomical structures common between ante mortem and post mortem radiographic examinations.

Such anatomical features might include:

- Crown morphology,
- Root shape, size and curvatures,
- Pulpal morphology, and
- The spatial relationship between the teeth.

The radiographic depiction of tooth morphology is highly dependent on image geometry. Small changes in horizontal or vertical beam angulation may result in critical differences in the radiographic appearance of comparators. Additionally, while it is reasonable to assume that some anatomical structures might not change with time (e.g. crown morphology, root dilaceration and taurodontism) others may change over time (pulp morphology **(Figs 4.7A and B)** and alveolar bone pattern). There have been no convincing long-term studies of the relative stability of individual anatomical dental features as seen on radiographs. Aside from relying on solitary dental anatomical observations it is possible to match antemortem to postmortem radiographic examinations using the spatial relationships of the posterior teeth one to another. This concept relies upon the alignment of Radiographically visible anatomical structures one to another. It requires no information from the crowns of the teeth, so it is also useful in macerated and partially incinerated remains where the clinical crowns may be damaged or lost.

The points of concordance are gained by evaluating the alignment of the periodontal ligament spaces, lamina dura, pulp chamber walls and root edges as seen on posterior films. Films are digitized and a horizontal section is "cut" from either the ante mortem or post mortem radiograph. It is then positioned over the corresponding anatomical area of its opposite radiograph.

The degree of concordance and points of discordance can then be assessed. With the advent of the desktop scanner and digital radiographs this process has been made easier. The technique is not usable in comparisons within or between the mixed dentition and other states of the dentition and orthodontic tooth movement or extractions in the antemortem to postmortem radiographic examinations may limit its use as may protracted antemortem to postmortem radiographic intervals.

When using the Digital Dental Radiographic Identification (DDRI) technique there are numerous occasions where it is difficult to recreate the ante mortem image geometry on the post mortem films. This may require numerous attempts

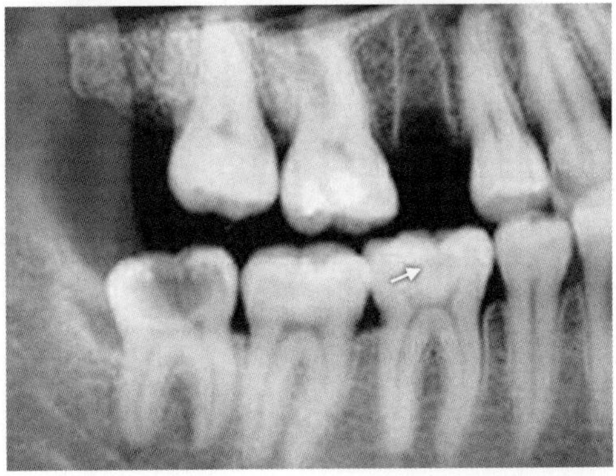

Fig. 4.7A: A bite wing radiograph showing the pulpal morphology

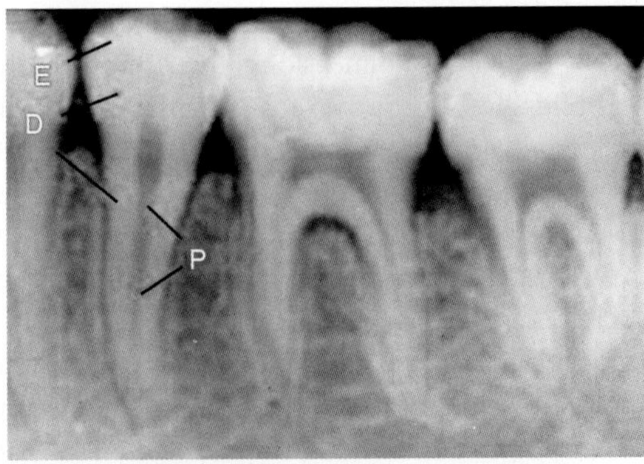

Fig. 4.7B: Trabecular pattern of mandibular bone, (E—Enamel, D—Dentin, P—Pulp)

using altered vertical and horizontal beam-angulations and object film placements. A device has been developed to aid in the recreation of the ante mortem image geometry for these spatial relationship issues or even in cases where the ante mortem images suggest a major differential from the norm.

Radiology in Reconstructive Dental Identification

Most agencies consider reconstructive identification only when there are no putative identification or antemortem records available. This often occurs in cases of found human remains where the body has been skeletonized or missing for long periods of time. Clinical and radiographic examinations can help to recreate a profile of the individual prior to death.

There are at least two other means by which oral radiological examination may aid in reconstructive identification. The first is to assess and define the angulation of anterior teeth that have been lost post mortem. The second is to examine reassembled macerated remains prior to facial approximation exercises. It is common for teeth to be lost following death. If remains are to be processed for facial approximation it is useful for the professionals involved to have information on the state of the dentition and the alignment of the anterior teeth. Radiographic examination of the dental sockets of anterior teeth in two dimensions (antero-posteriorly and occlusally) affords the reconstructive dentist or facial approximation scientist information as to the number and alignment of anterior teeth, the presence of periodontal bone loss and periapical disease that can make the facial approximation more accurate.

Occasionally skulls that have been macerated require reassembly. In these instances it is important that the forensic odontologist be consulted so that a thorough clinical and radiographic examination may be undertaken.

Another Aspect of Radiology in Identification-frontal Sinuses

Skeletal identification is recognized as a valid means of body identification in long bones. However, the facial bones are more difficult to use for radiological body identification because of their innate anatomical complexity, the comparative rarity of antemortem radiographic radiographs and the large number of overlapping structures in the radiographic projections of these structures. One maxillofacial anatomical structure that is amenable to comparison between antemortem and post-mortem radiographs is the frontal sinus **(Fig. 4.8)**. It may be used because it is commonly exposed in "sinus series" investigations; it is sandwiched between the internal and external surfaces of the frontal bone; the view commonly used to demonstrate it, the occipitomental or "Waters" view provides an excellent radiographic depiction of it since its shadow is cast over the flat posterior calvarium.

Culbert and Law performed the first radiographic comparison of paranasal sinuses in

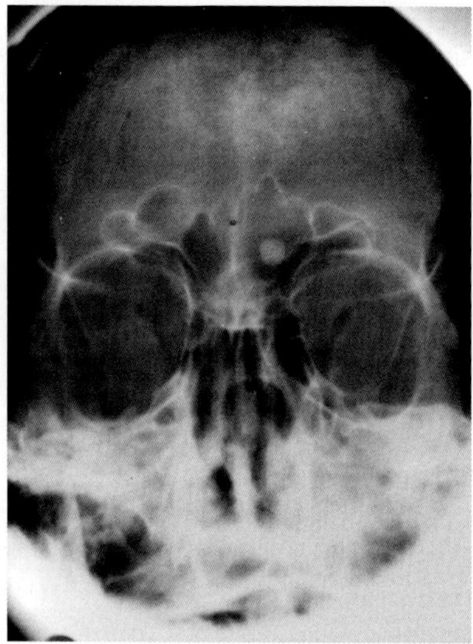

Fig. 4.8: AP view of the skull showing the frontal sinuses in detail

body identification although these were of the mastoid air cells and the identification was confirmed in part by the decedents dental restorations. Since then others have undertaken frontal sinus identification and have found that it has been highly useful. Christensen (2004) questioned the scientific validity and potential error rates of using frontal sinuses for body identification in light of the Daubert vs Merrel-Dow Pharmaceuticals decision by the United States Supreme Court. Perhaps it would be prudent to undertake an experiment in which a line-up of possible matches and definite mismatches was included with matching antemortem and postmortem radiographs.

The use of dry skulls and "pretend" antemortem and postmortem radiographs would not possess the requisite external validity of a decent clinical study. Alternately the potentially matching frontal sinus images could be examined by a qualified radiologist conversant in the radiographic anatomy of the region. In any case up to ten percent of persons may have no frontal sinuses to evaluate.

Radiography in Mass Disaster Victim Identification (DVI)

Dental radiography as objective evidence provides an invaluable means of person identification in mass casualty incidents. Dental identifications continue to be a rapid and accurate means of establishing identity in such situations. They provide objective data for reconciliation of antemortem and postmortem records. However, from a postmortem standpoint there are numerous factors that must be kept in mind:

a. In DVI incidents, the purpose of the radiographic examination is not to diagnose disease. Considerable latitude should be given therefore to the types of postmortem radiographic examinations to be undertaken. For example, bitewing radiographs, a simple procedure in the living, are much more difficult to perform than periapical radiographs in the deceased than posterior periapical radiographs of each quadrant. In life the bitewing radiographs might be of different angulation; however, in the deceased the film may be held in a position that allows almost exact duplication of bitewing image geometry.

   Occlusal size film is underutilized in all identification procedures but especially so in mass disaster where it can replace many views with one film. A common maxim applied to forensic photography is equally valid to forensic dental radiography "when in doubt max out." This means take more radiographs at the postmortem than the bare minimum. It is much simpler to expose a complete series of films at the first examination than it is to have to retrieve the body for further radiographic examination or alternately attempt reconciliation with minimal post mortem radiographic evidence. If the body is suspected to be a sub-adult or child a full mouth series of radiographs should be made in order that age-stratification can be accurate. Failure to do so will limit the forensic odontologist from later estimating age and may again necessitate body retrieval and re-examination.

b. If an assembly line approach is used for post mortem evaluation, dental radiographs should be exposed prior to the detailed dental examination and charting. If this is done, the examiners can use the radiographs in the charting and coding procedure up-front rather than modifying their charting or coding later.

c. If analog films are used it is extremely important that photographic chemistry be monitored, replenished and replaced regularly. Processors need to be emptied, cleaned and serviced regularly whether they are used or not. Photographic chemistry will deteriorate even if it is not being used. If a large number of radiographic examinations are done chemistry will need to be replenished more frequently.

Failure to do so will result in films that may look excellent at the time of the autopsy but deteriorate rapidly-perhaps prior to the reconciliation process. It would be prudent to digitize analog films on a flat bed transparency scanner and store them electronically.

d. If digital radiographs are to be used it is vital that they are "transportable" from location to location and stored in a common format such as JPEG or similar. Additionally, redundant back-up drives must also be available and updated regularly.
e. Whether analog or digital films are used it would be prudent to have a radiological quality control officer to catch errors such as cone-cuts, under or over exposure, under or over development and mounting errors. This person could also monitor processor function and maintenance and radiation safety issues. Few mass disasters are handled using dental office quality lead shielding and it is important that radiation safety aspects of gathering postmortem data be adequate. It is possible to "rescue" sub-optimal radiographs; however, the time to do this is not in the middle of a DVI incident.

Age Estimation and Dental Radiology

It is well recognized that in the sub-adult estimation of the age of subject, deceased or not may be attempted by examination of the maturation of the primary and permanent dentition. There are dozens of published papers on age determination. In cases where the sample cannot be destroyed, radiology is often used to assess age. It is obviously unethical to remove teeth from live persons so non-invasive techniques need to be used in those instances as well.

The goal of age determination in found human remains is to assist in the development of the biological profile of the deceased. If radiological examination demonstrates incomplete formation of the permanent dentition then the forensic odontologist can assist the investigation by narrowing down the population age group to which the deceased belonged. This being said it is just as important to avoid narrowing down the estimated age in a found set of remains so as to not cast too narrow a net and exclude possible matches from missing person files.

Pitfalls and Drawbacks in Age Determination

In those cases where a single live individual claims to be below the age of majority such as adult persons claiming to be juveniles, illegal refugee claimants, etcetera, radiological examination of the teeth might be used to try and pin-point the exact age. This is a far more difficult exercise in some cases such as in those persons who are very close to the legal age for being declared an adult. In age estimation in live individuals the goal may be to narrow the age range to a single point. This is very difficult. If we make the assumption that the radiological maturation of the teeth fits some form of normal distribution, and there is little evidence for this in many ethnic groups, then the following question might be legitimately posed:

Where does that Claimant Fit on that Normal Distribution?

Can we morally make life-changing decisions about that person based in part on dental radiographic features attributed to age?

There are other pitfalls in using radiology in age determination. The first one is the radiological examination used on the unknown individual that we are going to compare to the reference sample. There is a tendency to forget that panoramic radiographs, which are often used in this procedure are not plane radiographs. They are tomographs. As such they have a focal trough and anything that lies outside the focal trough will be blurred. It follows that if teeth that are being used to assess the dental age of a subject are out of the focal trough then there may be misestimation of the dental age.

Prior to any study in which panoramic radiographs are used, there should be a screening of the image by a radiologist for image quality. This is infrequently done. Even if a tooth lies within the focal trough, if it is tipped in a bucco-lingual direction its root end may lie outside the focal trough and provide a misleading radiological conception of the true clinical situation. There are numerous studies where third molar root development is used as a determinant of age; however, it is the most variable in its development and the study that forms the bedrock for the stages of root development is now over 30 years old.

There have been in excess of 100 papers since using Demirjian's stages or variants of his technique to different populations, a fact that may be invalid on the face of it because Demirjian's reference sample was, by and large, French-Canadian children developing in the 1960s and 1970s. It is reasonable to assume that both radiological techniques have changed since then and other ethnic and racial groups may have their own differing maturation rates. The other radiological variable that must be considered is the degree of overlapping soft tissue and hard tissue coverage in the radiograph of either the known reference sample or the unknown case. Estimation of the pulpal widths and height on intraoral radiographic films and to a lesser extent panoramic radiographs is influenced by the amount of hard and soft tissue present from the end of the collimator tube to the image plane. Simply put, a "thicker" or "denser" patient will have proportionally smaller pulp widths than a slender radiolucent one even though the pulps are of the same size. This is because radiographs are not photographs but rather two-dimensional representations of three-dimensional objects.

Evaluation of Cranial Trauma Using Radiological Methods

Radiology has been used to demonstrate fracture patterns in blunt-force trauma of the human calvaria. Post mortem radiography of skull fractures is complicated because of the amount of anatomical superimposition. Something as simple as a modified Parma radiographic approach in which the collimator of the dental unit is removed and the exit port of the dental X-ray unit is placed abutting the side contralateral to the skull fracture can provide excellent, simply produced radiograph depictions of calvarial fractures. If a putative weapon is found, the weapon can be compared to impressed injuries in the skull. This is difficult because it requires numerous comparisons; the use of CT scanning which is difficult to obtain in many mortuaries; if the weapon is metallic, which it invariably is, requires the production of models of the weapon in Type IV dental stone and on occasion either retention of the skull bones themselves or fabrication of the models of the skull. Further research in this area is likely to use such sophisticated imaging and may, in the future form part of virtual autopsy techniques.

Fraud, Claims and Dental Radiology

If a practitioner is going to commit fraud there is little that can be done to prevent it. In a study by Tsang et al, it was demonstrated that digital manipulation of radiographs to produce disease that was not present on the original films was successful in misleading third party insurers to provide care the patient did not need. Although the images in this study were digitally altered, the images submitted to the insurance companies were ultimately of the analog (film) variety. It has been since successfully argued that the same goal could have been accomplished using analog images of another patient; however, the fluidity of digital images should be of concern to honest practitioners, state funding agencies, third party insurers and patients themselves.

Radiographic evidence of caries and restorations may be readily added to radiographic images and this "evidence" of disease or treatment could subsequently be covered with restorations with nobody but the perpetrator any the wiser, just as troubling is the general lack of radiological knowledge of litigants in malpractice cases, their attorneys and even dental regulatory authorities. In the Western world there is an increasing number of patients who sue their dentist for actual or perceived negligence. There are only three pieces of evidence that will solve these cases: the written record, radiographs and other objective data such as models and photographs. If radiographs are used as evidence, it would be prudent to obtain the expert opinion of a dental radiologist. There are many studies that need to be undertaken in order to improve the scientific base from which forensic odontologists operate. These include the following:

a. There are no data on determining the stability of dental anatomical landmarks over protracted periods of time. A study such as this one could use radiographs of live individuals that are followed by a single practitioner or clinic. The antemortem and postmortem images could in actuality be substituted with high quality radiographic images exposed at specific time intervals established either prospectively or retrospectively. Such images could then be shown to a series of observers to determine the percentage that result in correct identification, inability to identify or false identification. Sensitivity, specificity and error rates from this process could thus be calculated.
b. There are no data on just how poor radiographic image geometry can be before it disallows identification. In order to calculate the influence of radiographic error on the ability to accurately determine the identity of a known antemortem case, studies could be done using restorations placed in cadaveric material in which various degrees of image geometry error are introduced. Such alterations would include changes in horizontal angulation; changes in vertical angulation; changes in both horizontal and vertical angulations; changes in the film plane (twisting of the film). The resultant images could then be shown to a series of observers to determine the percentage that result in correct identification, inability to identify or false identification. Sensitivity, specificity and error rates from this process could thus be calculated.
c. There need to be more populations studied for age determination to provide reference material for different ethnic groups and the ones currently used as base-line reference material need to be updated.
d. The technique of using CT scans for either blunt force calvarial trauma of sharp-force trauma where weapons are compared to wounds needs to be refined. It is unlikely that enough case material exists to support this at any one centre. For this reason either a cadaveric study, which carries with it the weakness that the bone was not vital at the time of the injury; or an in vivo animal study which might have associated ethical or anatomical problems makes this a problem. To design a study that is meaningful is large enough to calculate error rates, and possessing external validity is a daunting task.
e. For cases where age determination is required careful quality control of reference sample and unknown sample radiographs should be undertaken. Additionally further testing on the influence of soft tissue and hard tissue dimensions might need to be taken into account for techniques that primarily use radiological methods to assist age determination.

Contemplating Human Judgment

There is a tendency in light of Daubert and other decisions to give little credence to the concept of competent clinical judgment. There is also a tendency in clinical medicine towards evidence-based medicine. However, neither will wholly replace the clinical judgment of a competent practitioner — whatever the discipline. In a study evaluating the accuracy of age determination it was found that a study in which a practitioner made an educated guess of the age of the deceased was more accurate than more "sophisticated" technical methods.

Solheim and Sundnes performed age estimation very well using a relatively simple visual assessment. Ten Cate et al used yellow coloration of the root as a means of age estimation and found that trained observers performed this task quite well.

It is often implied that we need to perform some sort of a physical test on "something" in order to be assured that we are getting "the right answer". Radiologists make clinical decisions based on the interpretation of radiographic images on a daily basis. This author would like to see more investigation into the accuracy of the trained human observer in forensic cases as well as technical development. There are interesting technologies on the horizon such as automated dental identification systems; however, ultimately it is the clinician that has to sign off on the decision, whatever technique is used to arrive there. No technological advance can appear in court for cross-examination.

Limitations of Dental Radiography

A radiograph represents two-dimensional shadows of three-dimensional objects. Fillings on the cheek side of a tooth cannot be distinguished from those on the tongue side. Fillings can be obscured by superimposition of other fillings in the same tooth. The various metals used in dentistry cannot be distinguished; all are radiopaque. A dentist, however, would recognize outline patterns associated with the various metals. Radiolucent areas in teeth can represent decay, nonmetallic esthetic fillings, congenital defects, physical/ chemical injuries, or artifacts. Differentiation of these conditions is important yet radiographically difficult. Artifacts and disparities produced by improper angulation, orientation, exposure, processing, labeling, and storage present potential difficulties which must be controlled.

Bibliography

1. Cameriere R, Ferrante L. Accuracy of age estimation in children using radiograph of developing teeth. Forensic Science International 176.2008;173-7.
2. Maber M, Liversidge HM, Hector MP. Accuracy of age estimation of radiographic methods using developing teeth. Forensic Science International 159S.2006;S68-S73.
3. Wood RE. Review, Forensic aspects of maxillofacial radiology. Forensic Science International 159S. 2006;S47-S55.

Chapter 5

Age Estimation and Dental Methodology

Nitul Jain, Sohail Lattoo

Chapter Overview

- Historical perspective
- Need for age estimation
- Age changes in oral cavity
- Terminologies
- Chronology of human dentition
- Various methods for age estimation
- Steps of age estimation
- Commonly used dental developmental surveys

INTRODUCTION

Age is one of the essential factors in establishing the identity of the person. Estimation of the human age is a procedure adopted by anthropologists, archaeologists and forensic scientists. Examination of teeth in many ways form a unique part of human body e.g. they are most durable and resilient part of the skeleton. The science dealing with establishing identity of a person by teeth is popularly known as Forensic Odontology or Forensic Dentistry.

Forensic odontologists are often confronted with the problem of determining the age of unknown bodies, as well as living persons. Age estimation is of great importance for the identification of unknown bodies or skeletal remains of accidents and crimes as well in disaster victims. In the case of living people who have no acceptable identification documents, such as refugees, adopted children of unknown age, verification of chronological age is required in order to be entitled to civil rights and social benefits. In archaeological search, estimation of age at death for skeletal remains serves as an aid in palaeo-demography **(Fig. 5.1)**.

A forensic dentist carries a considerable responsibility, since his scientific opinion is frequently asked when all other paths of identification have been exhausted. There are instances in which teeth are the only preserved human remains and present the only means for age determination in order to narrow down the search within the missing person's file and enable a more efficient approach. In these cases final identification may depend on specific odontological matching of pre and postmortem dental data, DNA-typing and fingerprinting. Teeth have the benefit to be preserved long after other tissues, even bone, have disintegrated and also unlike bones they can be examined directly in living individual. However, one must not forget that the more parameters taken

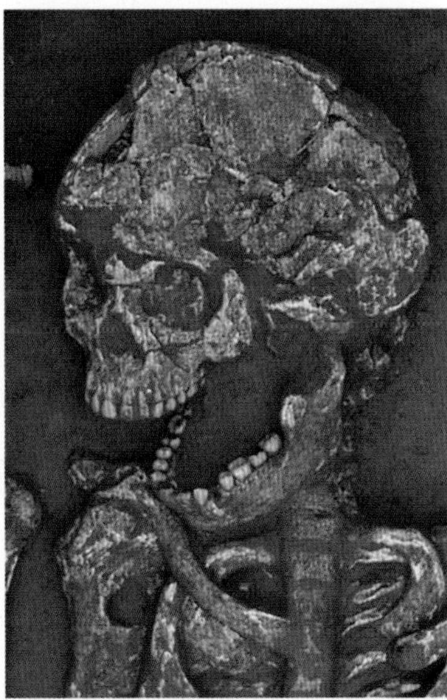

Fig. 5.1: Skeletal remains of the human may necessitate the approximate age estimation for paleodemography

into account the more accurate the determination of age is. For this reason clues from dentition must be correlated with clues found in the bones.

In this particular chapter, the important methods of age estimation are highlighted. The approach, the advantages and disadvantages of each technique are discussed giving an emphasis on the methods applied most. Then the steps that a forensic dentist should follow in order to estimate the age are presented. Finally the latest developments and speculations upon age estimation methods are also notified.

Historical Perspective

The use of teeth as age indicator dates back to 19th century. In Britain at that time the law decreed that children under seven years were not responsible for any crime they may have committed. Thomson (1836) a forensic medical expert stated: "If the third molar has not protruded, there is no hesitation in affirming that the culprit has not passed his seventh birthday". By the third molar he meant the permanent molar erupting after the two deciduous teeth.

The first known attempts which used teeth as an indicator of age originate from England. In the early 19th century, because of economic depression of the industrial revolution, juvenile work and criminality were serious social problems. The social legislation provided that no child under 9 years of age should be employed, while children under 13 should not work more than nine hours the day. The limit for criminal responsibility was seven years of age. However, there was not a registration of birth, thus making the proof of date of birth difficult. Up to this time the determination of age was based mostly on the calculation of height.

In 1836, AT Thomson who was one of the pioneers of medical jurisprudence claims that children, where the first permanent molars had not erupted, it was certain that they had not reached the age of seven. The first scientific study was presented in 1837 by Edwin Saunders, in which he points out that dentition is a more reliable standard than height for determination of age.

In 1872, Wedl made the first observations of changes with age in the permanent dentition and described fatty degeneration, calcification, colloid deposits, netlike atrophy and pigment deposits in the pulp tissue and a notable diminution in the size of the pulp cavity due to continued deposits of new dentine layers.

Need for Age Estimation

It constitutes an important part of the investigation of bodies or skeleton in forensic investigation and archeology, e.g. aborted fetus, a severely mutilated mass disaster victim.

Living person requiring age determination for:

- Birth certificate is not available or if records are suspected.
- To determine whether child has attained age of criminal responsibility.

- Assessment in case individual is either unwilling or unable to reveal his identity
- In case of disputed marriages, where, marrying couple are supposed to be below the legal permissible age limits.

Dead persons require age determination for
- In mass disasters to help identification
- In epidemiological surveys to know mortality indices of various diseases
- Age of aborted fetus

Age Changes in Oral Cavity

Following is the list of the changes that follow in the oral cavity as human being ages. Age changes in oral cavity may be divided into following three categories:
1. Soft tissue changes
2. Dental changes
3. Hard tissue changes

Soft Tissue Changes

- Epithelium becomes thinner and a flattening of the epithelium-connective tissue interface is seen.
- Marked Reduction in filiform papillae.
- Development of nodular varicose veins on undersurface of tongue
- Development of vascular nodules and nevi on lip and cheeks.
- Sebaceous gland of lip and cheek increases with age
- Minor salivary glands show marked atrophy with fibrous replacement.

Dental Changes (Figs 5.2A and B)

- Apical migration of dento-gingival junction and eventually the cemental surface of the tooth is exposed.
- Dystrophic calcification of central pulp

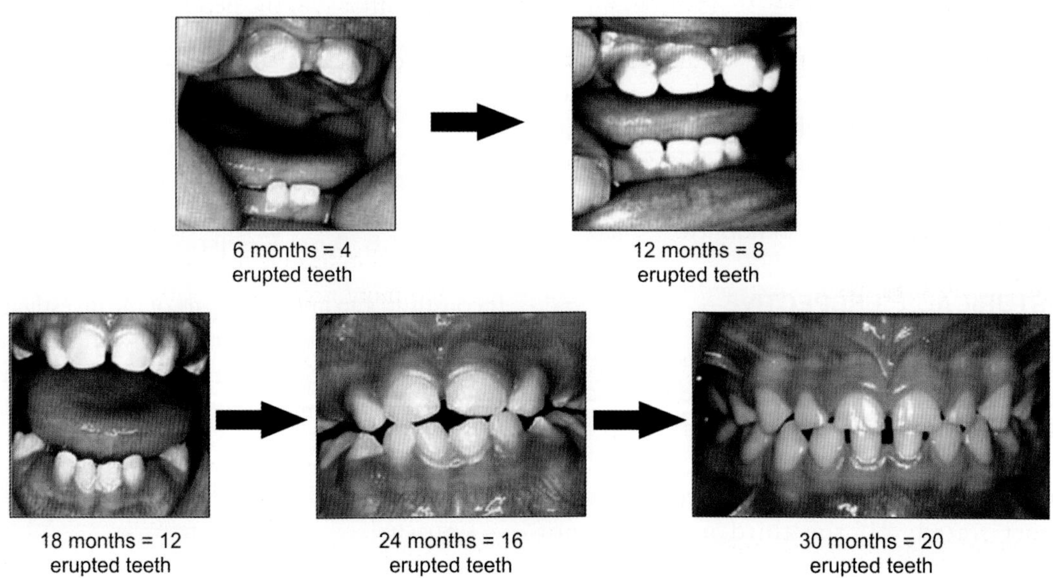

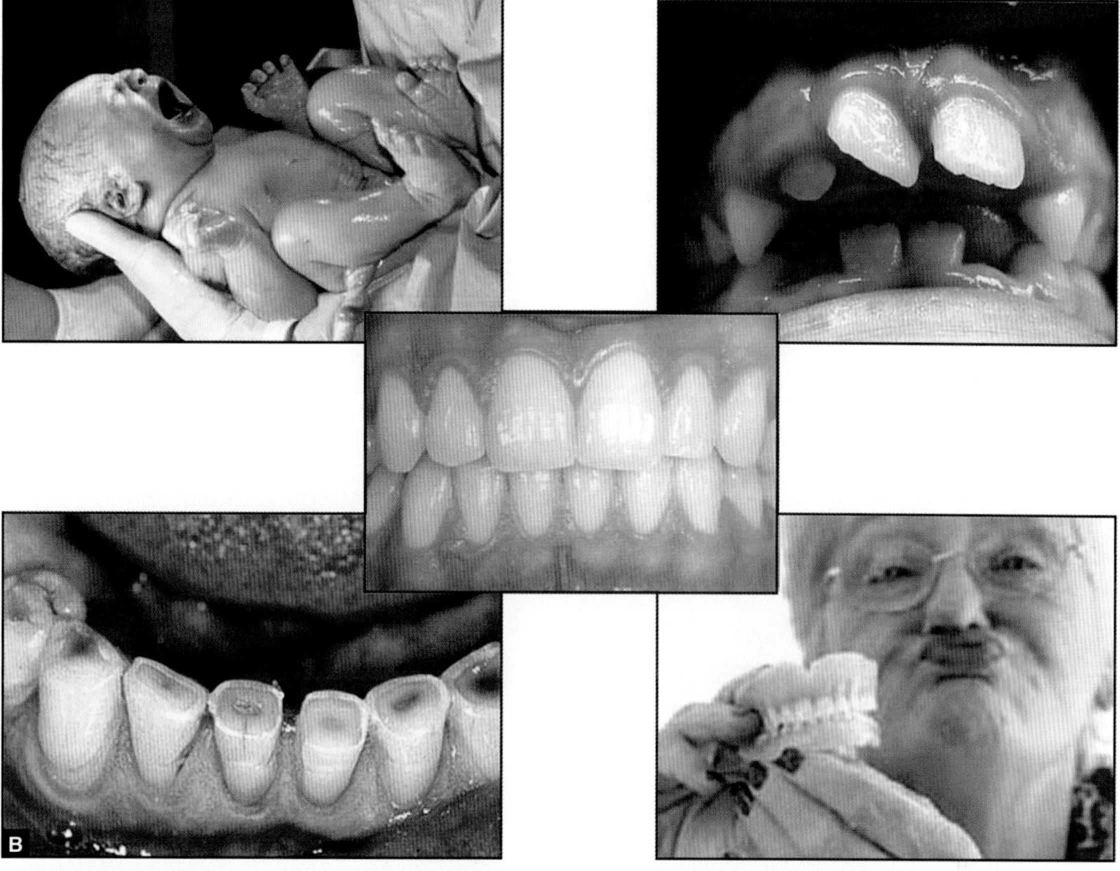

Figs 5.2A and B: Pictures showing the various changes in the dentition of a person throughout his life time

- Secondary dentin and dead tracts
- Attrition
- Gingival recession
- Cemental apposition

Hard Tissue Changes

- Articular eminence flattens.
- Condylar head rests more backward in glenoid fossa.
- Mental foramen comes close to upper border of mandible.
- Mandibular angle **(Figs 5.3A and B)**
  - At birth - obtuse (near 180°)
  - In adult age - about 90°
  - In old age - around 140°
- Mandible
  - Young - soft.
  - In adult - thicker and hard.
  - As age advances - thinner and brittle. Also, cortical bone of lamina dura becomes thicker and more irregular

TERMINOLOGIES

- Pathologic age: This is related to various conditions and disease process that results in deterioration of many tissues over time. Dental experts can estimate this by examining for
  - Arthritic changes in TMJ
  - Attritional wear of teeth
  - Root dentine transparency

Chronology of the Human Dentition

		Tooth	*First Evidence of Calcification*	*Crown Completed*	*Eruption*	*Root Completed*
Deciduous dentition	Upper jaw	Central incisor	3–4 mos in utero	4 mos	7½ mos	1½–2 yrs
		Lateral incisor	4½ mos in utero	5 mos	8 mos	1½–2 yrs
		Canine	5¼ mos in utero	9 mos	16–20 mos	2½–3 yrs
		First molar	5 mos in utero	6 mos	12–16 mos	2–2½ yrs
		Second molar	6 mos in utero	10–12 mos	20–30 mos	3 yrs
	Lower jaw	Central incisor	4½ mos in utero	4 mos	6½ mos	1½–2 yrs
		Lateral incisor	4½ mos in utero	4¼ mos	7 mos	1½–2 yrs
		Canine	5 mos in utero	9 mos	16–20 mos	2½–3 yrs
		First molar	5 mos in utero	6 mos	12–16 mos	2–2½ yrs
		Second molar	6 mos in utero	10–12 mos	20–30 mos	3 yrs.
Permanent dentition	Upper jaw	Central incisor	3–4 mos	4–5 yrs	7–8 yrs	10 yrs
		Lateral incisor	10 mos	4–5 yrs	8–9 yrs	11 yrs
		Canine	4–5 mos	6–7 yrs	11–12 yrs	13–15 yrs
		First premolar	1½–1¾ mos	5–6 yrs	10–11 yrs	12–13 yrs
		Second premolar	2–2¼ mos	6–7 yrs	10–12 yrs	12–14 yrs
		First molar	At birth	2½–3 yrs	6–7 yrs	9–10 yrs
		Second molar	2½–3 mos	7–8 yrs	12–13 yrs	14–16 yrs
		Third molar	7–9 mos	12–16 yrs	17–21 yrs	18–25 yrs
	Lower jaw	Central incisor	3–4 mos	4–5 yrs	6–7 yrs	9 yrs
		Lateral incisor	3–4 mos	4–5 yrs	7–8 yrs	10 yrs
		Canine	4–5 mos	6–7 yrs	9–10 yrs	12–14 yrs
		First premolar	1¾–2 yrs	5–6 yrs	10–12 yrs	12–13 yrs
		Second premolar	2¼–2½ yrs	6–7 yrs	11–12 yrs	13–14 yrs
		First molar	At birth	2½–3 yrs	6–7 yrs	9–10 yrs
		Second molar	2½–3 yrs	7–8 yrs	11–13 yrs	15–15 yrs
		Third molar	8–10 yrs	12–16 yrs	17–21 yrs	18–25 yrs

- Physiologic age: It is primarily determined by natural/expected changes that occur through growth and development, for example
  - Examination of development of roots (apical closure) and comparison with tables that record the amount of development vs age.
- Chronologic age (the time from birth to death): This is the age that investigators are most interested in.

Various Methods for Age Estimation

Basically there are two major means by which age of a person under consideration can be estimated.

These methods may be broadly divided into two categories:

1. Estimation of age by skeletal means
2. Estimation of age by teeth.

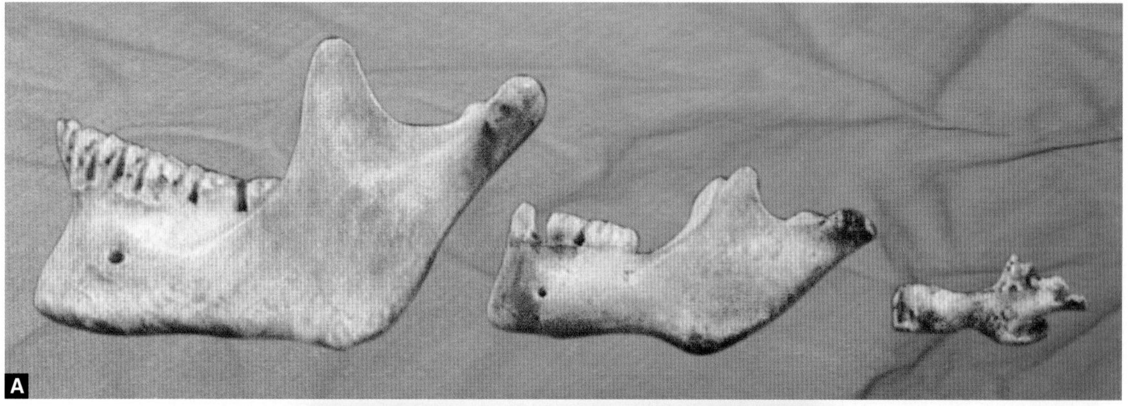

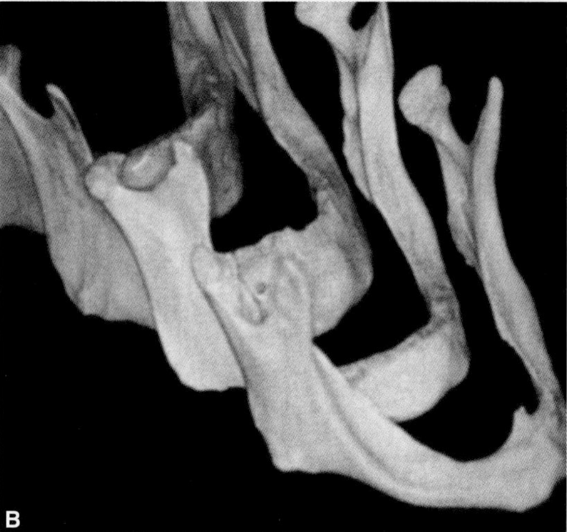

Figs 5.3A and B: Gradual changes in the mandibular bone of a person as he matures from a kid to fully mature adult and later on to an old age. Note the typical changes at angle of the mandible, height of alveolar process and width of ramus

Estimation of Age by Skeletal Means

The various methods for estimation of age by skeletal means are available, some of which are mentioned below. These procedures are quite elaborative, because of which it is beyond the scope of this title to give emphasis on each one. Mentioned below here are only the names of the procedures by which age can be estimated, details of these can be obtained from other relevant titles of the subject

A. Analysis of length of long bones.
B. Epiphyseal union.
C. Closure of frontanelle.
D. Ossification of hand and wrist bones **(Figs 5.4A and B)**
E. Closure of Skull sutures and palatine sutures (Later life).

Determination of age at time of death is an important step toward identification of unknown remains. Age can be established with considerable accuracy by roentgenography of the skeleton from the time of its appearance about the 20th week of gestation until early adulthood. This is possible due to the complex but dependable system by which the osseous framework of the body develops,

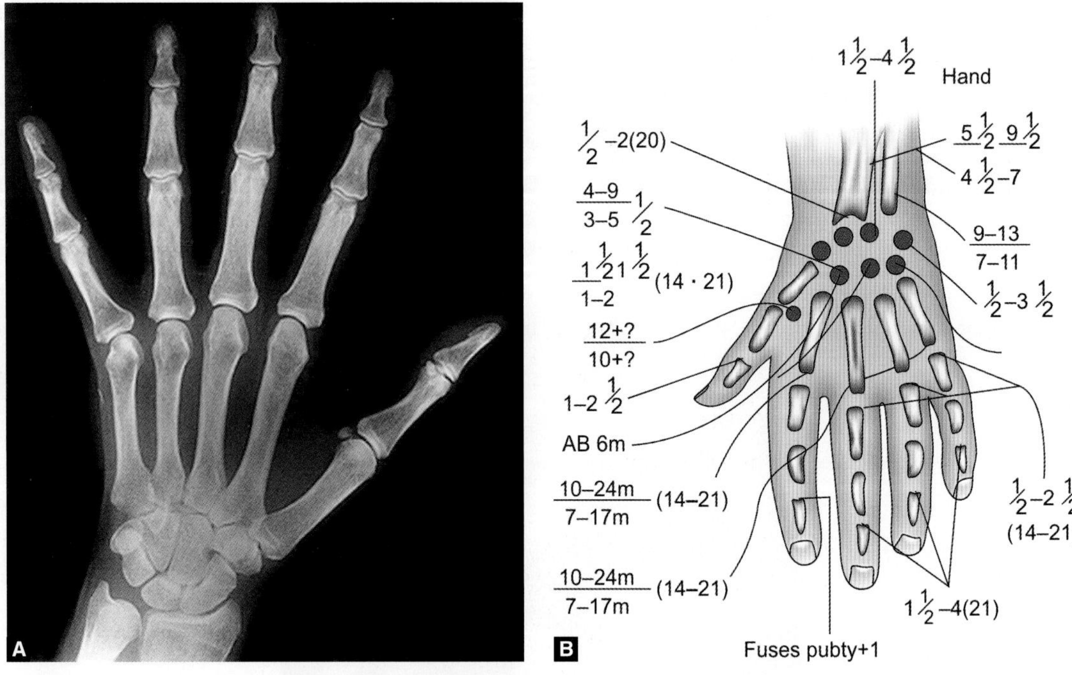

Figs 5.4A and B: (A) Radiograph of wrist bones, (B) Graphical diagram representing the typical timings and areas of ossification of wrist bones, whose assessment may give clues to the age of a person

grows, and matures. Most of the 206 bones of the human adult skeleton develop in cartilage precursors or anlagen from one or more primary centers **(Fig. 5.5)** of ossification (which make up the shaft or diaphysis of a long bone, the centrum of an axial or round bone) and secondary centers which develop the articular ends of the bones (epiphyses) or nonarticular processes (apophyses) for attachment of muscles, ligaments, and tendons. The appearance of these centers, and the fusion of secondary centers with the primary, follow a timetable allowing rather precise aging if appropriate skeletal parts are available for evaluation.

Estimation of Age by Teeth

- Most authorities have agreed that data derived from developing dentition is most accurate means of age estimation (*Garn et al.,1959; Stewart 1963; Liliequest and Lundberg 1971*).
- High survivability of teeth exposed to severe physical factors, such as fire and water immersion, make assessment of developing teeth the method of choice in forensic age estimation.

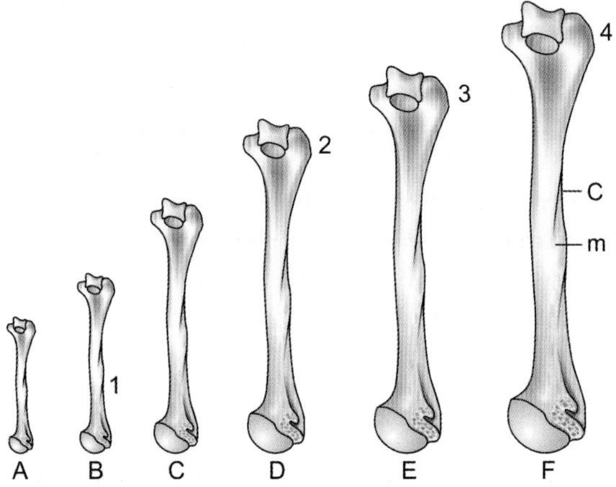

Fig. 5.5: Graphical picture representing the development and areas of ossification in the long bones

Further depending on the probable age group, we have different approaches for estimation of age of person under scenario, which can be broadly divided into five major groups.

1. Age assessment in prenatal child
2. Age assessment in neonatal and early postnatal child
3. Age assessment upto 14 years
4. Age assessment upto 21 years
5. Age assessment after 21 years.

Age Assessment in Prenatal Child

Various methods available are as following:

A. Haase's rule
B. Size of bones for age estimation
C. Krause and Jorden charts (1965)

A. Haase's Rule

- Age assessment is based on the fetal size (crown of the head to the heel of foot within body with body laid out straight).
- Fetal size = (No. of lunar months)2 = Up to 5th lunar month
- Fetal size = No. of lunar months X 5 = after 5th lunar month.

Fetal age can be measured by crown-rump measurements, fetal length, femoral length, biparietal diameter, or skeletal maturation. Fetal parts and soft tissues, if extrauterine, are small enough that radiological magnification will not be a major problem in view of the rather wide range of standard deviations for the various fetal measurements, most of which nowadays are based on real-time intrauterine measurements by ultrasonography.

Intrauterine fetuses imaged roentgenographically will be magnified. Under ideal conditions, the intrauterine fetal skeleton may be seen as early as the 10th week of gestation, but in practice it is not often visualized before the 18th or 20th week. The ossification centers that appear in the posterior elements of the spine often are the first skeletal components seen radiologically as a chain of densities or "string of beads" sometimes accompanied by tiny rib shadows. The base of the skull and long bones may be visualized between 20 and 25 weeks if not obscured by maternal gas, bones, or other tissues. The ossification center for the calcaneus appears between 24 and 26 weeks of gestation, followed in 2 weeks by the center for the talus. In the live fetus, intrauterine movement often obliterates the image of these small parts. Between 36 and 40 weeks the distal femoral epiphysis, followed by the proximal tibial epiphysis, will appear. Before obstetrical ultrasonography, this was the best method of determining fetal maturity. The distal femoral epiphysis will be found in 90 percent or more of term fetuses, the proximal tibial epiphysis in 85 percent or more.

B. Size of Bones for Age Estimation

I. *Based on basilar part of occipital bone*

Before 7 to 7½ lunar month: Sagittal length (In the midline from spheno-occipital synchondrosis to foramen magnum) > Width (between lateral tubercles).

After 7 to 7½ lunar month: Width > Sagittal length.

II. *Based on the temporal bone*

Before 7 lunar months: Temporal bone consists of 3 separate elements—squamous part, petrous part and tympanic ring.

After 7 lunar months fusion starts: At the end of 10 lunar months fusion is complete and may be taken as sign of full term fetus.

C. Krause and Jorden (1965)

Age Estimation at Neonatal and Early Post-natal Life

Incremental pattern of calcification of teeth:

- Calculated mainly by the histological technique, by using incremental pattern of calcification of individual developing teeth.

- Schour and Hoffman (1939) measured the rate of apposition of enamel and dentin and found this to be 16 μm per 24 hour period. Armed with this fact age can be estimated.
- The best known incremental disturbance is neonatal line **(Figs 5.6A and B)** present in deciduous teeth and permanent 1st molar. The amount of dentin deposited over this line can be taken as criteria to estimate the age. Also if neonatal line is present it indicates a live birth.
- Other methods:
  - Dry weight method of Stack (1960)
  - Radiographic interpretation of mineralization - Non mutilating.
  - Van der Linden and Duterloo (1976)—photographic standards of developing teeth.

Also at birth the primary ossification centers (diaphyses) of the long bones of the extremities, including the hands and feet, are present. The vertebral bodies and posterior elements have begun their process of ossification, as have the scapulae, pelvic, clavicles, base of the skull, calvaria, and facial bones.

Age Assessment up to 14 Years

- Sequence of eruption of both deciduous and permanent teeth are best way to acess age.
- Radiographical and histological means.
- Schour and Massler(1940) charts are the one commonly used.

Age Assessment up to 21 Years

- 3rd molar is only tooth on the eruptive path. **(Figs 5.7A and B)**
- Radiographical and eruption sequence observation can predict age.
- Commonly used—Schour and Massler(1940) chart and Gustafson (1971) table.
- Moorees et al. 1963, indicated that the crown formation stages for third molar tooth display less variation than root formation stages.

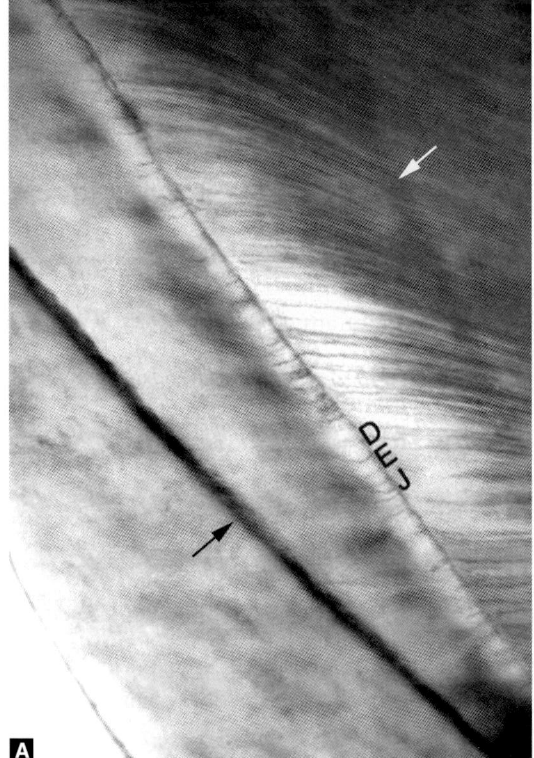

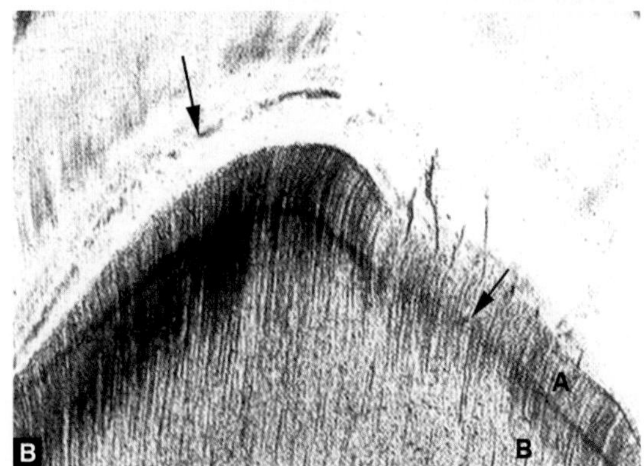

Figs 5.6A and B: Neonatal lines are shown in both enamel as well as dentin of the tooth structure, highlighted by the black and white arrows

Age Assessment after 21 Years

Several techniques are described in literature that addresses age estimation in adults. In general the

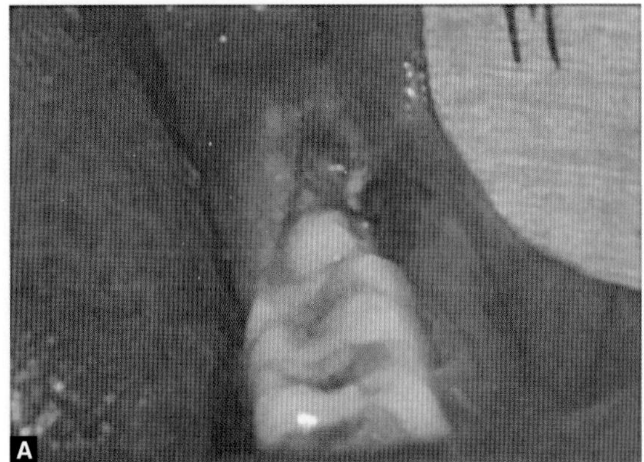

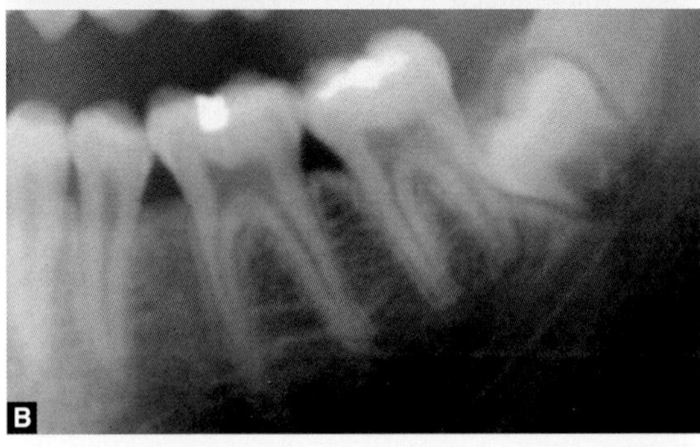

Figs 5.7A and B: Clinical and radiographic pictures showing the erupting third permanent molars, which is usually between 18 to 25 years of the age

methods are divided into three categories. The morphological, the radiological and the biochemical methods, which are all based on degenerative processes, observed in the dental structures. The methods described below are reproducible and rather accurate methods, some of which are non-destructive for the tooth substance.

The estimation of chronological age in living human beings and dead persons has been performed by forensic dentists for almost more than 50 years.

An optimum method for age determination in living individuals should fulfill the following conditions: age determination in all age groups and the procedure must not impair the health of the affected person. Tooth development and the sequence of eruption have been used extensively as a method of age estimation in children and adolescents.

In adults, following completion of the growth period, age estimation by morphological methods becomes difficult and particularly when nondestructive methods are used, it is not sufficiently accurate. Previously the methods of choice in adults were, theoretically, the method according to Gustafson and its modifications. These techniques are destructive, need extracted teeth and can be used only in dead. Gustafson's optimistic standard deviation of ±3.4 years has never been confirmed. Also Johanson's standard deviation of ±5.6 years seems to be too optimistic. Investigation has shown that a standard deviation of around ±10 years is normal for most methods, while others report that these methods have 95 percent confidence intervals of approximately ±12 years at best. The formulae are generally most accurate around 40 to 50 years and with increasing inaccuracy in younger and especially in older age groups. Also another difficulty is that there is a pronounced tendency for over estimation of younger persons and underestimation of older persons.

A. Morphological Methods

In the morphological methods belong all these that use morphological criteria. The samples can be observed sectioned or unsectioned with the eye. At this category belong the methods suggested by:

- Gustafson (1950),
- Dalitz (1962),
- Bang and Ramm (1970),
- Johanson (1971),
- Maples (1978), and
- Solheim (1993).

Gustafson (1950): The first technique for age estimation on teeth based on a systematic and statistical approach was published by Gustafson (1950). Once dental development is complete, through assessment of age and function, the dental structures undergo changes. Gustafson (1950) and Thoma (1944) described the age changes occurring in the dental tissues and noted attrition of the enamel, sclerosis of the dentin, denticles in the pulp, deposition of cementum, continuous eruption of the teeth and alternations in the perioodontal structures (periodontitis). After observing ground sections of adult human teeth, he designed diagrams of six changes related to age. These age-related changes were as following:

- Attrition of the meisal or occlusal surfaces due to mastication.
- Periodontitis.
- Secondary dentine.
- Cementum apposition.
- Root resorption.
- Transparency of the root.

Gustafson suggested the last two changes. In the method proposed each sign was ranked and allotted 0, 1, 2, 3 points **(Figs 5.8A and B)** according to degree of development. In forensic dentistry Gustafson's method of age estimation is the best known and most commonly referred to Kvall (2006).

Various codes given for assessment of above 6 values and their scoring criterions are enlisted here. **(Figs 5.8C to H)**

A = Attrition—loss of substances on the occlusal surface with teeth on the opposite jaw.
S = Amount of secondary dentin.
P = Periodontitis resulting in recession and exposure of root.
C = Apposition of cementum
R = Resorption
T = Transparency—dentinal canal are filled with mineralized tissue.

Attrition scoring sheet

A0.0 — No visible attrition on occlusal or incisal surfaces.
A0.5 — Minute attrition
A1.0 — Attrition only around the half of enamel thickness
A1.5 — Only a very thin layer of enamel is left with the dentin not exposed
A2.0 — The dentin has been attrited to a small extent
A2.5 — The attrition has reached halfway through the dentin
A3.0 — Attrition has reached through the whole layer of dentine and the original pulp cavity has been reached.

A_0 = No attrition	A_1 = Attrition within enamel	A_2 = Attrition reaching dentin	A_3 = Attrition reaching pulp
S_0 = No secondary dentin	S_1 = Secondary dentin has begun to form in upper part of pulp cavity	S_2 = Pulp cavity is half filled	S_3 = Pulp cavity is nearly of wholly filed with secondary dentin
P_0 = No periodontosis	P_1 = Periodontosis just begun	P_2 = Periodontosis along first one third of root	P_3 = Periodontosis has passed two-thirds of root
C_0 = Normal layer of cementum layer of cementum laid down	C_1 = Apposition a little greater than normal	C_2 = Great layer of cementum	C_3 = Heavy layer of cementum
R_0 = No root resorption visible	R_1 = Root resorption only on small isolated spots	R_2 = Greater loss of substance	R_3 = Great areas of both cementum and dentin affected

A

Fig. 5.8A

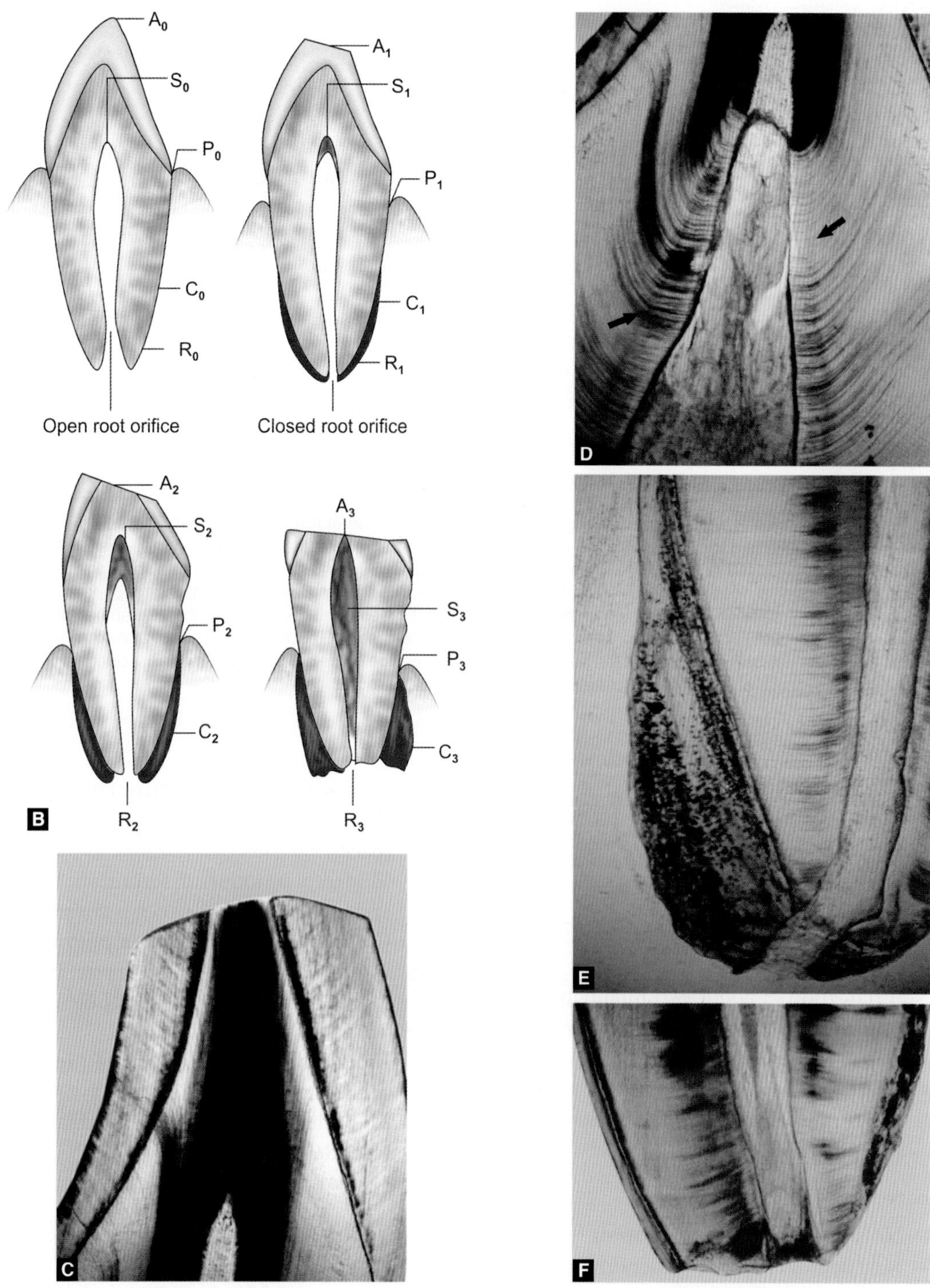

A_0
S_0
P_0
C_0
R_0
Open root orifice
A_1
S_1
P_1
C_1
R_1
Closed root orifice
A_2
S_2
P_2
C_2
R_2
A_3
S_3
P_3
C_3
R_3
B
C
D
E
F

Figs 5.8B to F

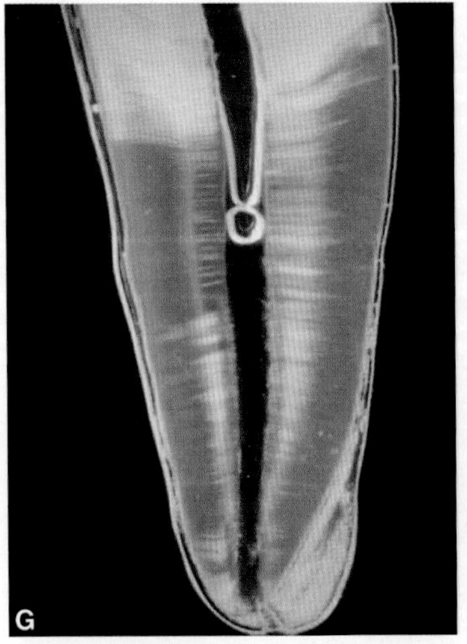

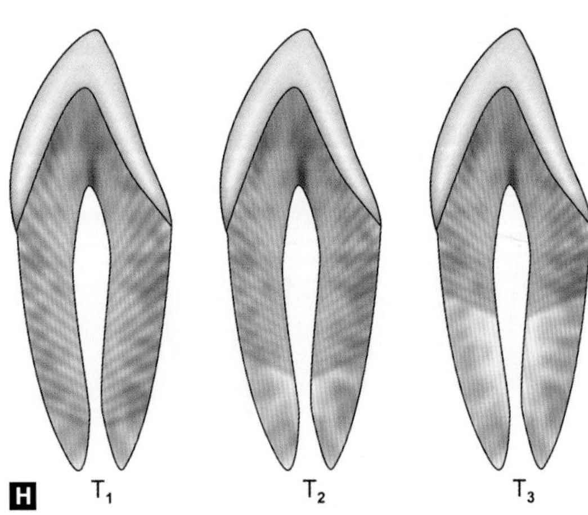

Figs 5.8G and H

Figs 5.8A to H: (A) Gustafson's grading and scoring criterion for determination of the age of a person based on regressive alterations of the teeth, as noted in the chart shown above; (B) Graphical representation of various regressive alterations of tooth to asses the score of Gustafson's scheme as shown in chart above; (C) Gground section of the tooth showing the attrition, physiological and mechanical wearing away of the tooth structure; (D) Picture showing the deposition of the secondary dentine, that is the dentin deposited after the completion of the root formation; (E) Cemental deposition at the peri-apex of the tooth; (F) Ground section of the tooth showing the root resorption at the peri-apical areas; (G) Root transperacncy arising in the ground section of the tooth because of the sclerosis of the dentinal tubules (deposition of the calcium salts within the dentinal tubules); (H) Graphical representation of the tooth structure to acess the degree of root transparency in the ground sections

Gingival recession scoring chart/periodontitis

- That is the distance from CEJ to the gingival attachment.
- It is done with the help of a periodontal probe.

P0.0 — Normal periodontium
P0.5 — A small retraction from cemento-enamel-junction
P1.0 — A retraction of about two millimeters
P1.5 — A retraction of about 4 to 7 mm
P2.0 — About 10 mm
P2.5 — About 15 mm
P3.0 — Only some millimeter of the root is still surrounded by a periodontium

Secondary dentin scoring chart

S0.0 — No secondary dentin formation
S0.5 — Mild degree of secondary dentin deposited at the roof of the pulp chamber, Covering 1/4 of the crown portion of the pulp space.
S1.0 — Moderate amount of secondary dentin at the roof of the pulp chamber which is covering half the crown portion of pulp space.
S1.5 — Moderate amount of secondary dentine at the pulp chamber which is covering the Complete crown portion of pulp space.
S2.0 — The entire crown portion of pulp space as well as some root portion of pulp space is filled with secondary dentin.
S2.5 — Almost half of pulp space is filed with secondary dentin.
S3.0 — More than two third of pulp is filled with secondary dentin

Cemental apposition chart

C0.5 —Very mild cemental thickening at the apical area
C1.0 —Cemental thickening which is 1/4 of the root length area

C1.5 — Cemental thickening of about 1/3 of root length area
C2.0 — About 1/2 of root length, cemental apposition seen
C2.5 — Cemental apposition is more than 1/2 but less than 2/3 of root length area
C3.0 — More than 2/3 of root length area is affected by cemental apposition

Root resorption scoring chart

R0.5 — Small resorptions on only one place
R1.0 — Resorption on two or more places without getting very deep
R1.5 — Extensive resorptions
R2.0 — Deep and wide resorption
R2.5 — Resorption practically over the whole surface
R3.0 — Resorption going into the dentin

Root transparency scoring chart

T0.0 — No transparency
T0.5 — Very mild amount at the apex
T1.0 — Mild areas of transparency less than 1/4 of root length
T1.5 — Transparency is less than 1/3 of root but more than 1/4
T2.0 — More than 1/3 and less than 1/2 of root length
T2.5 — More than 1/2 of root length and less than 2/3
T3.0 — More than 2/3 of root shows transparency.

The point values of each age-change are added according to the following formula:

$$A_n + P_n + S_n + C_n + R_n + T_n = \text{points}$$

It was found that an increase in points corresponded to an increase in age and that it was possible to draw a regression line for the correlation between age and points. In order to estimate the age of an individual, the point value is entered in the graph and the corresponding age is found **(Fig. 5. 9)**.

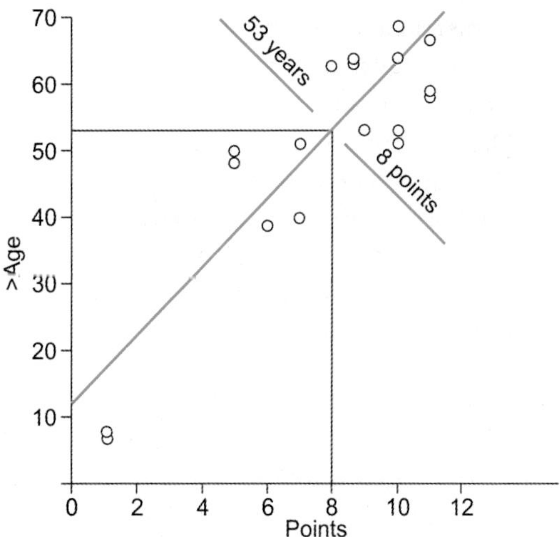

Fig. 5.9: The chart to obtain the age of person under investigation by calculating the scores of all changes as notified by the Gustafson and plotting them against the standard graph

The exact equation calculated was: $y = 11.43 + 4 - 56x$, where y = age and x = points according to the formula above. The error of estimation as calculated by Gustafson (1950) was ±3.6 years (Gustafson, 1947).

Gustafson's method has for many years been used by forensic odontologists in actual cases. At the same time it has been criticized for a number of reasons.

Disadvantages:

1. It can not be used in living person, only in dead when extraction of a tooth is allowed.
2. The assessment of the scores is the result of a subjective evaluation of the changes.
3. Too many age related changes needed to be considered making the method time-consuming.
4. Periodontitis is often impossible to determine due to decomposition of soft tissue.
5. One regression line is given for all teeth ignoring eruption time and morphological differences for the various teeth.

6. The method assumes that all six criteria are age changes of equal importance. Also it ignores any possibility of interrelationship between the criteria themselves.
7. Another problem stated was that the size of the material was small and consisted of only 40 teeth, while many of them originated from the same patient. Since, the variation of age-related changes in teeth from the same individual is evidently less than in teeth form different individuals, this affects the statistical analysis and contributed to even more favorable deviation. Also the regression formula was incorrectly calculated. Malpes and Rice (1978), Dalitz (1962) found the new formula: Y = 13.45 + 4.25 X.

Dalitz (1962): Dalitz in 1962 re-examined Gustafson's method and suggested a 5 point system from 0 to 4, give a slightly greater accuracy. His results showed that root resorption and secondary cementum formation could be disregarded. The other criteria, attrition, periodontitis, secondary dentine deposition and transparency of the root of the 12 anterior teeth, are related appreciably to age and to a similar degree. Dalitz suggested that it is preferable to use up to 4 of the 12 anterior teeth from the one individual for age estimation, but if using a greater number of teeth does not necessarily increase the accuracy of the determination. This over-ruled Gustafson who considered that his error in estimation would decrease when more teeth are examined. Dalitz's method results in a standard deviation in age determination of ±6 years.

The regression equation suggested by Dalitz (1962) was:

$$E' = 8.691 + 5.146A' + 5.338P' + 1.866S' + 8.411T'$$

Disadvantages:

The improvement is that Dalitz used weights for each factor. One of the problems is that it does not take into account bicuspids and molar teeth. This is critical for the application of the method since in many cases the only teeth left are molars and bicuspids as a result of severe external force.

Johanson: Gustafson's technique had been improved first by Dalitz in 1962 and finally by Johanson in 1971. The improvements implemented by Johanson are actually the most appreciated among forensic odontologists. He differentiated for seven different stages **(Fig. 5.10)**; instead of four originally and evaluated for the same six criteria, mentioned earlier, attrition (A), secondary dentine formation (S),

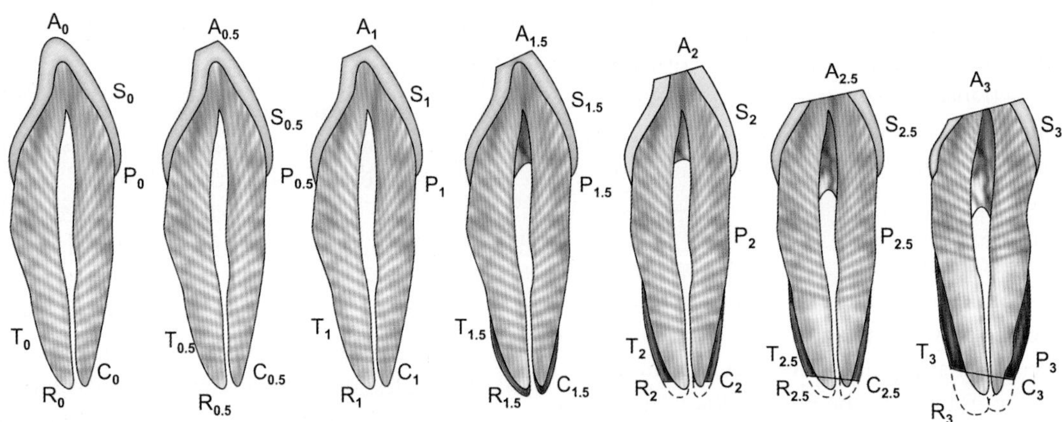

Fig. 5.10: The graphical picture depicting the calculation of various scores as per of Johnson's method of age determinations

periodontal attachment loss (P), cement apposition (C), root resorption (R) and apical translucency (T). Johanson made a more detailed study of the root transparency and stated that it is more clear when the thickness of the ground section of the tooth was 0.25 mm. The following formula was recommended:

$$Age = 11.02 + (5.14*A) + (2.3*S) + (4.14*P) + (3.71*C) + (5.57*R) + (8.98*T)$$

Bang and Ramm (1970): Bang and Ramm (1970) suggested a totally new approach in age estimation. They found that the root dentine appears to become transparent during the third decade starting at the tip of the root and advancing coronally with age.

This alteration is believed to be caused by a reduction of the diameter of the dentinal tubules caused by increasing intratubular calcification. The examination of the teeth is done in two ways. First the teeth were examined unhurt and then, 400 micrometer thick labio-lingual sections were cut. The total length of the root was measured buccally in the midline from the cemento-enamel junction to the apex. The transparent root dentin was measured from the apex of the root in coronal direction to the borderline between transparent and opaque dentin.

From the material collected, they found that it was difficult to make accurate measurements in molars and bicuspids and thus the survey included only incisors and cuspids. In spite the difficulties a small number of molars and bicuspids were examined. The mesial and distal roots showed good correlation in the degree of root transparency. However, there was difference between mesial, distal and palatal roots.

For practical reasons Bang and Ramm (1970) recommend the exclusion of upper first premolars and all the molars in order to arrive at the best estimation. They also suggest 2 different equations, one when the transparent length is less than or equal to 9 mm and a second when it exceeds 9 mm.

Advantages:

1. A great advantage of the method is that good results are obtained by measuring intact roots only.
2. The measuring of one factor-degree of root transparency-makes the method simple and rather fast compared to previous methods.
3. It is an objective method because it is not based on a point system but on measurements.
4. It can be applied without previous extensive training or expensive equipment. Also no differences were found between living and dead persons in the degree of root transparency and storage of specimens in 10 percent neutral formaldehyde caused no significant changes.

Various studies have been made about the influence of different conditions upon the degree of root transparency. Gustafson (1947) and Nalbandian et al. pointed out that root transparency is less influenced by pathological processes, while Bang and Ramm found the opposite. Kvaal (2005) states that studies in archaeology show root transparency to be reduced in the presence of metal. Also according to Reppien (2006) root transparency increases in diabetes and drug addicts Maples (1978).

Maples (1978): Maples (1978) suggested the use of only two criteria of the total six Gustafson recommended-secondary dentine formation and root transparency, in order to make the method more simple and accurate. The results of his research showed that root resorption was negatively correlated to age. Elimination of root resorption improved the results and the error of the estimate was reduced 20 to 30 percent. Periodontitis was not used because it was difficult to determine it long after soft tissue decomposition. In the same way attrition was excluded because differences among populations were found as a result of diet habits or abnormal occlusion.

Advantages:

1. As said before the method requires the scoring of secondary dentin and root transparency. This means that teeth with broken crowns, no evidence of periodontal attachment and lost cementum may still give accurate age estimates.
2. Also the technique can be used on other populations, contemporary and prehistoric, with less fear that dietary differences will decrease the estimation. Since, secondary dentin and root transparency; are easy to evaluate, observer error may be lessened.

Solheim (1993): For age estimation Solheim (1993) used five of the changes that Gustafson recommended (attrition, secondary dentin, periodontitis, cementum apposition and root transparency) and added another three new changes which showed significant correlation in different types of teeth. The three new age-related changes were surface roughness, color and sex. Solheim after examining a collection of 1000 teeth, excluding molars came down to good correlation between age and the whole number of changes. He found that mandibular canines and second premolars had the weakest relationship between the parameters and age, so when possible it was recommended to avoid the use of these teeth. Two sets of formulas were presented, one including sex and color and the other without them, because these factors were not always determinable in deceased individuals.

In Solheim's (1993) study there was a variety of origin of teeth (cadavers, forensic cases, living) which might better reflect the biological variation. Compared with teeth from living individuals, teeth removed from deceased bodies were darker, possibly owing to the changes or reactions to the environment after death. The finding indicates the need for cautiousness in using color as a factor in estimating the age of a corpse and this depends upon the condition of the teeth. In order to estimate color a shade guide is needed. Regarding sex as factor depends upon the condition of skeletal remains. The reported formulae are recommended for deceased bodies for identification purposes (unsectioned teeth) and in archeology.

B. Radiological Methods

Dental radiographs have been used quite recently in dental age estimation methods for adults. Kvaal and Solheim were the pioneers on this subject. They estimated the age of an adult from measurements of the size of the pulp on full mouth dental radiographs, without tooth extraction and destruction. The size of the dental pulp cavity is reduced as a result of secondary dentine deposit, so the measurements of this reduction can be used as an indicator of age.

Kvaal and Solheim presented a method where radiological and morphological measurements are combined in order to estimate the age of an individual. Using the radiographs they measured pulp length and width as well as root length and width. Then different ratios between the root and pulp were measured. These ratios were found to be significant correlated with age. They also found inclusion of the length of the apical translucency and penodontical retraction in some types of teeth. The results showed the strongest correlation with age to be in the ratio between the width of the pulp and the root.

This may indicate that the rate of deposition of dentine on the mesial and distal walls is more closely related to age than that on the roof of the pulp cavity. However, the correlation between age and the ratios between pulp and the root length was significant for only maxillary cuspids and premolar. The method is non-destructive and can be applied in living people or dry skeletal material, where single-rooted teeth are often loose in the jaw or can be removed easily. It can be employed when the preservation of the material is requested, as in archeological studies and in forensic investigations. Formulae for premolars showed a stronger correlation with age and this may be an advantage, because these teeth are less prone to damage by trauma or fire and also more often retained in skeletal material. Also the measurements require a fairly short time compared to methods where the teeth have to be sectioned.

Kvaal (1995) however proposed a method based totally on radiographic measurements (periapical radiographs) and did not depend on other factors such as root transparency and periodontal retraction, thus not requiring extraction of teeth. Measurements on dental radiographs may be a non-invasive technique for estimating the age of adults, both living and dead in forensic work and in archaeological studies.

Regression formulae for all six teeth together was proposed and also for each one of the 6 different teeth (11/21, 12/22, 15/25, 32/42, 33/43, 34/44). According to the survey there was a better age estimation when several teeth were included. Maxillary first premolars and molars were excluded because accurate measurements were difficult to perform. In order to compensate for differences because of magnification and angulation on the radiographs, ratios of measurements were used. Also correlation between age and the ratio of tooth to root length was insignificant to all types of teeth, indicating that attrition on the occlusal surface was so weak that it could not be related to age. As in the previous survey the width ratio was found to have a stronger correlation than the length ratio.

Bosnians et al (2005) applied the original formulas of Kvaal's technique (1995) using measurements made on panoramic radiographs instead from the typical periapical radiographs as originally described. The age estimations were comparable to those based on the original technique.

Kvaal states that when dealing with radiographs several complicating factors are encountered since the curved arch of the jaws is projected on to a flat film thus giving a certain amount of distortion. When periapical radiographs must be taken, the parallel technique should be used, because if the film is at an angle to the root the ratio will be influenced resulting in wrong estimation. For this reason when dealing with orthopantomographs (OPG) the patient should be correctly positioned to the X-ray machine. In many cases the bone overshadowed the apical third of the tooth, so that the width from this area of the tooth could not be measured with sufficient accuracy. This necessitates the use of a stereomicroscope. Rotated teeth, teeth with enamel overlap, teeth with restorations, cavities, attrition and periapical pathological processes cannot be used. With all the restrictions mentioned above in the older age groups it was difficult to find patients who retained all the six teeth that were measured in their study.

Vandevoort et al reported a morphometric method pilot study using microfocused computer tomography (CT) on extracted teeth to compare pulp-tooth ratios in the determination of age. Yang et al. (2006) using cone-beam CT scanning acquired the 3D images of teeth in living individuals. Using the 3D images the ratio of pulp/tooth volume can be calculated. Promising results for age estimation based on the pulp/tooth volume ratio were obtained

C. Biochemical Methods

Racemization of aspartic acid in human teeth: The biochemical methods are based upon the racemization of amino acids. The racemization of amino acids is a reversible first-order reaction and is relatively rapid in living tissues in which metabolism is slow. Aspartic acid has been reported to have the highest racemization rate of all amino acids and to be stored during aging. In particular, L-aspartic acids are conversed to D-aspartic acids and thus the levels of D-aspartic acid in human enamel, dentine and cementum increase with age. The D/L ratio has been shown to be highly correlated with age.

Helfman and Bada were the first that reported studies that focused on the racemization of amino acids and obtained a significant correlation between age and ratio of D-/L-enantiomers in aspartic acid in enamel and coronal dentine. Ohtani and Yamamoto (1987) showed that even higher correlations were obtainable using longitudinal sections of whole dentine. Ohtani et al (1995) applied the racemization method to cementum, which has higher water content.

The racemization rates of the cementum, enamel and dentine samples showed that cementum had the fastest reaction, followed by dentine and then enamel. This may be because cementum is surrounded by periodontal tissue and dentine and possibly has a highly environmental temperature, which would speed up the rate of reaction, as well as a known higher water content. Also the cementum was found to have a relative irregularity of the increase in the D/L ratio compared with that of dentine. As dentine is covered with cementum, enamel and periodontal tissue, it is presumably exposed to a relatively constant environment. In addition, the D/L ratio in dentine is assumed to increase linearly with aging (Ohtani et al. 1995). Although, cementum showed the fastest reaction, dentine showed the highest correlation with actual age. The results show that in cementum the racemization reaction proceeds in a relatively constant manner and that cementum is, like dentine, a tissue that has low metabolism. As a result the racemization method with cementum is, as with dentine, sufficiently useful for precise age estimation.

Ritz et al (1995) used the racemization method in dentinal biopsy specimens in order to estimate the age of living individuals. This method emerged from the need to identify the age of living individuals without extracting teeth. In Germany for example extraction of a tooth exclusively for age estimation when it is not medically indicated is regarded as ethically and legally problematic. The results were hopeful and showed a close relationship between the extent of aspartic acid racemization in dentinal biopsy specimens and age, thus facilitating age estimation. However, for accurate results the performance of biopsies must occur under strictly standardized conditions.

The specimens taken by the biopsy technique were approximately 1mm in diameter and 1 mm long. Specimens were taken from posterior teeth (molars). These amounts of dentine proved sufficient for the determination of the extent of aspartic acid racemization in all cases. The cavities were then treated with conventional filling materials. The only cases in which the technique was not applicable were in teeth with extensively destroyed crowns. In these cases, the biopsies had to be taken in deeper dentine layers, often close to filling materials or carious lesions.

As said before, in order to use the formulas proposed by Ritz et al. (1995), the biopsies must be taken from a specific region of the tooth. The study showed that the biopsy layer had a significant influence on the results, since the extension of aspartic acid racemization is higher in deep layers. The biopsy technique is a low-risk procedure that causes only minor discomfort to the affected person.

Others

Incremental lines analysis: The premise for incremental line analysis in identification efforts is based on the fact that these lines have the same pattern in an individual whose enamel formed at the same time in a given dentition. The different teeth developing in one individual give the same pattern of incremental lines which is distinct from that of another individual, in effect creating a "fingerprint" of enamel development specific to the individual. Incremental line analysis is usually done on ground sections of longitudinally sectioned dentition which results in the destruction of the dental structures. The Skinner and Anderson study is unique in that ground sections were not used. Reconstructed crowns were embedded in crystal clear polyester casting resin with Fiber-tek catalyst and allowed to cure. They were then longitudinally sectioned at 180 to 200 μm with a Buehler-Isomet low-speed saw with a diamond wafering blade. The mounted sections were examined and photographed at × 20 magnification with ordinary and polarized light. Composite photographs were then created showing the entire labial/buccal enamel to homologize striae between teeth. Limitations in incremental line age determinations appear age dependent. Lipsinic et al. studied the correlation of age and incremental lines in the cementum of human teeth and found that direct predictions of age based on these lines generally underestimated the age of older specimens. There was, however, correlation between the number of lines and age. These authors concluded that such studies would have greater usefulness if a large enough population group was studied and that a computer-generated formula resulted.

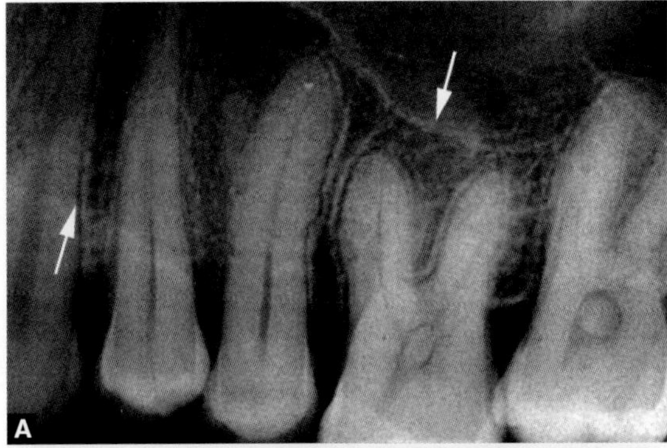

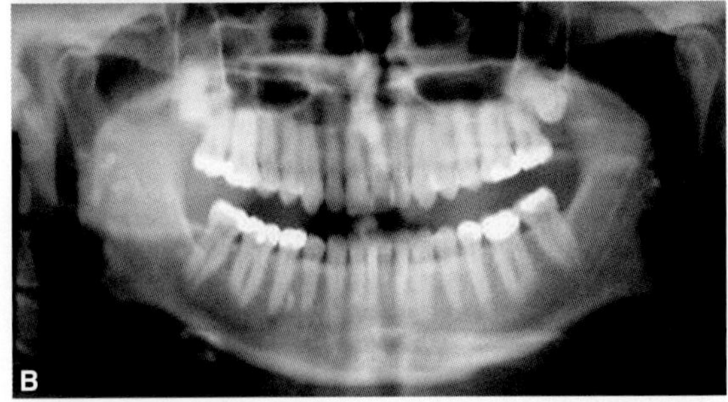

Figs 5.11A and B: IOPA and OPG are mainly used for calculation of the age as per of radiographic means of age determination

Steps of Age Estimation

Kvaal (2006) describes the approach using different methods in order to reach to relatively accurate estimation.

Visual Assessment

Initially a gross "clinical" examination ought to be performed which include the condition of the soft tissues as well as the dentition. Dental attrition, tooth colour and stains, periodontal status as well as quantity and quality of dental restoration may be employed. From this visual impression an experienced dentist may give a good estimate of chronological age.

Radiographs (Figs 5.11A and B)

Periapical radiographs or orthopan-tomographs (OPG) will give additional information in the size of the pulp. In cases of fragile tissue e.g. burnt bodies or skeletal remains from archaeological excavations the radiographs ought to be made with minimal handling of the remains to avoid further destructions of tissue.

Extraction and Preparation of Single Teeth

Age estimation methods that cause irreversible destructions of tissues are used last. Different methods require single intact teeth, half sectioned teeth, or ground sections **(Fig. 5.12)**.

It is recommended that age is calculated using preferable two independent scientific methods. This may either be one method using the whole dentition, selected teeth from the dentition or the same method applied to two or more teeth from the same dentition (Kvaal, 2006). In all cases repetitive measurements should be made in order to verify the reproducibility of the calculations performed. The final age estimate ought to be based on the results of the methods and the initial visual age assessment.

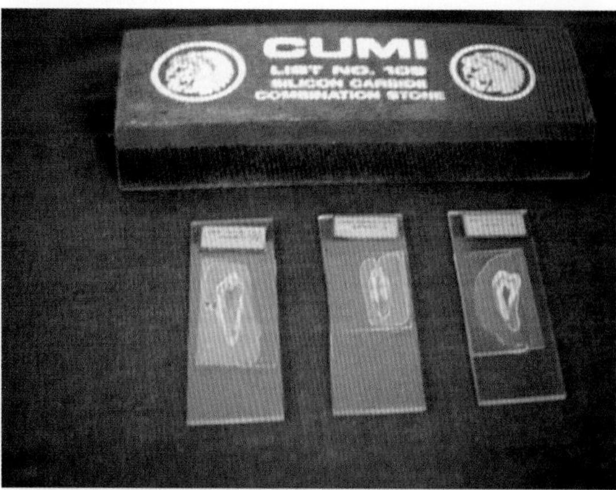

Fig. 5.12: Picture showing the stone and methods to prepare the ground sections of the teeth

To this direction the following software program was developed. Dental age calculating software. Willems, in year 2000 developed a software program in order to automate dental age calculations. The program is named "Dental Age Estimation". It includes the most accurate and often referenced morphological and radiological techniques that are reported in literature and which demand extensive calculations. The great advantage of the program is the immediate dental age estimation results and the avoidance of calculating errors. All that is needed is to measure the required parameters and enter their values into the program. Also it enables the forensic odontologist to apply different techniques and not to stick to one age estimation technique thus providing a more reliable result.

Following **(Table 5.1)** are the recommended dental Age estimation procedures in adults (ASFO, 2007)

Dental Age Estimation by Means of Commonly Used Developmental Surveys

By these methods, dental age is estimated by comparing the dental development status of a person of an unknown age with published developmental survey. It basically consists of three necessary steps:

A. Collection of appropriate data
B. Use of Appropriate dental development survey
C. Evaluation

Collection of Appropriate Data

- Thorough history (living) and antemortem data (for dead individuals).
- Clinical examination (in both living and dead individuals)
  1. General examination of person
  2. Examination of oral cavity and dentition.
- *Radiographic examination:* Radiographs taken should enable one to use the method that he/she has decided to use.
- Histological examination

Table 5.1: Recommended dental age estimated procedure in adults (ASFO, 2007)

Status	*Examination type*	*Specific techiniques of methods*
Living	Radiographs/Morphological	Kroad and softenin (dental radiographs)
	Extracted tooth-biochemical	Aapartic acid racenization
	Post-formation changes	Johanson sectioning
	Post-formation changes	Lamindin *et al.* (1992)
Deceased	Biochemical	Aspartic acid recemization
Anthropological/Historical Collection		
Skeletal	Non-Destructive	Kvaal/Solheim Intact Methods

ASFO: American Society of Forensic Odontology

- Other relevant information
  - Impression for study model
  - Dental photography

Appropriate data should be obtained from the subject ideally in a form similar to that used in the development survey chosen

Appropriate Dental Development Survey

- Use as many appropriate parameters as possible.
- Use methods as originally described in the literature.
- Use as many teeth as possible.

Evaluation

- Assess if the methods are appropriate in relation to the individual.
- Assess factors which may have influenced tooth development or ageing.
- Assess especially if pathologic factors or other may have influenced the findings
- Make a final complete assessment of the most likely chronologic age

Commonly Used Dental Developmental Surveys

The most commonly used dental developmental surveys are outlined here, with their descriptive charts as well.

1. Schour and Massler method (1940)
2. Moorees method (1963)
3. Demirijian seven-tooth system for age estimation
4. Gustafson method (1966)

Schour and Massler Method (1940)

- Published numerical development charts for deciduous and permanent tooth.
- Periodically updated by ADA.

Figure showing development of deciduous teeth **(Fig. 5.13)**.

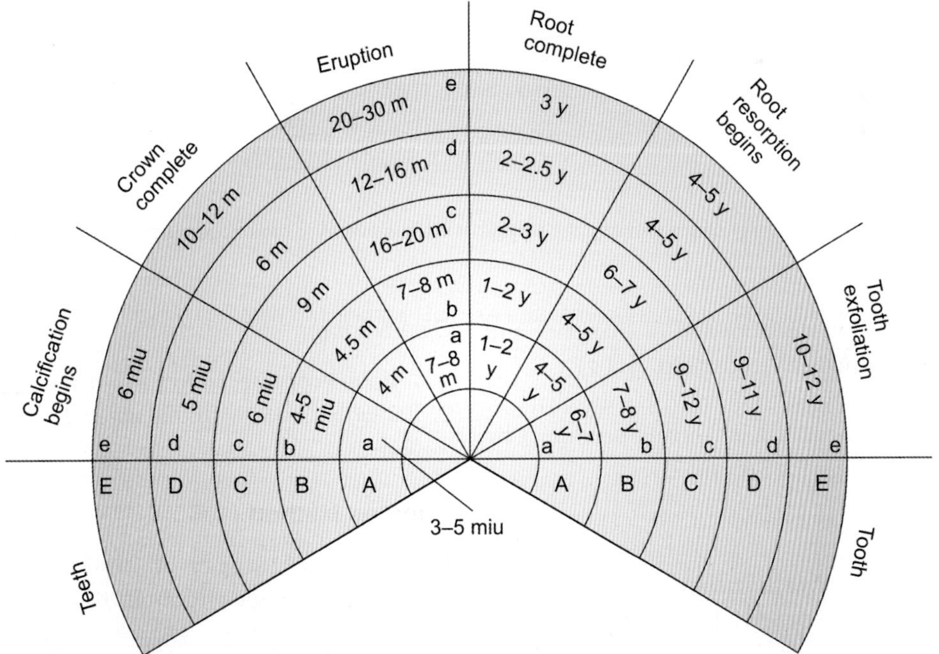

Fig. 5.13: Schour and Massler charts showing the timings of various events in morphogenesis of deciduous dentitions

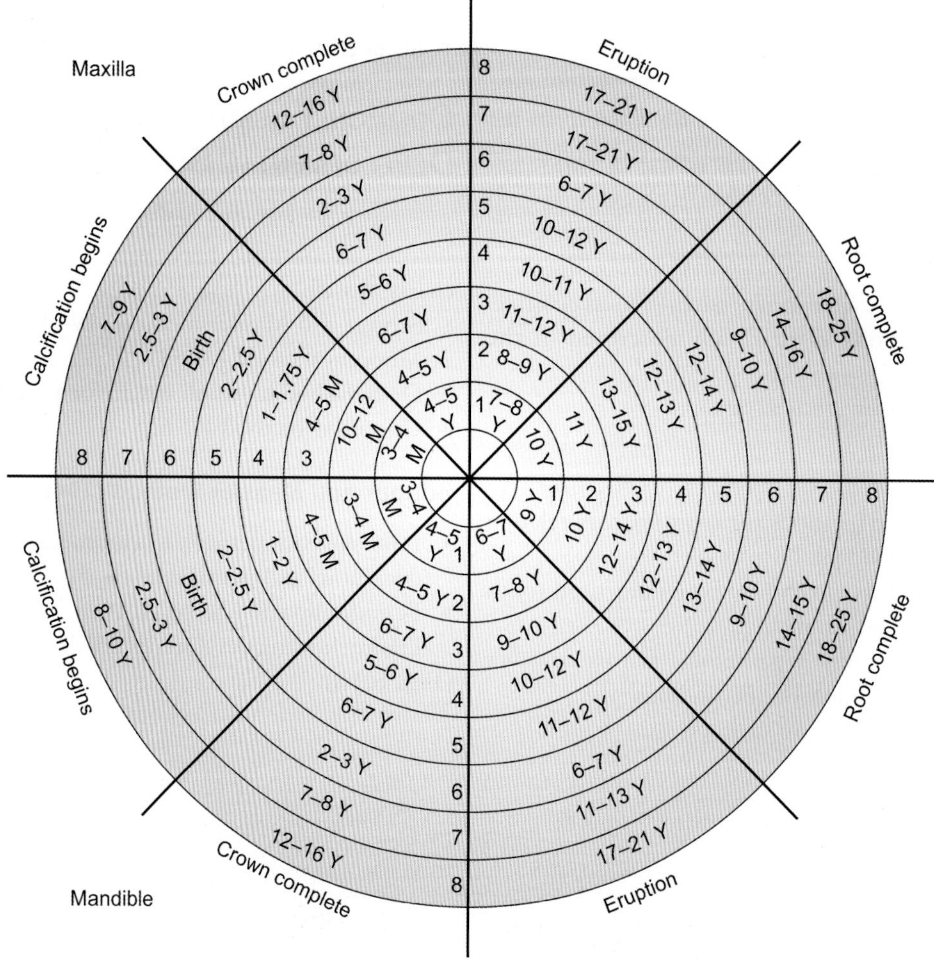

Fig. 5.14: Schour and Massler charts showing the timings of various events in morphogenesis of permanent dentitions

Figure showing development of maxillary and mandibular permanent teeth **(Fig. 5.14)**.

Figure showing Schour and Massler chart of dental development. Chart shown produced by ADA (1982) **(Figs 5.15A and B)**.

Advantages

Easy comparison with either radiographs or individually removed developing teeth.

Disadvantage

1. It do not separate survey for males and females.
2. Range obtained with this survey is from 2 to 15 years.

Moorees Method (1963)

- Defined 14 stages of mineralization for developing single and multi-rooted permanent teeth.

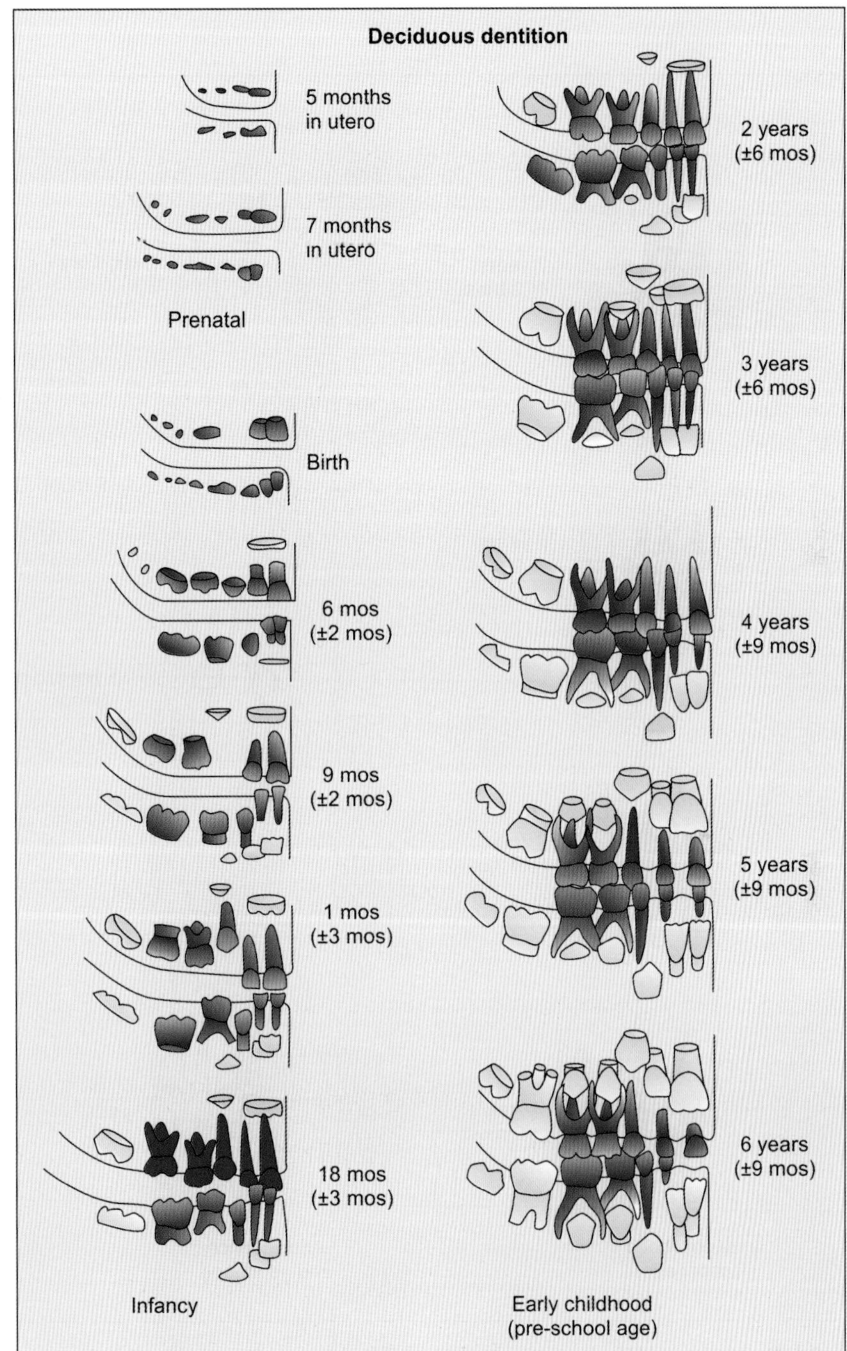

Fig. 5.15A: Schour and Massler (as produced by ADA) charts showing the timings of eruptions of deciduous dentitions and a corresponding age calculation

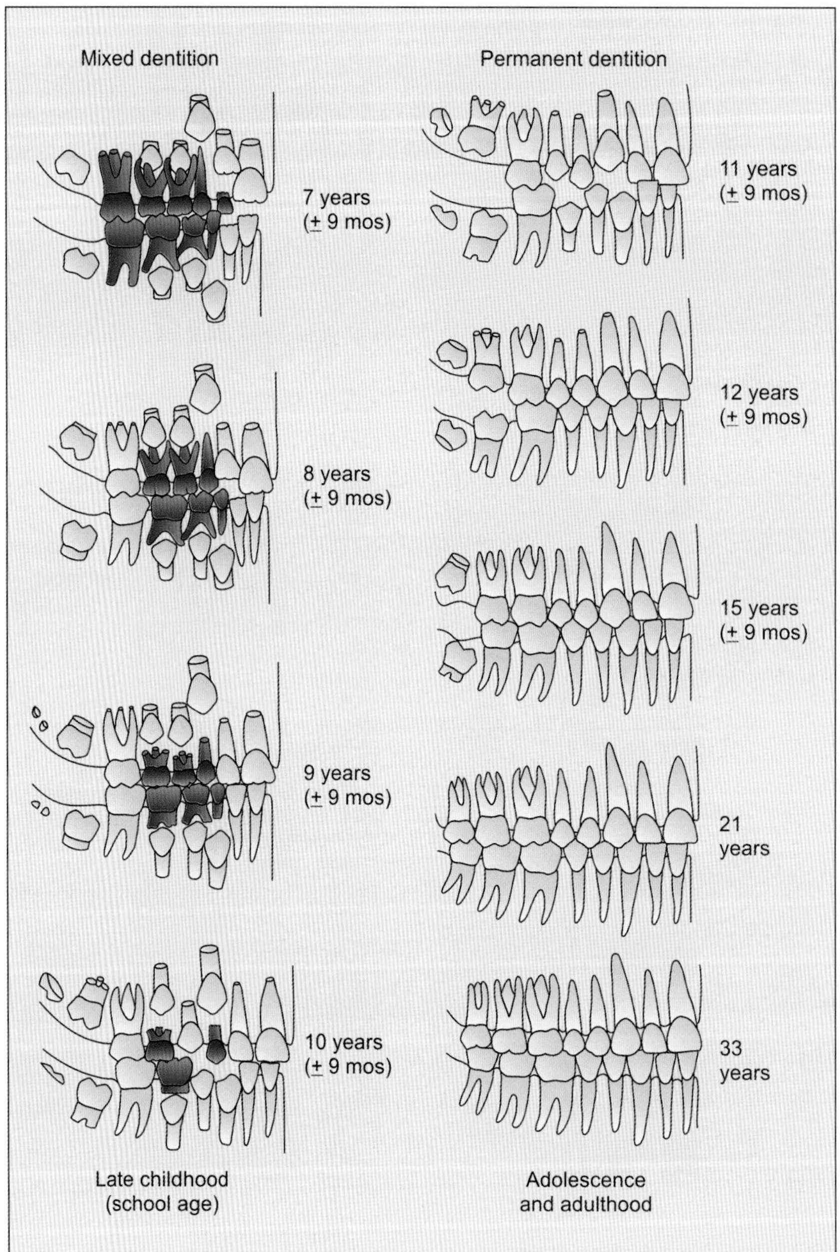

Fig. 5.15B: Schour and Massler (as produced by ADA) charts showing the timings of eruptions of permanent dentitions and a corresponding age calculation

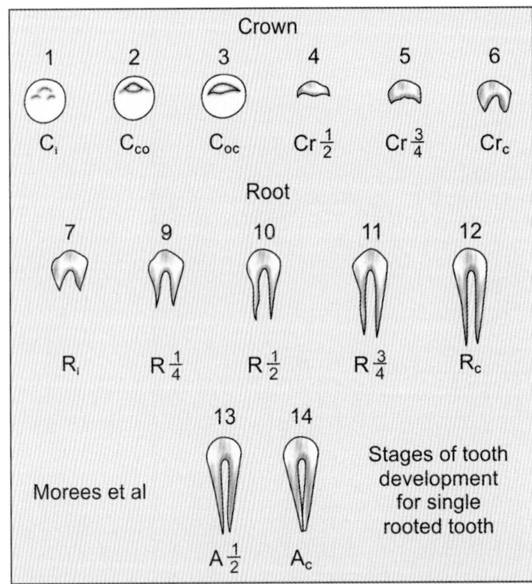

Fig. 5.16: Stages of development of a single rooted tooth as shown by Morees et al

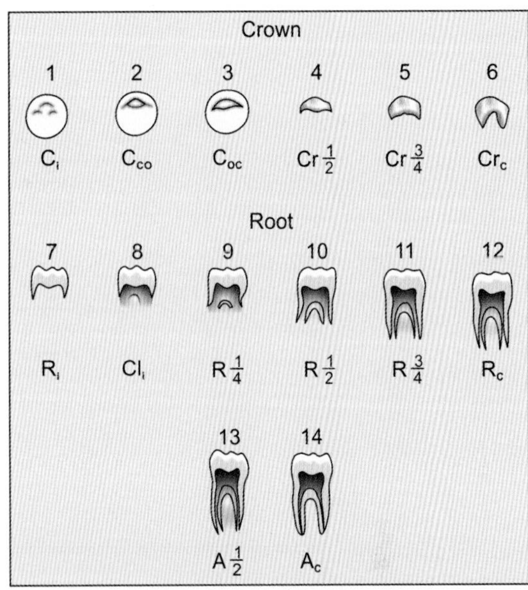

Fig. 5.17: Stages of development of a multi-rooted tooth as shown by Morees et al

Figure showing stages of tooth formation for single rooted teeth (Moorees et al 1963) **(Fig. 5.16)**.

Note: Abbreviations stand for

Ci	Initial cusp formation
Cco	Coalescence of cusps
Coc	Cusp outline complete
Cr1/2	Crown half complete
Cr3/4	Crown ¾ complete
Crc	Crown complete
Ri	Initial root formation
R1/4	Root length one quarter
R1/2	Root length one half
R3/4	Root length three quarters
Rc	Root length complete
A1/2	Apex half closed
Ac	Apical closure complete

Figure showing stages of tooth formation for multi-rooted teeth (Moorees et al 1963) **(Fig. 5.17)**.

Note: Code symbols are same as for single rooted dev. with addition of Cli initial cleft formation.

Highlights of the Moorees method (1963)

- Earliest age of survey is 6 months.
- Includes development of mandibular third molar.
- Has a standard deviation of ± 2
- Teeth emerged clinically at R3/4 stage
- Difference in crown formation between sexes are minimal.
- In case of root development female developed ahead of males.
- Greatest sexual dimorphism is expressed in the mandibular canines, females being upto 11 months ahead of male in development

Figure showing development of female incisors from Moorees et al. 1963 with mean age standard deviation ± 2 **(Fig. 5.18)**.

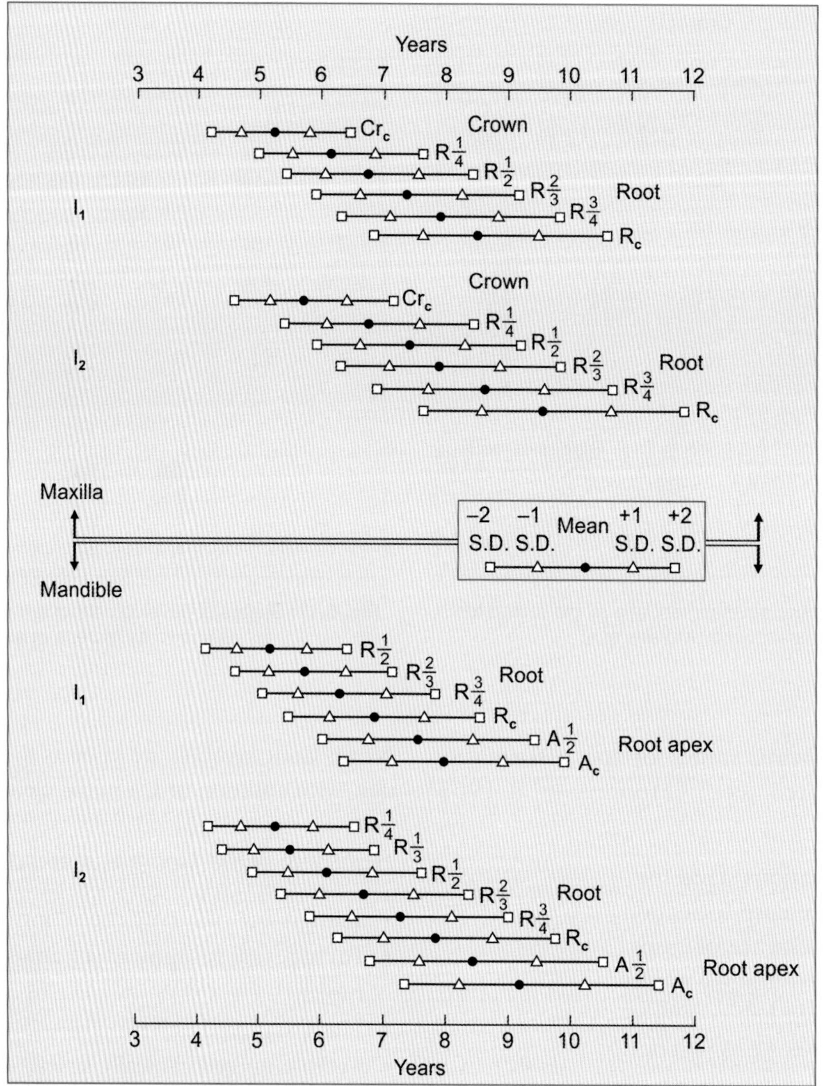

Fig. 5.18: Development of incisor as per of the chronology of the events told by Morees et al

Demirijian Seven-tooth System for Age Estimation

Technique: Following procedure needs to be followed in order to calculate the age of a person using this particular technique.

Radiographs

Take an IOPA of left and right mandibular incisors, canines, premolars, 1st and 2nd molars OR

Right and left oblique radiographs together with right and left lower occlusal oblique films OR

Rotational tomographs.

Calculation of Maturity Score

Seven teeth must be used, i.e. mandibular left or right incisors, canines, premolars, 1st and 2nd molars. In case of any tooth missing corresponding tooth of opposite side should be substituted. Use

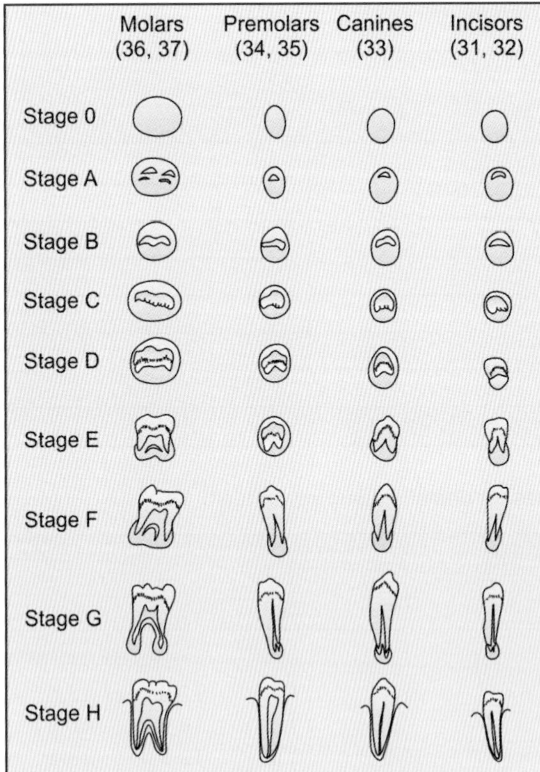

Fig. 5.19A: Graphical pictures showing the stages of tooth development as per of Dermijian

pictorial guide together with reference to written criteria, determine the mineralization stage of tooth.

Figure showing pictorial guide to mineralization assessment **(Fig. 5.19A)**.

Figure showing mineralization assessment of development teeth **(Fig. 5.19B)**.

A. Mark X in appropriate square of chart for recording mineralization stages (or zero if mineralization is absent) as shown here in the following table **(Table 5.2)**.

B. For each completed square, convert X into number using self weighed score table for dental stages and add the numbers to find the total score i.e. the maturity score, as shown in table below **(Table 5. 3)**.

Add the numbers to find the total score i.e. the maturity score

Stage		*Description*
A		In both uniradicular and multiradicular teeth, a beginning of calcification is seen at the superior level of the crypt, in the form of an inverted cone or cones. There is no fusion of these calcified points.
B		Fusion of the calcified points forms one or several cusps, which unite to give a regularly outlined occlusal surface.
C	a	Enamel formation is complete at the occlusal surface. Its extension and convergence toward the cervical region is seen.
	b	The beginning of a dentinal deposit is seen.
	c	The outline of the pulp chamber has a curved shape at the occlusal border.
D	a	The crown formation is completed down to the cementoenamel junction.
	b	The superior border of the pulp chamber in uniradicular teeth has a definite curved form, being concave toward the cervical region. The projection of the pulp horns, if present, gives an outline like: an umbrella top. In molars, the pulp chamber has a trapezoidal form.
	c	Beginning of root formation is seen in the form of a spicule.
E		*Uniradicular teeth.*
	a	The walls of the pulp chamber now form straight lines, whose continuity is broken by the presence of the pulp horn, which is larger than in the previous stage.
	b	The root length is less than the crown height.
		Molars
	a	Initial formation of the radicular bifurcation is seen in the form of either a calcified point or a semilunar shape.
	b	The root length is still less than the crown height.
F		*Uniradicular teeth*
	a	The walls of the pulp chamber now form a more or less isosceles triangle. The apex ends in a funnel shape.
	b	The root lengrh is equal to or greater than the crown height.
		Molars
	a	The calcified region of the bifurcation has developed further down from its semi lunar stage to give the roots a more definite and distinct outline, with funnel-shaped endings.
	b	The root length is equal to or greater than the crown height.
G	a	The walls of the root canals are now parallel (distal root in molars).
	b	The apical ends of the root canals are still partially open (distal root in molars).
H	a	The apical end of the roor canal is completely closed (distal root in molars).
	b	The periodontal membrane has a uniform width around the root and the apex.

Fig. 5.19B: Chart showing the detailed illustrations of the various stages of tooth development as per of the graphical picture shown in previous figure by Dermijian

Table 5.2: Showing the chart to record the mineralization stages

Stage	*Mandible*						
	I1	I2	C	PM1	PM2	M1	M2
A							
B		×					
C							
D							
E							
F							
G							
H							

Table 5.3: Showing self-weighed scores for dental stages, seven teeth

Tooth	*Stages*								
	0	A	B	C	D	E	F	G	H
Boys									
M2	0.0	1.7	3.1	5.4	8.6	11.4	12.4	12.8	13.6
M1				0.0	5.3	7.5	10.3	13.9	16.8
PM2	0.0	1.5	2.7	5.2	8.0	10.8	12.0	12.5	13.2
PM1		0.0	4.0	6.3	9.4	13.2	14.9	15.5	16.1
C				0.0	4.0	7.8	10.1	11.4	12.0
I2				0.0	2.8	5.4	7.7	10.5	13.2
I1				0.0	4.3	6.3	8.2	11.2	15.1
Girls									
M2	0.0	1.8	3.1	5.4	9.0	11.7	12.8	13.2	13.8
M1				0.0	3.5	5.6	8.4	12.5	15.4
PM2	0.0	1.7	2.9	5.4	8.6	11.1	12.3	12.8	13.3
PM1		0.0	3.1	5.2	8.8	12.6	14.3	14.9	15.5
C				0.0	3.7	7.3	10.0	11.8	12.5
I2				0.0	2.8	5.3	8.1	11.2	13.8
I1				0.0	4.4	6.3	8.5	12.0	15.8

Reading Graph

- Locate maturity score on y axis of graphs
- Locate the intersection of maturity score with 50th percentile curve.
- Drop a perpendicular to the x axis to locate the median age.
- Repeat for other percentile curves.

Figure showing graph with locating of score on Y axis of the graph **(Fig. 5.19C)**.

Figure showing graphs giving percentiles for age and maturity score for girls **(Fig. 5.19D)**.

Figure showing graphs giving percentiles for age and maturity score for boys **(Fig. 5.19E)**.

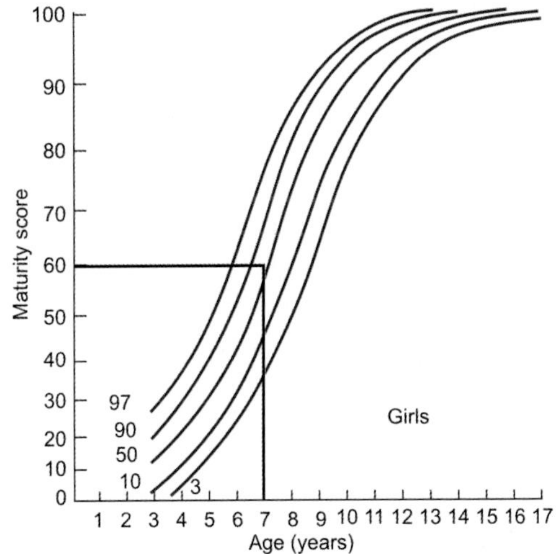

Fig. 5.19C: Figure showing Graph with locating of score on Y axis of the graph

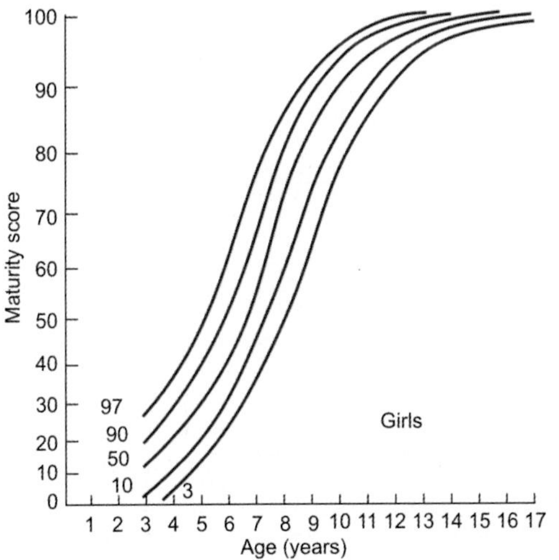

Fig. 5.19D: Figure showing Graphs giving percentiles for age and maturity score for girls

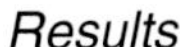

Results

Record the results in the form of table **(Table 5.4).**

Drawbacks of the Demirijian Seven-tooth System for Age Estimation:

1. Developmental difference between males and females are not usually apparent until 5 years. of age.

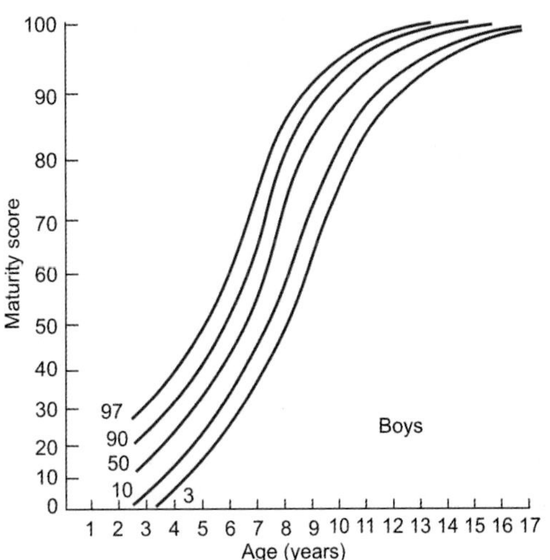

Fig. 5.19E: Figure showing Graphs giving percentiles for age and maturity score for boys

Table 5.4: Showing format for entering age determinant results

Percentile	*Age*
97	
90	
50	
10	
5	

2. Inter-observer variation may be as high as 20 to 25 percent.
3. Mandibular teeth are required for this particular process and also 3rd molars are not included in this study

Gustafson (1966) Mehod for Estimation of the Age

a. Gustafson developed a comprehensive compact chart of dental development. However this chart does not differentiate between male and female. He divided the dental development into the following four stages.

b. 4 stages of development
  I. Mineralization starts
  II. Crown completes
  III. Eruption
  IV. Root complete

Figure showing Gustafson's (1966) chart of formation and eruption of deciduous and permanent teeth (excluding 3rd molars) **(Fig. 5.20)**.

Other Less Commonly Used Methods for Estimation of Dental Age

Objective Measurement of Dental Color for Age Estimation by Spectroradiometry

Tooth color estimation is also of interest in forensic odontology. Several authors have reported that teeth tend to darken with age. In the method for dental age estimation suggested by Solheim, who proposed 10 formulas for different teeth, dental color contributed to 7 of these formulas. In addition, changes in tooth color have been observed in human populations of different postmortem intervals. The most common method to estimate dental color is to compare color in the specimen with dental shade guides. Nevertheless, the use of tooth color for age estimation in forensic odontology is limited by difficulties with objective measurements. In an attempt to develop a more objective method, various scientists have used a spectroradiometry technique to measure dental color changes in order to avoid the bias inherent

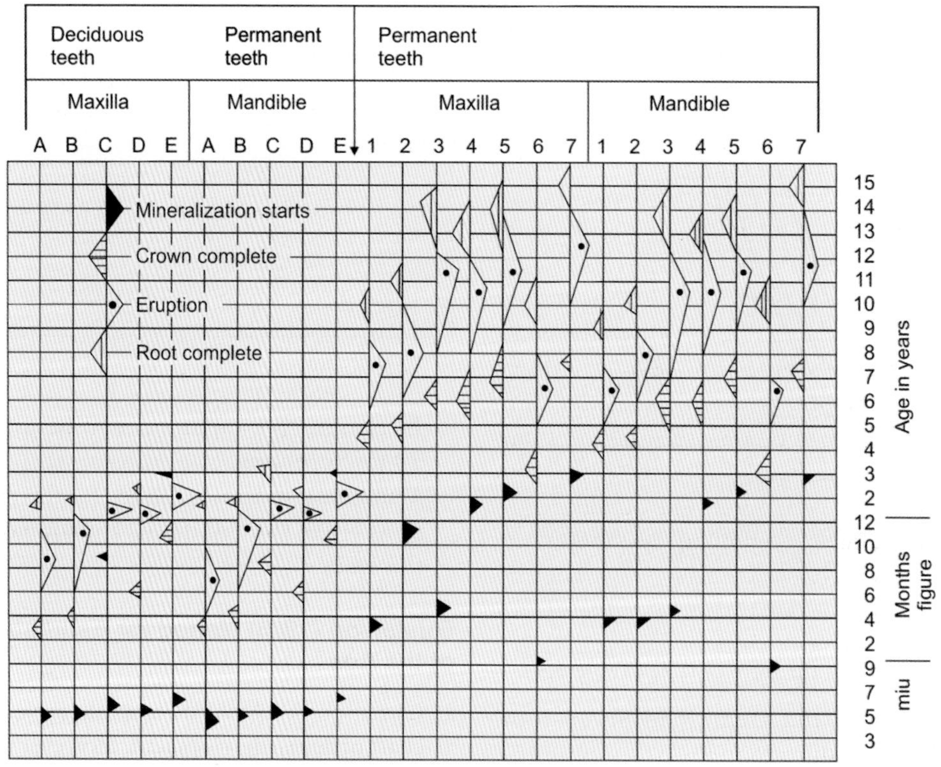

Fig. 5.20: Figure showing Gustafson's (1966) chart of formation and eruption of deciduous and permanent teeth (excluding 3rd molars)

in observer subjectivity. Of particular interest are differences in dental color depending on the condition of the body and the postmortem interval. S. Martin-de las Heras et al have concluded that spectroradiometry may be an objective and useful tool to determine dentine color, and may provide forensic odontologists with a complementary method to calculate the chronological age in recent corpses. Moreover, determination of dentin color by spectroradiometry could be used in combination with other morphological methods in order to improve the accuracy to estimate the age.

SUMMARY

Age is one of the essential factors in establishing the identity of the person. Age estimation is a sub discipline of forensic sciences and should be an important part of every identification process, especially when information relating to the deceased is unavailable. Different factors have been used for age estimation but none has withstood the test of time. Teeth are considered as optimal for this purpose. Examination of teeth in many way form a unique part of human body as they are most durable and resilient part of the skeleton.

The estimation should be as accurate as possible since it narrows down the search within the police Missing Persons files and enables a more efficient and time saving approach. Age estimation is of broader importance in forensic medicine, not only for identification purposes of deceased victims, but also in connection with crimes and accidents.

In addition, chronological age is important in most societies for school attendance, social benefits, employment and marriage.Denial maturity has played an important role in estimating the chronological ages of the individuals because of the reported low variability of dental indicators.

Different techniques and numerous studies have been published for age estimation, each one demonstrating various accuracy, precision and reliability. In all cases reproducible and reliable estimation results are possible when the appropriate methods for each case are properly applied and used. Error is present in every approach. For this reason when investigating a case the forensic odontologist should apply different techniques available and perform repetitive measurements and calculations in order to reach to reliable conclusion. Research into age estimation is ongoing. Forensic odontologists should continually watch the scientific presentations and journals that report new developments and validate or challenge existing techniques.

BIBLIOGRAPHY

1. Cameriere R, Ferrante L. Accuracy of age estimation in children using radiograph of developing teeth. Forensic Science International. 2008;176:173-7.
2. Gustafson G. Age determination from teeth; Journal of American Dental Association. 1980;41: 45-54.
3. Lipsinic FE, Paunovic F, Houston GD, Robinson F. Correlation of age and incremental lines in the cementum of human teeth, J. Forensic Sci. 1986;31:982-9.
4. Maber M, Liversidge HM, Hector MP. Accuracy of age estimation of radiographic methods using developing teeth. Forensic Science International 2006;159S:S68-S73.
5. Meinl A, et al. Comparison of the validity of three dental methods for the estimation of age at death Forensic Science International. 2008;178:96-105.
6. Mesotten K Dental age estimation and third molars: a preliminary study Forensic Science International. 2002;129:110-5.
7. Phrabhakaran N. Age estimation using third molar development. J. Pathol. 1995;17:31-4.
8. Pillai PS, Bhaskar G. Age Estimation from the teeth using Gustafson's method-A Study in India; Journal of Forensic Science 1974;3:135-41.
9. Singh A. Age estimation from the physiological changes of teeth. JIAFM. 2004;26(3).

Chapter 6

Bite Marks

Nitul Jain, Soniya Adyanthaya

Chapter Overview

- Historical aspects
- Legal admissibility
- Skin as registration material
- Classification of various bite marks systems
- Typical presentation and composition of bite marks
- Bite marks recognition
- Difference in bite patterns of child and adults
- Bites, bite wound infections, prevention and management

INTRODUCTION

Although bites and biting have been around as long as animals with teeth have inhabited the planet, the science of bite mark identification is comparatively new and potentially valuable. Identifying human remains by dental characteristics is a well established component of forensic sciences with a definite scientific basis.

However, the whole arena of bite marks is a recent and still controversial pat of this discipline. In mortal combat situations, such as the violence associated with life and death, struggles between assailants and victims, the teeth are often used as a weapon. Indeed, using the teeth to inflict serious injury on an attacker may be the only available defensive method for a victim **(Fig. 6.1)**.

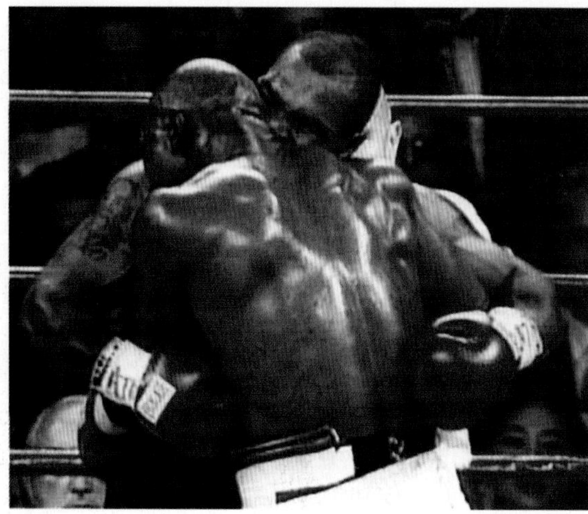

Fig. 6.1: The ear bite inflicted by Mike Tyson during the sports of wrestling to his competitor

Alternatively, it is well known that assailants in sexual attacks, including sexual homicide, rape and child sexual abuse, often bite their victims as an expression of dominance, rage and animalistic behavior. The teeth are a significant component of our natural arsenal. It is suspected that many dentists have seldom considered their patients' teeth as such effective weapons!

Teeth are often used as weapons when one person attacks another or when a victim tries to ward off an assailant. It is relatively simple to record the evidence from the injury and the teeth for comparison of the shapes, sizes and pattern that are present. However, this comparative analysis is often very difficult, especially since human skin is curved, elastic, distortable and undergoing edema.

In many cases, though, conclusions can be reached about any role a suspect may have played in a crime. Additionally, traces of saliva deposited during biting can be recovered to acquire DNA evidence and this can be analyzed to determine who contributed this biological evidence. If dentists are aware of the various methods to collect and preserve bite mark evidence from victims and suspects, it may be possible for them to assist the justice system to identify and prosecute violent offenders.

This form of forensic evidence demonstrates how human bite marks are used by courts to answer important questions that may arise during the prosecution of accused suspects. Currently, there is no agreement among forensic odontologists about the individuality (uniqueness) of the dentition or the behavior of human skin during biting. Although these issues have never been proven scientifically, much research is currently underway in an attempt to prove the suspicion that each human dentition is unique. The sizes, shapes and pattern of the biting edges of the anterior teeth that are arranged in the upper and lower dental arcades are thought to be specific to that individual. This is mainly caused by the sequence of eruption of anterior and posterior teeth. Canines must force their way into the dental arch, which often results in bodily movement, rotation and displacement of other teeth. The resulting configuration of the dentition produces an identifiable pattern that may be compared with similar patterns found on bitten objects to determine the likelihood that a specific individual has left their calling card. The importance of bite marks as an invaluable tool in criminal assaults and victim forensic identification lies in fact that *no two dentitions are identical* (**Fig 6.2**).

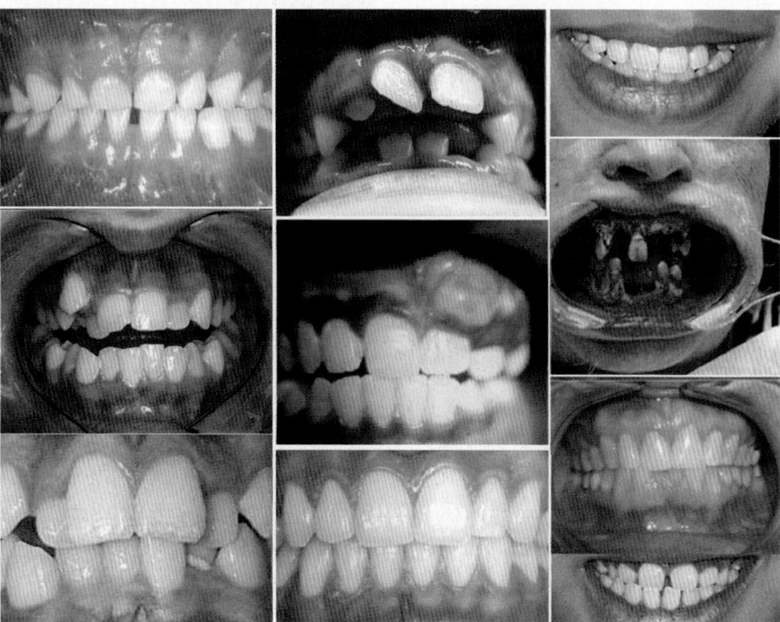

Fig. 6.2: Composite pictures showing the various types of dentition in human beings, reflecting the uniqueness in each

A pattern injury: Bite marks are patterned injury that is any injury in which the instrument of injury can be determined and possibly may be individualized as the weapon making the injury. A bite mark is an injury to skin in which the instruments of the injury are teeth. In contrast to finger prints, which leave a definite ridge marks, bite marks leave blurred contusions, which tend to leak in surrounding tissues **(Figs 6.3A and B).**

- It may be caused by humans or animals
- Must be differentiated from animal bite
- May be on tissues, food items or other objects
- It is a Primititive type of assault, which may highlight;
  - Aggressive or sexual behavior,
  - Form of self-defense,
  - In children, biting is a form of expression when verbal communication fails,
  - Playground altercations or sports competition.

According to Dr Brown, investigating bite marks is greatest technical challenge to forensic dentists.

Historical Aspects

Wax Seal: William the Conqueror reportedly validated royal documents by biting into a wax with his characteristic dentition.

Indentured Servants: Debtors coming from Britain or Europe to America to work as servants verified their agreements by biting the seal on the pact in stead of a signatures and became known as so.

The Doyle Case: Even though using bite mark evidence began around 1870, the first published account involving a conviction based on bite marks as evidence was in the case of Doyle vs State, which occurred in Texas in 1954. The bite mark in this case was on a piece of cheese found at the crime scene of a burglary. The defendant was later asked to bite another piece of cheese for comparison. A firearms examiner and a dentist evaluated the bite marks independently and both concluded that the marks were made by the same set of teeth. The conviction in this case set the stage for bite marks found on objects and skin to be used as evidence in future cases.

Another landmark case was People vs Marx, which occurred in California in 1975. A woman was murdered by strangulation after being sexually assaulted. She was bitten several times on her nose. Walter Marx was identified as a suspect and dental impressions were made of his teeth. Impressions and photographs were also taken of the woman's injured nose. These samples along with other models and casts were evaluated using a variety of

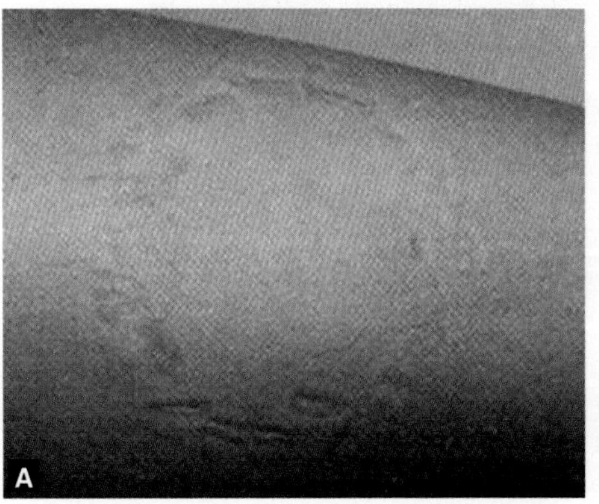

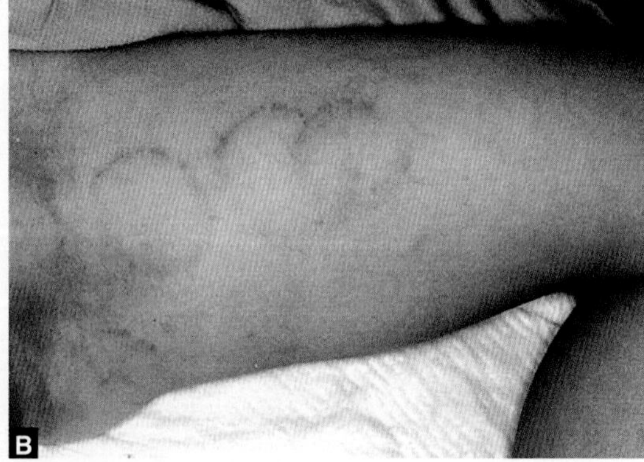

Figs 6.3A and B: Bite marks appearing as blurred contusions on some of the incidences of bite marks

techniques, including two-dimensional and three-dimensional comparisons, and acetate overlays. Three experts testified that the bite marks on the woman's nose were indeed made by Marx and he was convicted of voluntary manslaughter.

The first person to whom real credit must be given for having published an analysis of a bite-mark case is Sorup, in 1924. The method used he called "odontoscopy" analogous to the fingerprint identification called "dactyloscopy".

Presumably the first case involving a bite mark that led to a conviction sustained on appeal was a 1972 rape case, Illinois vs Johnson. Several famous cases, most notably Theodore "Ted" Bundy's serial murder trial, **(Fig. 6.4)** made bite marks a high-profile item with excessive media attention.

The Legal Admissibility

The relevance and admissibility of new forms of scientific evidence depend upon their general acceptance in the scientific community. Identification by fingerprint comparison was accepted first in USA courts in 1911 only on the basis of its general and common use and acceptance. In 1923, the justification for admitting scientific evidence was established as a standard that became known as "Frye Test". Frye test required 3 components for admissibility; these were:

- The principle must be demonstrable
- It must have been sufficiently established
- It must have gained the general acceptance of experts working in the particular scientific field (s) to which the evidence belongs.

1st case involving admissibility of bite mark evidence was 1954 Texas case, Doyle vs State. In a landmark 1975 case, People vs Marx, the California Court of Appeals concluded that, bite mark analysis was generally acceptable in the proper scientific community and thus admissible, in spite of the court's acknowledgement that "there is no established science of identifying a person from bite marks".

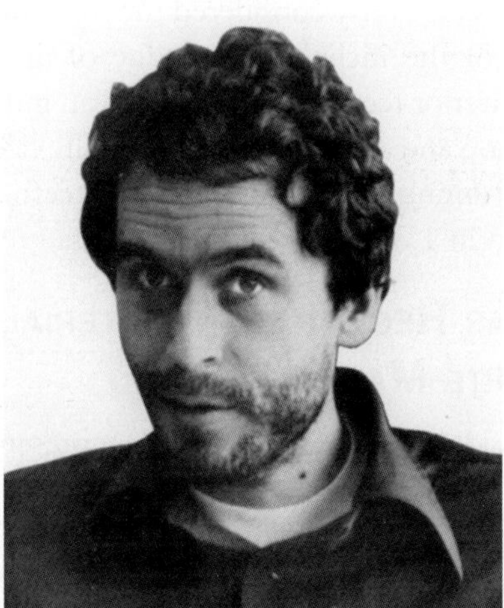

Fig. 6.4: The famous and most notable serial killer Ted Bundy whose bite marks on the victims led him to behind the bars

The definitions of bite marks by various authors:

MacDonald:

A mark caused by the teeth either alone or in combination with other mouth parts.

ABFO: (American Board of Forensic Odontology)

A physical alteration in a medium caused by the contact of teeth.

Or

A representative pattern left in an object or tissue by the dental structures of an animal or human.

The Overlying Principle

Bite mark analysis is based on two postulates:

a. The dental characteristics of anterior teeth involved in biting are unique amongst individuals, and
b. This asserted uniqueness is transferred and recorded in the injury.

The debate over the uniqueness of human teeth is probably one of the fiercest in current forensic dental discourse. Many forensic dentists, appellants, and lawyers have questioned the validity of dental uniqueness determination and demand to know from testifying experts, the relative frequency of dental features identified in bite marks.

The first article to consider the statistical nature of dental uniqueness was published by MacFarlane and Sutherland in 1974. The authors began by differentiating between "positive" and "negative" features of the dentition. A positive feature was described as the presence of a tooth with a certain rotation or other individualizing feature. A negative feature was the absence of a tooth. This study concentrated on the positive features that occurred on the anterior teeth (canine to canine, maxillary and mandibular). Patients were selected from an outpatient clinic and in total 200 study casts (maxillary and mandibular) were produced. The authors only studied the dental casts, not bite marks that would have been produced by such casts.

The investigators noted the number and shape of each tooth, the presence of any incisal restoration, relationship of teeth to arch form, and tooth rotation (four categories). The amount and degree of detail recorded in the bitten surface may vary from case to case. And, even if it is assumed that the dentition is individual enough to warrant use in forensic contexts, it is not known if this individuality is recorded specifically enough in the injury. In situations where sufficient detail is available, it may be possible to identify the biter to the exclusion of all others. Perhaps more significantly, it is possible to exclude suspects that did not leave the bite mark.

Also, every member of the dental clinic team — from the receptionist and assistant to the dentist should become familiar with the appearances and presentations of bite-mark evidence. These injuries are often associated with physical and sexual abuse of children, spouses and elders. Moreover, the evidence is usually easily observed in the dental office during regular patient visits. Recognition and reporting of such injuries to specific authorities that are equipped to investigate such suspicions may end the episodic pattern of abuse and stop the cycle of violence from which many victims are not able to escape.

A distinction must be drawn from the ability of a forensic dentist to identify an individual from their dentition by using radiographs and dental records and the science of bite mark analysis. Dental identification, as opposed to bite mark identification, utilizes the number, shape, type, and placement of dental restorations, root canal therapies, unusual pathoses, root morphology, trabecular bone pattern and sinus morphology.

Bite marks are important because of the following properties bite marks possess:

1. More unique than DNA
2. Identical twins share the same genetic makeup, but their dental impressions will differ.

"There are 28 teeth, plus four wisdom teeth, in an adult's dentition", Delattre says "Each tooth has five surfaces, for a possible total of 160 surfaces. Each surface has its own characteristics and may have fillings, crowns, extractions, bridges, etc. In addition to the teeth we see in our mouths, the roots and bone around them are specific to each person." Given all of these parameters, it is safe to say that the physical make-up of each person's dentition is unique.

Fellingham and coworkers have calculated that there are 1.8×10^{19} possible combinations of 32 teeth being intact, decayed, missing or filled.

Sweet and Pretty considered the size, shape and pattern of the incisal/biting edge of upper and lower anterior teeth to be specific to an individual.

Rawson and associate mathematically calculated that the biting edge of 12 anterior teeth can be arranged in 1.3×10^{26} different ways.

Skin as Registration Materials for Bite Marks

The considerable variation of bite mark presentations on human skin brings the accuracy of skin as a registration material into doubt. While many studies have examined the accuracy of bite marks on other substrates, such as cheese, apples, sandwiches, and soap, studies pertaining to human skin are relatively scarce. This represents both the most debated area of substrate accuracy and the most commonly bitten material.

Skin is a poor registration material since it is highly variable in terms of anatomical location, underlying musculature, or fat, curvature, and looseness or adherence to underlying tissues. Skin is highly visco-elastic, which allows stretching to occur during either the biting process or when evidence is collected.

In 1971, DeVore issued a preliminary report describing studies performed on the variability of bite marks found on skin. The experiment involved the inking of human skin (living volunteers) using a stamp with two concentrically placed circles with intersecting lines. Following the analysis of the photographs it was found that in all cases there was an expansion or shrinkage of the stamp, with a maximum linear expansion of 60 percent at one location. The design of the stamp permitted the investigators to examine the distortion in both size and direction. DeVore concluded that, due to the level of distortion found, photographic images of a bite mark in comparative analysis should be used only if the exact position of the body can be replicated. The placement of a body in such a position is usually impossible, as the exact position of the body during an attack is rarely known. DeVore stated that further research to investigate the effect of postmortem changes on skin distortion were required.

In 1974, researchers from the Bioengineering Unit of the University of Strathclyde examined the features of the biting process likely to impact upon the appearance of bite marks on human skin. They described the differing characteristics of skin from a variety of anatomical locations; e.g. Langer's Lines represent directional differences in the degree of extensibility of skin. Like DeVore, they emphasized the importance of body location during biting as the directional variations or tension lines will alter with movement. The report also described distortion that can occur in skin after biting. The edematous response of skin to trauma is likely to stiffen the area, thus rendering it more stable. However, the subsequent resorption of this fluid will cause a large amount of distortion. They concluded that the changes in bite mark appearance are likely to be greater as the injury grows older. This was found equally applicable to both living and dead victims.

Classification of Various Bite Mark Systems

The various systems have been proposed depending upon; biting agent, material bitten, and degree of biting. Along with these, there are other systems proposed by Cameron and Sims, MacDonald and Webster.

Depending upon biting agent, bite marks may be caused by:

- Human
  - Children
  - Adults
- Animal
  - Mammals
  - Reptiles
  - Fish
- Mechanical
  - Denture
  - Saw blade tooth marks
- Others

Depending on material bitten

- Skin
  - Human
  - Animal
- Perishable items
  - Food items
- Non-perishable
  - Object

Depending on degree of biting

Definite bite marks: Direct application of pressure by biting edges causing tissue damage.

Amorous bite mark: Made in amorous situations, tend to be made slowly with absence of movement between teeth and tissues.

- Lower teeth marks— when teeth are pressed into tissue with a gradually increasing pressure.
- Upper teeth— forms a series of arches where the tissue is sucked into mouth and pressed against back of the teeth with tongue.

Aggressive bite marks: Shows scraping, tearing or avulsion

- Usually involves ears, nose or breasts
- Difficult to interpret.

Cameron and Sims classification: It is relatively simple, and broad encompassing, it classifies bite marks in two categories, that is:

Depending on the Agents

- Human
- Animal

Depending on the materials bitten

- Skin, body tissue
- Foodstuff
- Other materials

MacDonald's classification: It is one of the most cited, mainly pertinent to human bite marks.

Tooth pressure marks: Marks produced on tissue as a result of direct application of pressure by teeth.

Tongue pressure marks: When tongue presses the tissue against rigid area such as lingual surfaces of teeth and palatal rugae. There is a combination of sucking and tongue thrusting involved.

Tooth scrape marks: Marks caused due to scraping of teeth across the bitten material. Usually present as scratches and abrasions.

Webster's classification: This system classifies bite marks made in foodstuffs **(Figs 6.5A to C)**.

Type I: Food item fractures readily with limited depth of tooth penetration, e.g. hard chocolate.

Type II: Fracture of fragment of food item with considerable penetration of teeth, e.g. bite marks in apple and other firm fruits.

Type III: Complete or near complete penetration of the food item with slide marks e.g. cheese.

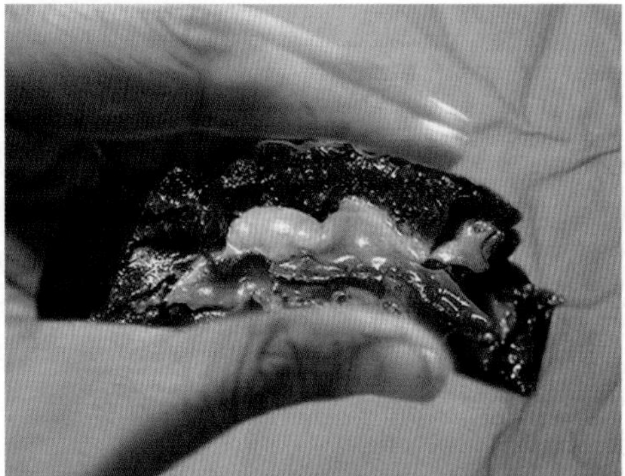

Fig. 6.5A: Bite marks left on chocolate cake. Note the penetration of the teeth

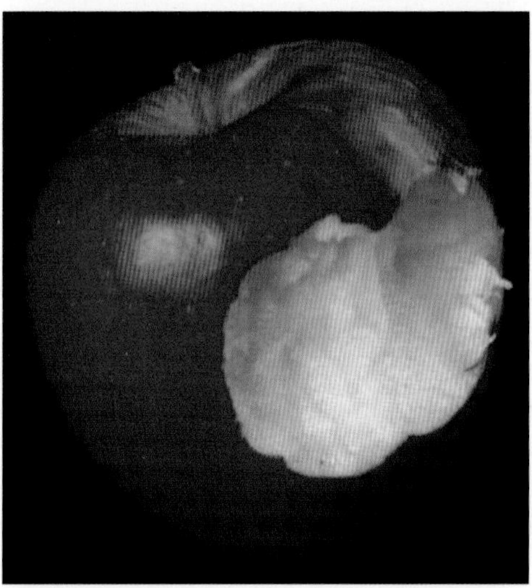

Fig. 6.5B: Bite marks on hard food stuff like apples

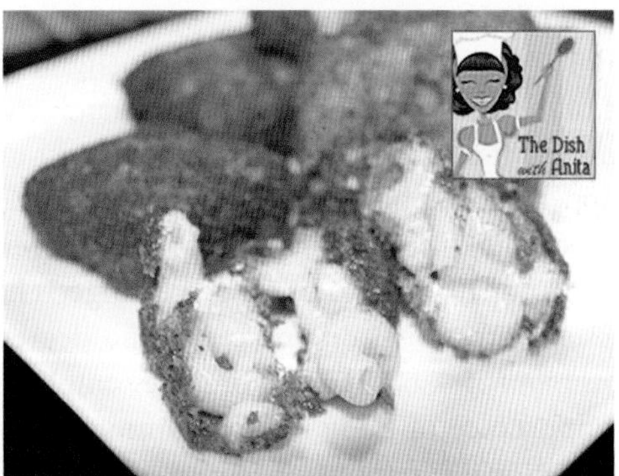

Fig. 6.5C: Bite marks penetrating through the full thickness of softer materials like cheese

Typical Presentation and Composition of Bite Marks

Any discussion on recognition should be preceded by a brief review of the classification of characteristics observed within the injury. Evidence is often compared with tool mark evidence when attempting to show a narrowing of the focus from the big picture (i.e. a patterned injury on skin) to the smallest details discovered (i.e. defect for an individual tooth).

Component Injuries Seen in Bite Marks

Abrasions (scrapes), contusions (bruises), lacerations (tears), ecchymosis, petechiae, avulsion, indentations (depressions), erythema (redness) and **(Figs 6.6A and B)** punctures might be seen in bite marks. Their meaning and strict definitions are found in medical dictionaries and forensic medical texts and should not be altered. An incision is a cut made by a sharp instrument and, although mentioned in the bitemark literature, it is not an appropriate term to describe the lacerations made by incisors.

The term latent injury or wound was preferred over occult or trace wound when referring to an injury which is not visible but can be brought out by special techniques.

A characteristic, as applied to a human bite mark, is a distinguishing feature, trait or pattern within the bite mark and is delineated as a class or an individual characteristic.

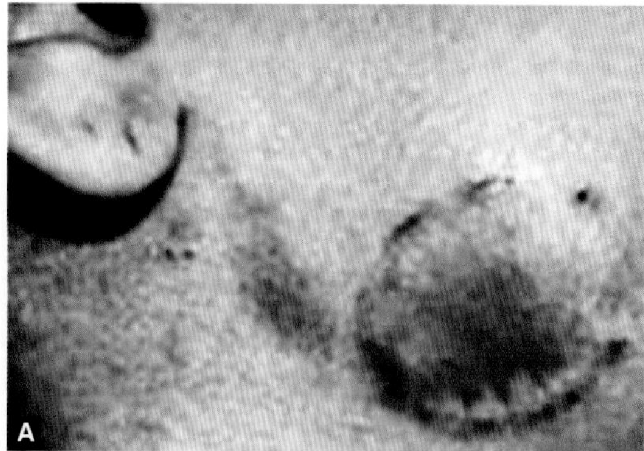

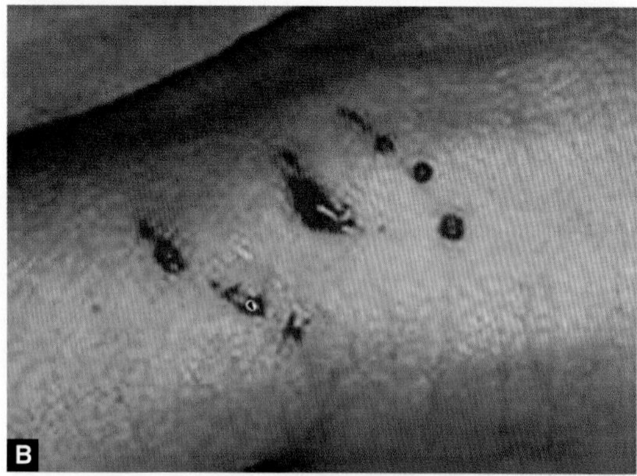

Figs 6.6A and B: Various components in a bite marks, reflecting bleeding, contusions, ecchymosis and lacerations

Characteristics to look for

Class characteristics: A feature, trait or pattern preferentially seen in, or reflective of, a given group. For example, the finding of linear or rectangular contusions at the midline of a bite mark arch is a class characteristic of human incisor teeth. "Incisors" represent the class in this case. The value of identifying class characteristics is that, when seen, they enable us to identify the group from which they originate. For instance, the class characteristics of incisors (rectangles) differentiates them from canines (circles or triangles) **(Fig. 6.7)**. If we define the class characteristics of human bites, we can differentiate them from animal bites. Via class characteristics, we differentiate the adult from the child bite or mandibular from maxillary arch. The original term "class characteristic" was applied to tool marks and its definition has been modified to make it more applicable to bite marks. So these features allow ascertaining whether bite mark produced is formed by:

- An adult vs a child bite
- Maxillary from mandibular arch
- Human vs animal/non-dental

Next is to determine which teeth are present in the pattern, as each tooth has class traits of its own like

- Incisors — rectangular marks,
- Canines — triangular or rectangular,
- Bicuspids often with figure of '8' and
- Molars —spherical or point-shaped.

Individual characteristics: Individual characteristic: a feature, trait or pattern that represents an individual variation rather than an expected finding within a defined group. An example of this is a rotated tooth **(Fig. 6.8)**. The value of individual characteristics is that they differentiate between individuals and help identify the perpetrator. The number, specificity and accurate reproduction of these individual characteristics determine the confidence level that a particular suspect made the bite mark. In a nutshell, these are the deviations from standard class characteristics and may be grouped as underlined.

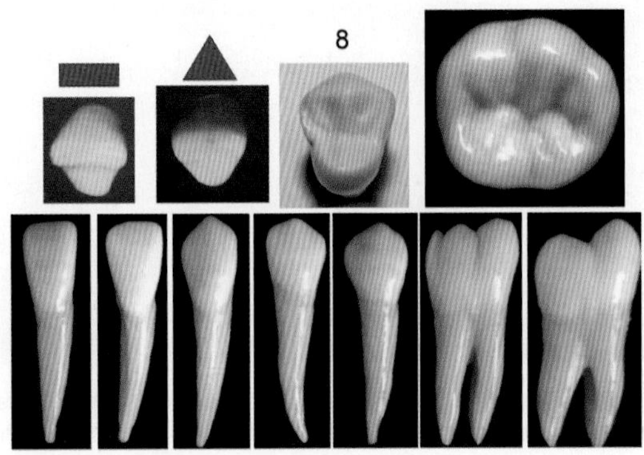

Fig. 6. 7: The class characteristics of the teeth of the occlusal surfaces appearing in bite marks, incisors—square shaped, canine—triangular, and premolars/ molars appearing in fig of eight

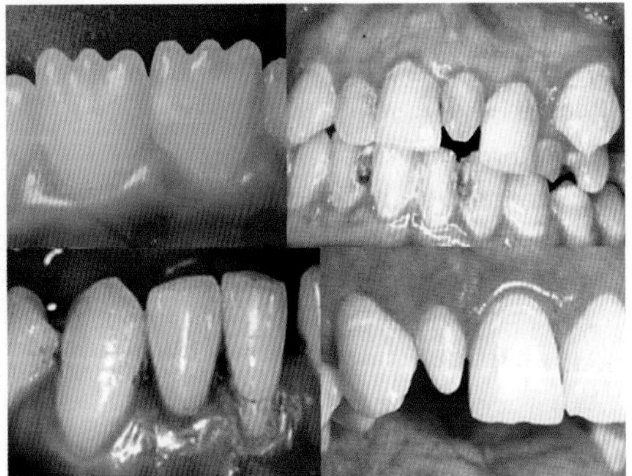

Fig. 6.8: The individual variation of teeth in various humans, like diastema, spacing, crowding, rotated tooth, mammelons etc.

- Anatomical,
- Physiological,
- Iatrogenic,
- Traumatic

For example, dental characteristics such as enamel fractures, rotated tooth, talon cusps or restorations. The principle is similar in someway to the forensic anthropology osteobiography approach to a skeleton, in that an individual's life history or, perhaps more appropriately, medical history is written in their bone.

Location of Bite Marks

Human bite marks are most often found on the skin of victims, and they may be found on almost all parts of the human body. Females are most often bitten on the breasts and legs during sexual attacks, whereas bites on males are commonly seen on the arms and shoulders. In defensive circumstances, as when the arms are held up to ward off an attacker, the arms and hands are often bitten. Following are the most common location of the bite marks in various types of crimes **(Fig. 6. 9)**.

Sexual crimes: Breast, abdomen, nipple, thigh, back and shoulders

Fight and violence: Extremities, any area of body

Animal bites: Exposed skin surfaces, extremities

Self defense: Extremities.

Homosexual activity: Axillary bites and bite patterns on the back, shoulder and genitalia.

Child abuse: Bitten in areas of the face, particularly cheek, ears and nose.

The Classic Appearance

The injury commonly present as circular/elliptic pattern injury, divided into two distinct halves representing both arches. Following the periphery of the arches are a series of individual abrasions, contusions, and/or lacerations reflecting the size, shape, arrangement, and distribution of the class characteristics of the contacting surfaces of the human dentition. Petechiae, punctures, erythema and avulsions may be seen as well, but when present usually are concurrent or superimposed with the bruise or abrasion appearance **(Fig. 6.10)**.

Commonly there is an area of Ecchymosis contained within the defining shape of bite mark either at centre or periphery. This extravascular bleeding is caused by pressure from the teeth as they compress the tissue inward from the perimeter of the mark. Individual arches most frequently are produced by anterior six teeth, but may be by all as well. Occasionally a double bite can be observed. Pattern of clothing or interposing material may be superimposed. Size of pattern must fit within known parameters of human dentition (from pediatric to mixed to adults).

The diameter of the injury typically ranges from 25 to 40 mm. But because of reaction within tissues, shrinkage in deceased victims or putrefactive swelling in others, a reliance on size may give false negative conclusions.

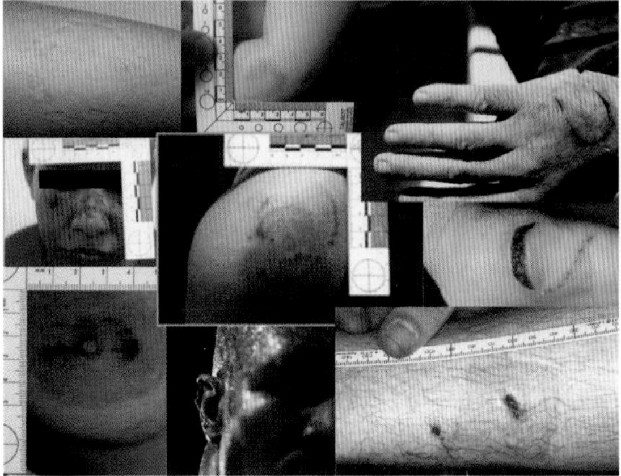

Fig. 6.9: Composite picture showing the various locations of bite marks, which may be on any body surfaces or parts depending on the type of the assaults

Variations of the Prototypical Bite Mark

Variations include additions, subtractions and distortions.

A. *Additional Features*

Central ecchymosis (central contusion) — When found, these are caused by two possible phenomena:

a. Positive pressure from the closing of teeth with disruption of small vessels.
b. Negative pressure caused by suction and tongue thrusting.

Linear abrasions, contusions or striations — These represent marks made by either slipping of teeth against skin or by imprinting of the lingual surfaces of teeth. The term drag marks is in common usage to describe the movement between the teeth and the skin while lingual markings is an appropriate term when the anatomy of the lingual surfaces are identified. Other acceptable descriptive terms include radial or sunburst pattern.

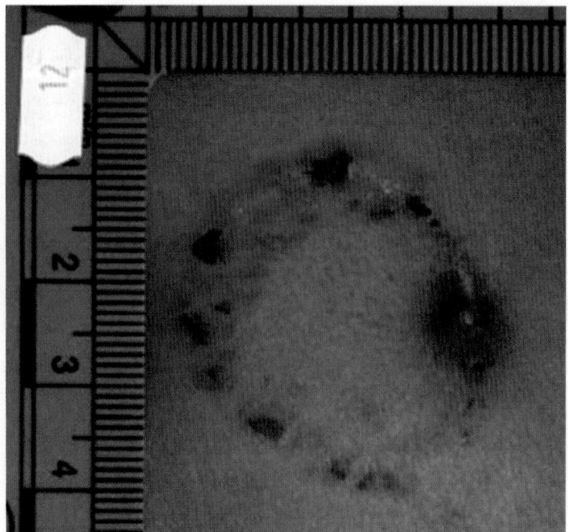

Fig. 6.10: A picture of classic bite on human tissue showing two semicircular arches with various teeth occlusal morphology present

Double bite — A "bite within a bite" occurring when skin slips after an initial contact of the teeth and then the teeth contact again a second time.

B. *Partial Bite marks:* These types of bite marks may be produced by one-arched (half bites) or one to few teeth. Apart from this unilateral (one-sided) marks may also be produced due to incomplete dentition, uneven pressure or skewed bite.

C. *Indistinct/Faded bite marks:* these are formed by fused Arches — collective pressure of teeth leaves arched rings without showing individual tooth marks.
   Solid-ring pattern is not apparent because erythema or contusion fills the entire center leaving a filled, discolored, circular mark.

D. *Superimposed or Multiple bites.*

E. *Avulsive bites.*

Bite Mark Recognition

Recognition is of paramount importance. Many injuries go undiscovered. Victims might fear repercussions that reporting such incidents may bring. It may present in a variety of ways. Although the prototypic or textbook bite mark can be described, it does not exist in real practical sense. No bite mark containing all ideal features that experts might agree on collectively has been demonstrated/published till date. The old adage, "one can not ever have enough evidence" applies to all forensic applications, especially the forensic bite mark analysis.

Aging/Changes Over Time

In 1973, Harvey stated that the external physical appearance of bite marks changed with time. It should be the standard operating procedure for the collection of evidence to continue for as long as it shows change. The healing dynamics of bruising observed has not been studied sufficiently, so poorly understood. Langolis and Gresham concluded that it would seem unlikely that a bruise could be reliably aged upon from appearance alone.

Variables Affecting Appearance of Bruises

1. *Structure and vascularity:* depending upon the area of tissue bitten and its vascularity and anatomy, the appearance of bite marks may differ significantly for example eyes and palms have different vascular dynamics and hence wound dynamics will also be different. Vascular tissue over bone bruises more and where as children and elderly bruise more easily, because of loose delicate skin in former and loss of SC tissue in latter. Also a deep subcutaneous tissue injury may prolong bleeding time.
2. *Metabolic rate:* It is often seen that females bruise more than males, and also obese people do bruise more than leaner people.
3. *Victim's state of health:* Victims of attack if having hypertension, coagulation disorder, or taking medication (Aspirin, Steroids— delay healing) also bleed significantly more than apparent normal healthy counter parts. Sometimes bruise may appear at instant or take as long as 48 hours, related to time required for extravascular blood to reach surface (AM injury may be revealed at PM).
4. *Skin pigmentation:* Affects observation.
5. *Environmental conditions:* Lights, temperature, interpretation.

Ageing/changes over time as determined by color of the bruise after infliction of bite mark injury (Fig. 6.11)

Published findings on color changes in bruises

Time	Camps	Glaister	Poison & Gee	Smith & Fiddes
Hrs 0-24	R	V	R	R
Hrs 24-48	P/			P/
Day 3				
Day 4-5	G			G
Day 5-7		G	G	
Day 7-10	Y		G	Y
Day 8-10		Y		
Day 13-18		Resolution		
Day 14-15	Resolution		Y	Resolution
Up to day 30			Resolution	

Fig. 6.11: The chart showing the various published findings on color changes in injured human tissue as a result of bite marks

Keys to color coding

- R—red,
- P—purple,
- G—green,
- Y—yellow,
- V—violet,
- P/—black

Range of Bite Mark Severity—The Bite mark Severity and Significance Scale (Figs 6.12A to F)

a. Very mild bruising, no individual tooth marks present, diffuse arches visible, may be caused by something other than teeth — *Low forensic significance*
b. Obvious bruising with individual, discrete areas associated with teeth, skin remains intact—*Moderate forensic significance*
c. Very obvious bruising with small lacerations associated with teeth on the most severe aspects of the injury, likely to be assessed as definite bite mark— *High significance*
d. Numerous areas of laceration, with some bruising, some areas of the wound may be incised. Unlikely to be confused with any other injury mechanism— *High forensic significance.*
e. Partial avulsion of tissue, some lacerations present indicating teeth as the probable cause of the injury—*Moderate forensic significance.*
f. Complete avulsion of tissue, possibly some scalloping of the injury margins suggested that teeth may have been responsible for the injury. May not be an obvious bite injury—*Low forensic significance.*

Distortion in Human Bite Marks

The occurrence of distortion in human bite marks is well recognized. A forensic classification of distortion is suggested which is based upon the causative factors and their inter-relationships.

There are several factors that contribute to the character of the bite mark. These include the resiliency of the matter bitten, the degree of pressure applied during the bite, the time lapse between when the bite is produced and the examination, whether the person is living or deceased.

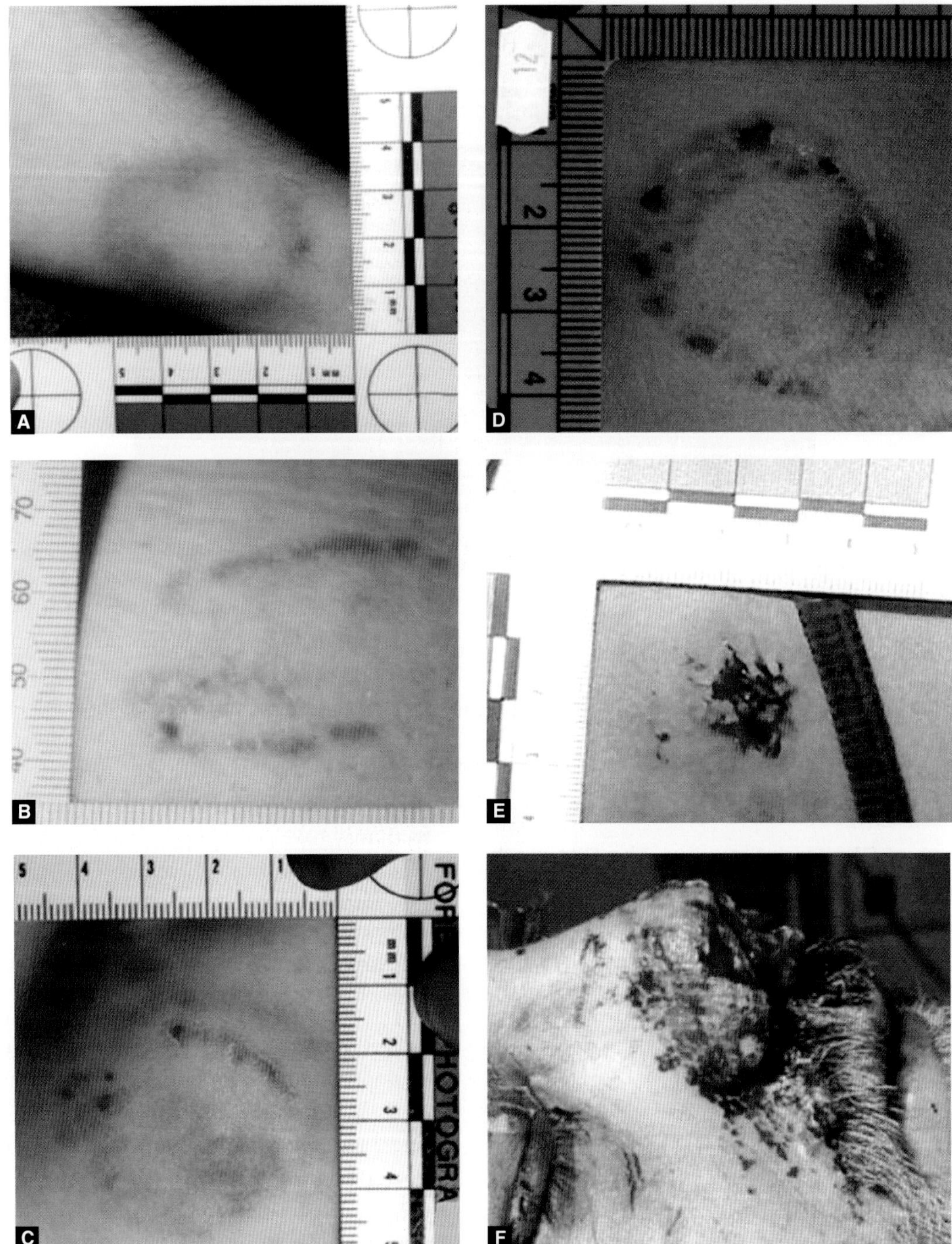

Figs 6.12A to F: The range of severity of bite marks on human tissue on a grade scale of 1 to 6, along with their forensic significance

A recurring difficulty in analysis arises from the distortion, which is a variable feature of bite marks. In the context of a bite mark, distortion may modify the appearance of a bite, or the photo-graphs of a bite, such that it is not an exact mirror image of the features of the mouth of the biter. Distortion may complicate or even preclude proper comparison of the bite mark and the causal dentition.

Distortion can occur at different stages in the causation and the investigation of bite marks. It may occur at the time of biting defined as primary distortion. Distortion may occur subsequent to the bite being made or introduced at the stage when the bite mark is being examined or recorded which is defined as secondary distortion.

Primary Distortion

The two main components of primary distortion are the dynamics of the biting process (dynamic distortion) and the detailed features of the tissue being bitten (tissue distortion). Dynamic and tissue distortion are complex and unpredictable phenomena, which are closely related because of their simultaneous occurrence during the episode of contact between the dentition and the skin. Distortion may be produced by the dynamics of the action of biting **(Fig. 6.13)**. The degree of movement between the teeth and the bitten tissue can range from essentially nil in static bite marks to extreme in tooth scrape marks. Dynamic distortion is proportional to the degree of movement. The dynamic event is composed of multiple component movements by the assailant and/or the victim during the episode of contact between the dentition and the skin. Every episode of contact is a unique event. Accordingly, a dentition can produce bite marks, which exhibit variations in appearance. In cases of multiple bite marks produced by a single dentition in one victim the bite marks vary in appearance due to the unique dynamics of each biting episode.

Skin is an elastic medium capable of distortion due to pressure and reconstituting to its original contour when the pressure is removed. Skin tension, due to elastic fibers in the dermis, varies depending on age and anatomical location. The phenomenon of stretching and relaxing produces a variable degree of tissue distortion in all bite marks. Tissue distortion can also arise due to edema produced in response to biting. The quantity of tissue available for biting is also a contri-butory factor in tissue distortion. When a quantity of tissue is taken into the mouth, this may produce "tenting" of the tissue, which results in dimensional changes in the skin.

Secondary Distortion

There are three categories of secondary distortion. Time-related distortion occurs when a bite changes with time elapsed subsequent to the bite being made. The other two categories of secondary distortion, posture distortion and photographic

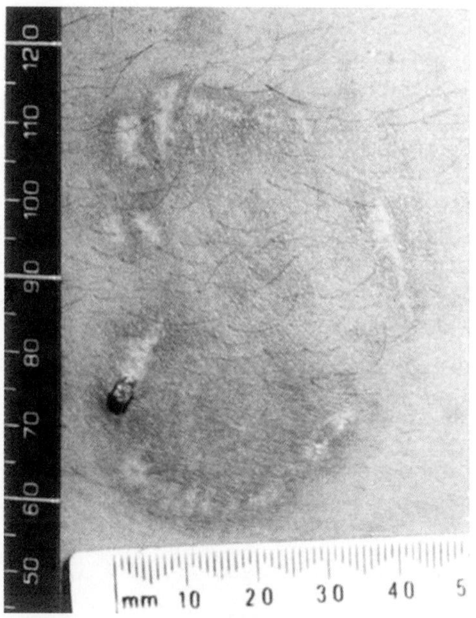

Fig. 6.13: The primary distortion of bite marks (for details see the text)

distortion occur during examination and evidence recording.

Time-related distortion can take different forms. Where there is a laceration or where a segment of tissue has been bitten off, the subsequent healing can involve changes, particularly tissue contraction, which can modify the dimensions and detail of the bite. Bruise changes with time can result in migration of part of the bruise to a slightly different anatomical location. The bruise may also diffuse variably giving an altered shape.

Posture distortion occurs when the bite mark is viewed or recorded in a position, which is different from the position of the tissue at the time of biting **(Figs 6.14A and B)**. The degree of posture distortion depends on the variation in body position and anatomical location. The greater the variation in body positions between the time of biting and evidence recording, the greater the likely degree of posture distortion. Different anatomical locations potentially demonstrate varying degrees of posture distortion. Marked posture distortion can be observed in a limb depending on the degree of flexion and extension and in the female breast depending on the arm position and body position. Posture distortion during photography, is necessary to attempt to reconstruct the victim's body position at the time of biting. Clearly this ideal is not always possible and if not, it is suggested that bite marks are photographed in a range of positional possibilities.

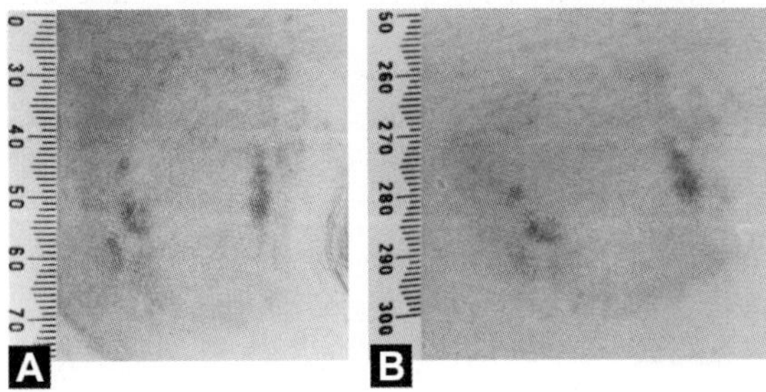

Figs 6.14A and B: The secondary distortion of bite marks (for details see the text)

Reconstruction of the victim's known body position at the time of biting or the reconstruction of a range of positional possibilities is most applicable to the live victim. In cases involving a dead victim, the body position is unknown and the reconstruction of a range of body positions is not so readily achieved. Therefore, the potential occurrence of posture distortion may be more difficult to account for in dead victims.

Distortion may be produced by the photographic method of recording the bite mark. Photographic distortion arises as a result of the influence of the angle of the film to the mark and body curvature. The ideal photographic angle is 90 degree with the camera perpendicular to the center of the bite mark. This angle produces parallelism between the film plane and the bite mark plane and consequently photographic distortion is insignificant. Variation from the perpendicular will produce photographic distortion in proportion to the extent of the variation. In effect, moving the camera to one side or the other of the bite mark creates photographic parallax.

There are four categories of photographic distortion:

Type I distortion

This occurs when the scale and bite mark are on the same plane, but the camera is not parallel to them. This is also called off-angle distortion (perspective distortion). This type of distortion can be corrected digitally.

Type II distortion

If the scale is not on the same plane as the bite mark, rectifying the scale adversely affects the proportions of the injury pattern.

Type III distortion

In some cases, one leg of a two dimensional scale has perspective distortion, but the other leg does not. In this situation, only the non-distorted leg of the scale is used for the rectification and resizes procedures.

Type IV distortion

In type IV distortion, the scale itself may be bent or skewed. There can be forensic value if the scale is relatively flat in the area directly adjacent to the bite mark.

The American Board of Forensic Odontology (ABFO) Bite Mark Guidelines Committee suggested that a circular scale should be included in photographs, to permit accurate calculations of the photographic angle and to allow correction for any distortion caused by improper angulations. If the roundness of the circular scale was re-established in the superimposition process, then the photographic distortion in the bite mark was also corrected. This suggestion resulted in the development of the bite mark standard reference scale — ABFO No. 2. The plane of the scale must be parallel to the bite mark plane and on the same level. For more detailed discussion on phtotgraphy in bite marks cases, readers are advised to see the chapter titled "Dental Records and Forensic Photography".

According to Rawson et al a curved body surface, which allows visualization of the entire bite mark, has a surface angle too small to produce significant photographic distortion. This statement can only be made if the entire bite mark can be visualized from one direction. If the body curvature is so great as to obscure part of the bite mark, then the surface angle is large enough to cause significant photographic distortion and multiple photographs would have to be taken of the various parts of the bite mark.

The degree of distortion present in a bite mark is variable and affects arch size and shape. Clearly, size-matching techniques are only applicable to bite marks exhibiting minimal distortion. The incidences of discrete morphological points of comparison or distinctive features in a bite mark are the most significant criteria in bite mark analysis. This is partly due to their relative immunity to distortion. As the degree of distortion increases, bite mark analysis relies progressively more on distinctive features. The role of superimposition techniques is to ensure that there is sufficient correspondence between the sizes and positions of the teeth of an accused.

All types of distortion complicate the process of matching marks to dentition, thus making it important to understand the distortion.

General Principles Behind Identification of Bite Marks

The scientific basis is rooted in the premises of the individuality of human dentition and belief that no two humans have identical dentitions in regard to size, shape and alignment. Similar to fingerprint and DNA analysis, with one major exception, that they can be expressed quantitatively as a numerical probability based on databases, while individuality of dentition is commonly observed, there is no database to express it quantitatively.

As mentioned earlier, the first person to whom real credit must be given for having published an analysis of a bite mark case is Sorup. The method used he called "odontoscopy," analogous to the fingerprint identification called "dactyloscopy." By this method, plaster casts of the teeth of the suspect are obtained, dried, and varnished, after which the incisal edges and occlusal surfaces are coated with printer's ink. Upon this inked surface a sheet of moistened paper is pressed, and a print is transferred from it to transparent paper. This print is placed over a life-size photograph of the bite mark and compared.

During the process of bite mark analysis, the unique characteristics of a suspected biter's dentition are compared with patterns observed in the bitten skin, two simultaneous and opposite paths develops.

Inclusive path: Strong and consistent linking in tooth by tooth and arch by arch comparison between suspect and the victim.

Exclusive path: Suspected biter's dentition show no linking with the patterns recorded.

Various author's experience suggests that exclusionary pathway is accomplished more frequently and easily.

Human skin is not fixed and rigid; one must acknowledge that the dynamics of biting process together with the location of bite on the body affects the pattern of resulting injury and its usefulness in the process. Also skin is not a good impression medium and that the skin distortion occurs at the movement bitten, investigator should be mindful about the level of distortion.

It has been suggested by the experts that the forensic dentist charged with collection of bite mark evidence should not be the same dentist that makes the impression of the suspected biter. Stone dental models should be referred to using letters or numbers instead of names. If dentists are aware of the various methods to collect and preserve bite mark evidence from victims and suspects it may be possible for them to assist the justice system to identify and prosecute violent offenders. Conclusions can be reached about any role a suspect may have played in a crime. It is important not to inflate its value in attempting to increase its significance to the trier of the fact.

ABFO's Recommended Procedure and Guidelines: Bite Mark Analysis Guidelines

The following chain and custody of events reflects the opinion and procedures to be followed in a manner whenever a dentist/forensic odontologist is called upon for an investigation of the case involving bite marks. It should consist of three major steps:

1. Evidence collection from the bite victim, first consisting of:
   - First aid
   - Preliminary examination and documentation
   - Photographs
   - Saliva swabs
   - Impression
   - Excision of bite mark in deceased victim.
2. Evidence collection from the bite suspect
   - Clinical examination
   - Photographs
   - Impressions
   - Bite-sample.
3. Bite mark analysis and scoring.

Evidence Collection from the Bite Victim

In private general practice we do not often have the opportunity to deal for collecting evidence from bite victims. It is the detectives at the scene of the crime, pathologists at autopsy or medical personnel who find most bites. But since physical and biological evidence from a bite mark begins to deteriorate soon after the bite is inflicted, all dentists should be familiar with the general principles of evidence collection. This is especially true for dentists that deal with patient populations that may potentially contain victims of domestic violence, in which bites are often discovered. Practitioners should make every effort to accurately and precisely preserve the evidence as soon as it is discovered using the following techniques, and not wait until others with more experience can be consulted or summoned. The best or only opportunity to collect the evidence may be when it is first presented and observed. If a dentist finds a patterned injury that is suspected to be a bite mark, it should be reported to the police or social welfare agency with local jurisdiction. Then, the dentist should complete the following list of procedures to properly collect the evidence:

a. The first aid

The best or only opportunity to collect the evidence may be when it is first presented and observed. Prompt medical attention should be provided for the living victim since human bites have a higher potential for infection (HIV, Hepatitis –B), than animal bites (rabies). Injuries that disrupt the integrity of the skin's surface should be treated as soon as possible. If suspected, it should be reported to the police or social welfare agency. Then, the dentist should complete the following list of procedures to properly collect the evidence.

b. Preliminary examination and documentation: The dentist should record and describe:

Identification data
Case number, agency, name of examiner(s)
Location of bite mark
Anatomical location or object bitten
Surface contour (e.g. flat, curved or irregular)
Tissue characteristics (elasticity, vascularity)
Shape, color, and size of the injury
Type of injury, e.g. cuts, bruises, abrasion, contusion, avulsion
Other Information as indicated.

Along with above said features dentist should also determine that can the difference between marks from the upper and lower teeth be made. Three-dimensional characteristics, and any other unusual conditions found should also be described. Vertical and horizontal dimensions of the bite mark should be noted, preferably in the metric system.

Bite marks with high evidentiary value that can be used in comparisons with the suspect's teeth will include marks from specific teeth that accurately record distinct traits. It is possible to identify specific types of teeth by their class characteristics. For example, incisors produce rectangular injuries and canines produce triangular injuries. But it is necessary to have individual characteristics recorded in the bite mark to be able to identify positively the perpetrator. Use, misuse and abuse of the teeth result in unique features that are referred to as accidental or individual traits. Such characteristics include fractures, rotations, attritional wear, congenital malformations, etc. When these are recorded in the injury it may be possible to compare them to identify the specific teeth (person) that caused the injury. If these individual characteristics are not present in the teeth, or if they are not recorded well in the injury, the overall forensic significance of the bite mark is reduced.

It is very important during initial examination of the injury to be certain that an artefact, such as an ECG electrode applied by emergency medical personnel, did not cause the pattern or that some object other than teeth has caused a circular or elliptical injury. Some authors have witnessed burns from the end of a hair curling iron **(Fig. 6.15)** and patterns from the end of a lead pipe that closely resembled bite marks. These could be differentiated by the absence of class characteristics caused by human teeth in each case.

The injuries caused by teeth can range from bruises to scrapes and cuts or lacerations. Certainly, it is possible for enough force to be generated to allow penetration of the biting edges of the teeth into the deep layers of the skin. If much time elapses from the moment of injury to the time of discovery, the diffuse nature of bruises and the changes associated with injuries over a period of time may further diminish the evidentiary value. This is especially true in the case of living bite victims but also in deceased individuals.

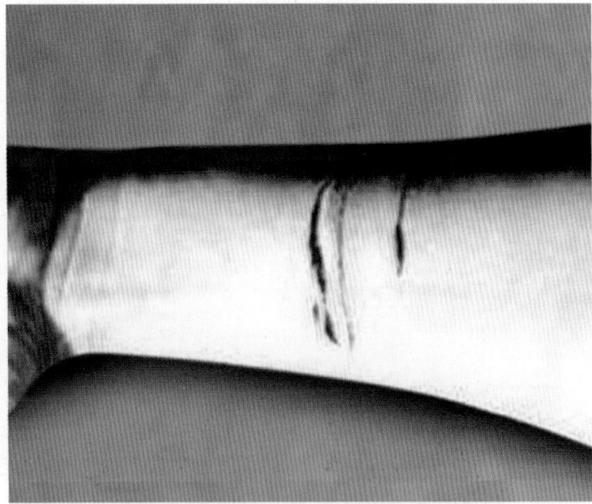

Fig. 6.15: The artifactual marks left on the fore arm by a hair curling iron rod

c. Photographic documentation of the bite site: Guidelines of the ABFO Digital Enhancement Committee

The bite site should be photographed using conventional photography and following the guidelines as described in the ABFO Bite mark Analysis Guidelines. The actual photographic procedures should be performed by the forensic dentist or under the odontologist's direction to insure accurate and complete documentation of the bite site.

Using 35 mm film, start with general orientation and move on to close-up photographs using an intraoral camera with a macro lens and take both color and black-and-white photos, as color may block eyes to see subtle changes that may be seen in black and white. Take extensive orientation and close-up photographs **(Figs 6.16A to E)**. Color or specialty filters may be used to record the bite site in addition to unfiltered photographs. Alternative methods of illumination may be used. Video/digital imaging may be used in addition to conventional photography. A tripod, focusing rail, bellows or other devices may be utilized.

The ABFO no. 2 **(Fig. 6.17)** reference ruler is recommended in bite mark photography. The placement of the scale should follow the guidelines as established in the ABFO Bite mark Analysis Guidelines. Be certain that the camera is positioned directly over the injury site. The long axis of the lens should be perpendicular to the bitten skin to reduce perspective distortion in the photographs.

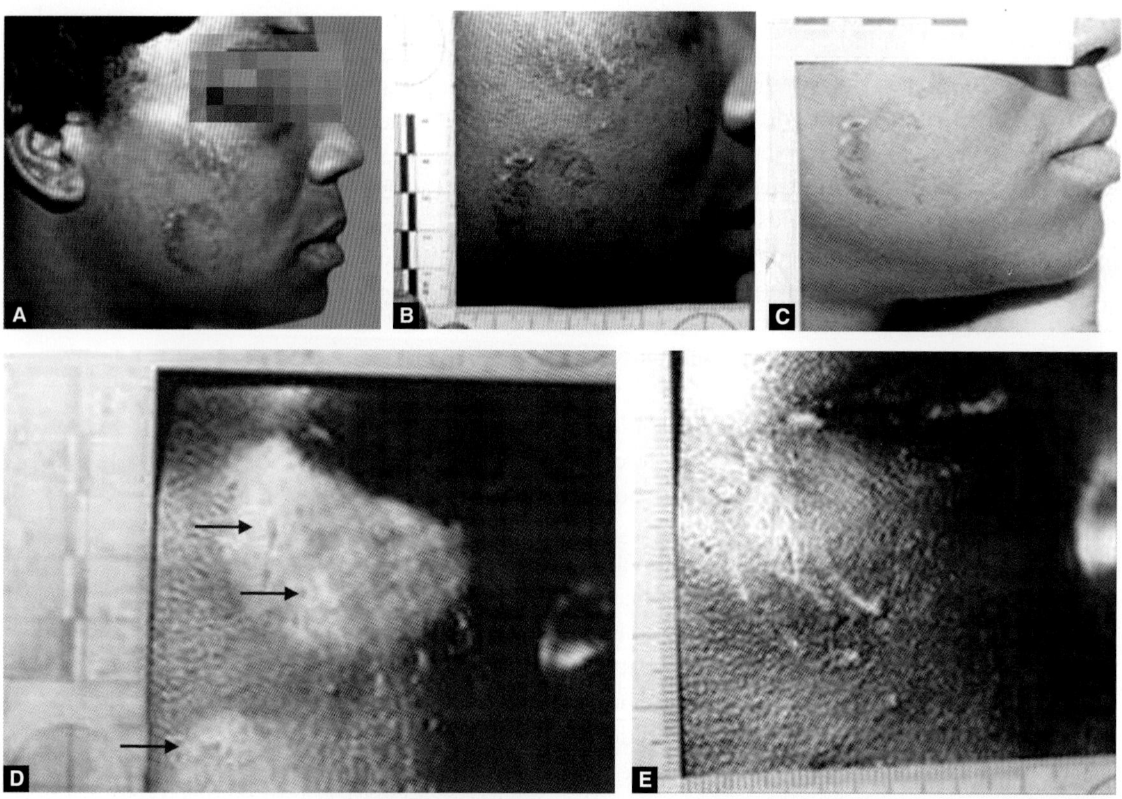

Fig. 6.16A to E: The ABFO recommended pictures of a bite mark victim, including his orientation; close up, black and white, color and special photographs

With living victims, serial pictures are taken over several days for documentation of healing of the wound. For more details readers are advised to please go through the chapter devoted to forensic photography for better understanding of the subject.

Lighting

Off angle lighting using a point flash is the most common form of lighting and should be utilized whenever possible. A light source perpendicular to the bite site can be utilized in addition to off angle lighting; however, care should be taken to prevent light reflection from obliterating mark details in photograph due to "wash out" due to light reflection. A light source parallel to the bite site can be utilized in addition to off angle lighting. A ring flash, natural light and/or overhead diffuse lighting can be utilized to off angle lighting.

Special photographs: Generally visible light photography is used in practice with slowest film of speed < 100 (ASA speed< 100), because of high grain density and sharper details even at enlargement.

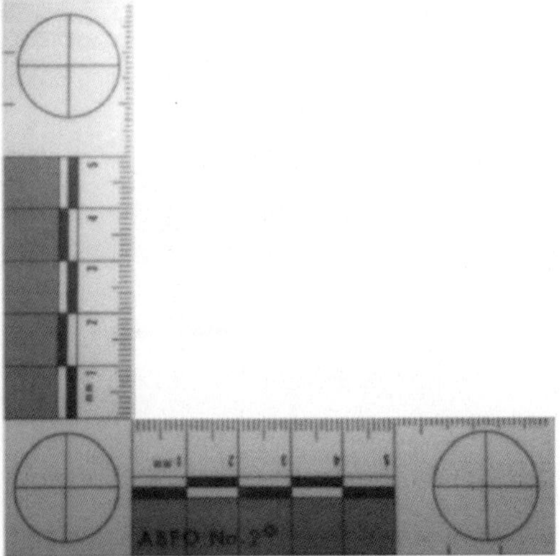

Fig. 6.17: The ABFO Scale No. 2, to be used for measurement of a bite mark size

Digital photography is used only as an adjunctive, as their legal admissibility is doubtful and limited. In certain cases of extensive tissue damage special photographs are used in order to reveal deep wound patterns and detailed surface topography of the wound.

Non-visible light photography: UV light: Do not penetrate deep in skin and is reflected back as a highly detailed surface image of skin, containing additional data about teeth

Infra red: Does penetrate skin for a few mm. with this, it is possible to create an image of injury as it appears below the surface of skin. Infra red photography captures bleeding pattern below skin.

d. Saliva swabs

Saliva will have been deposited on the skin during biting or sucking and this should be collected and analyzed, the aim being solely the collection of cells for DNA. Swabs should be taken as soon as possible after the bite is inflicted and before the area is cleaned or washed. If it can be determined that the bite was inflicted through clothing, attempts should be made to seize the clothing for DNA analysis. The following technique will maximize the amount of DNA recovered.

Double swab method

First, a cotton swab moistened with distilled water is employed to wash the surface that was contacted by the tongue and lips using light pressure and circular motions to wash the dried saliva from the surface over a period of 7 to 10 seconds. Then, a second swab that is dry is used to collect the remaining moisture that is left on the skin by the first swab. Both swabs are thoroughly air-dried at room temperature for at least 45 minutes before they are released to police authorities for testing.

The two swabs must be kept cool and dry to reduce the degradation of salivary DNA evidence and the growth of bacteria that may contaminate the samples and reduce their forensic value. Then they should be submitted to the laboratory as soon as possible for analysis. If the time until submission is protracted, it is recommended that the swabs be stored in a paper evidence envelope or box that will allow air to continue to circulate around the swab tips. (The swabs should not be sealed in plastic bags or plastic containers). They are kept at room temperature if submitted within 4 to 6 hours, or refrigerated (not frozen) if stored longer than six hours.

A DNA sample must also be collected from the victim at this time to provide the opportunity for comparison with the sample from the bite mark. This sample could consist of a buccal swab or a sample of whole blood. The victim's DNA profile will enable analysis of any mixtures that are found in the sample from the bite, which may involve contributions from the depositor and the victim.

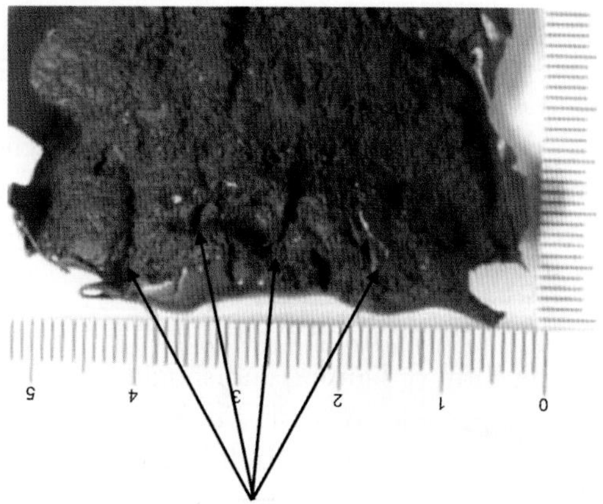

Fig. 6.18A: A sequence depicting the of recording of registering a bite mark case Impression of a bite mark of the culprit

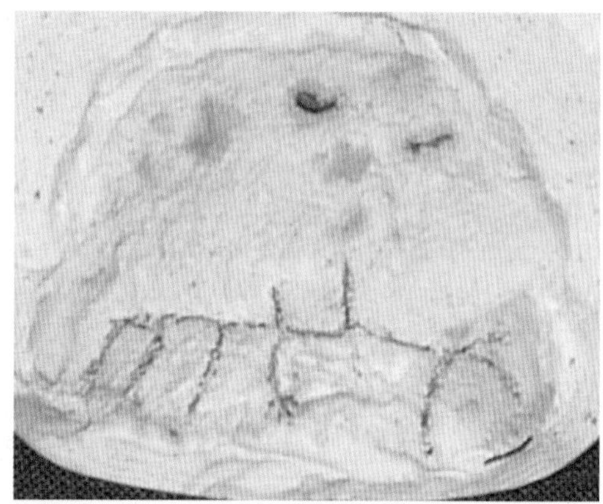

Fig. 6.18B: Pouring of master cast and looking for the details recorded

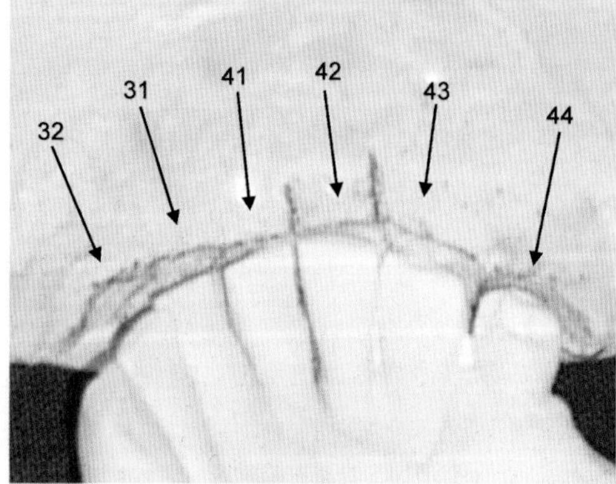

Fig. 6.18C: Comparison of cast of the suspect with the indentation marks left on the victim

e. Impression

Indicated when indentations, depth or a 3-D quality could be seen in injury. Fabricate an accurate impression **(Figs 6.18A to C)** of the bitten surface to record any irregularities produced by the teeth, such as cuts, abrasions, etc. Use Vinyl polysiloxane, Polyether or other impression material available in the dental office that is recommended for fixed prosthetic applications. Dental acrylic or plaster can be used as a rigid support for the impression material; this will allow the impression to accurately record the curvature of the skin. Make two casts always, one working and another virgin. When a self-inflicted bite is possible, impressions of the individual's teeth should be made.

f. Tissue Samples: Excising bite area

In the deceased, tissue specimens of the bite mark should be retained whenever possible. The skin and underlying muscle and adipose tissue with one inch margins is removed for trans-illumination analysis **(Fig. 6.19)**. Most of the authors dealing with examination of bite marks in human corpses have called attention to the possibility of shrinkage by rigor mortis and the considerable shrinkage (nearly two-thirds) after the tissue with the bite marks has been cut out.

This shrinkage takes place in spite of immediate fixing of the skin flap in five percent formalin. Before excision, an acrylic support ring should be secured to the tissue sample to prevent tissue shrinkage. Excised tissue can be transilluminated by a shining light from dermal/inner side, it may illustrates fine bleeding patterns.

Buhtz and Erhardt, therefore, have recommended that not only the skin flap but the whole area with the underlying tissue should be cut out. In the case of a bite mark left in the breast of a female, the whole breast is to be removed. In the case of a bite mark left in an arm or a leg of a corpse, it is not sufficient to remove the actual tissue area to the bone; instead, one must transect the arm or leg and include a broad margin on both sides of the bite mark.

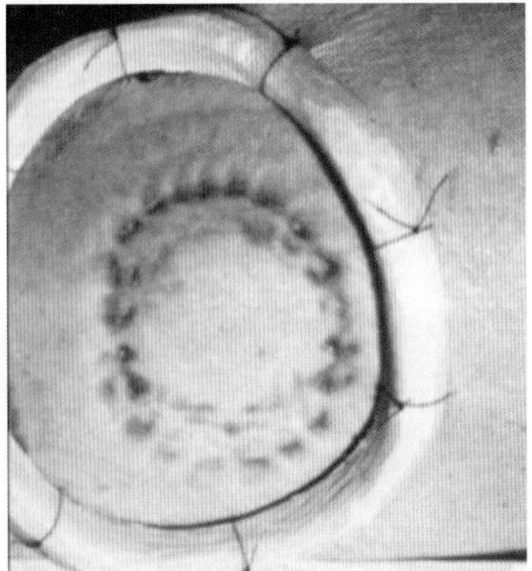

Fig. 6.19: An excised bite mark from a dead person in order to preserve the bitten tissue and in order to perform the test of trans illumination. Note the acrylic ring tighten all around the excised tissue

Evidence Collection from the Bite Suspect

Evidence collection from the bite suspect: As said earlier this chain of events must include clinical examination, photographs, impressions and bite sample. The collection of dental exhibits for forensic uses has been deemed to be an invasive procedure. Thus, dental impressions and bite samples that are seized from a suspect are susceptible to strict rules of evidence. Another dentist should always perform these events to eliminate any arising bias. A search warrant, court order or legal consent may be required before evidence is collected form the suspect. So they must be obtained either using a court order (warrant) or with a signed and witnessed informed consent. Generally, suspects are usually quite cooperative during the collection of physical exhibits. However, this is not always the case and most commonly, the suspect is in custody and the dental examination takes place away from the practitioner's dental office, perhaps in a jail or remand facility. So the dentist who is requested to assist authorities to collect evidence should see that provisions to ensure their personal security are in place.

North American Courts have ruled that collection of this type of evidence does not violate the individual's rights against self-incrimination because he is not being required to testify against himself, only to provide physical evidence that will be used in a comparison. If the suspect refuses to provide exhibits for comparison purposes, he may be held in contempt until he complies. The Court might issue an order in this instance to authorize the use of force to obtain the exhibits. In the United Kingdom, court orders are not available to collect evidence by force. A jury is left to develop their own conclusions if the suspect refuses to submit to dental evidence collection procedures. The following exhibits and items of physical evidence are recovered during examination of the bite mark suspect.

a. Clinical examination

The extraoral and intraoral structures are examined and significant findings are noted on a dental chart. Special attention is focused on the status of the general dental health, occlusion and mandibular articulation. Results of a specific examination of such things as:

- Maximum mouth opening
- Tooth mobility,
- Periodontal pocketing,
- Dental charting of restorations,
- Diastema, fractures, caries and
- Function of masticatory muscles are documented

b. Photographs

Full facial and profile photographs are produced in addition to intra-oral exposures to depict the upper and lower dental arches and frontal and lateral views of the teeth in occlusion **(Fig. 6.20)**. A reference scale to enable measurements to be taken from the photographs should be included in the same plane as the teeth.

c. Impressions

It is necessary to produce extremely accurate study casts of the teeth that record all of the physical traits and characteristics of the dentition. Accurate dental impression materials, such as vinyl polysiloxane or polyether should be used, although custom special trays are seldom fabricated for the suspect. It is recommended that two sets of study casts be produced using a hard stone, such as dental die stone. All of the materials, including the trays, impressions and casts are maintained in secure storage for eventual release to police authorities. The specific instructions for product handling and material mixing that are recommended by the manufacturer must be closely followed. Buccal swabs from the suspect's oral cavity is also taken.

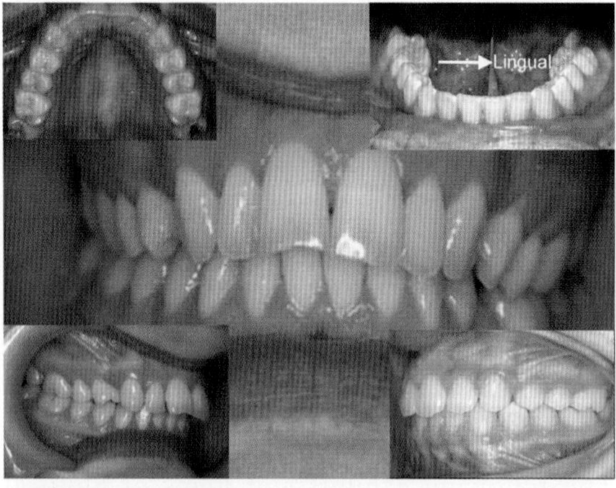

Fig. 6.20: A composite highlighting the various photographs of the suspect to be taken during the course of investigation, viz. maxillary, mandibular arches separately, and in occlusion with frontal and lateral views

d. Bite sample

Collect test bites from all suspects including victim, if bite mark occurred in an area of body where victim could have bitten himself. Aluwax, base plate wax, Styrofoam may be used **(Fig. 6. 21)**. In case of avulsive injury, use thicker textured material like partially set impression material. It can also be taken from stone model's of biter's teeth. This exhibit should be photographed immediately after it is recorded. This will provide an opportunity for future comparison of the photograph and the exhibit to verify that no distortion has occurred. The suspect should be held in custody until the quality and accuracy of all of the exhibits is determined to be satisfactory.

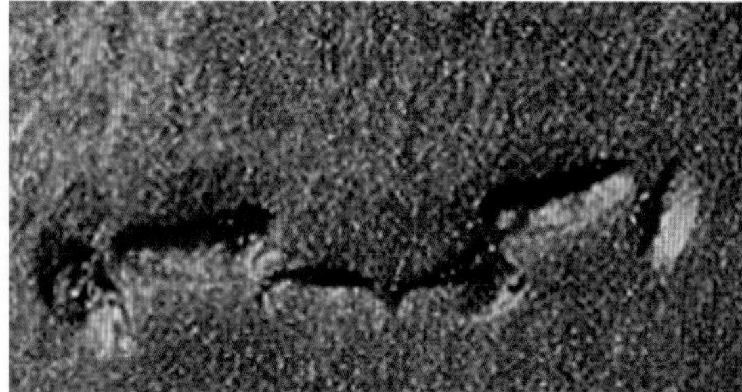

Fig. 6.21: A typical bite mark left on the styrofoam of the suspect. Styrofoam is commonly used for registration of the bite sample

Bite Mark Analysis and Scoring

An essential component of the determination of the validity of bite mark analysis is that the techniques used in the physical comparison between suspect dentition and physical injury have been assessed and found valid. One of the fundamental problems with this task is the wide variety of techniques that have been described in the literature. Techniques using confocal, reflex and scanning electron microscopes, complex computer systems, typing of oral bacteria, special light sources, fingerprint dusting powder and overlays have all been reported. It is a widely held belief that while methods that are more esoteric exist, the dominant technique for comparison of exemplars is transparent overlays.

The lack of direction from the forensic dental organizations, both European and American, complicates this matter. The American Board of Forensic Odontology (ABFO) has reported advice and guidance on many aspects of bite marks and yet one of the most pivotal questions, i.e. what is the best comparison technique to use, has not been addressed.

Transparent overlays utilize materials found in any dental office. The vast majority of forensic dentists use techniques that utilize materials that are inexpensive and easily obtainable, hence the popularity of overlays **(Figs 6.22A and B).** There are numerous techniques for the fabrication of transparent overlays. Of all the techniques, an examination of case reports and experiments reveals that the xerographic and radiographic techniques are the most popular.

The computer technique **(Fig. 6.23)** represents the most accurate fabrication method with respect to representation of rotation and area of the biting edge. Various authors have concluded that the fabrication methods that utilized the subjective process of hand tracing should not be used in favour of techniques that are more objective. The use of computer-generated techniques was advised over any other method.

Dr Rawson, a forensic dentist, two dental students, and a statistician wrote arguably the most cited and well-known bite mark paper describing an empirical experiment. In an attempt to prove finally the uniqueness of the anterior segment of human teeth, Rawson examined 397 bites and applied a statistical probability theory to the results.

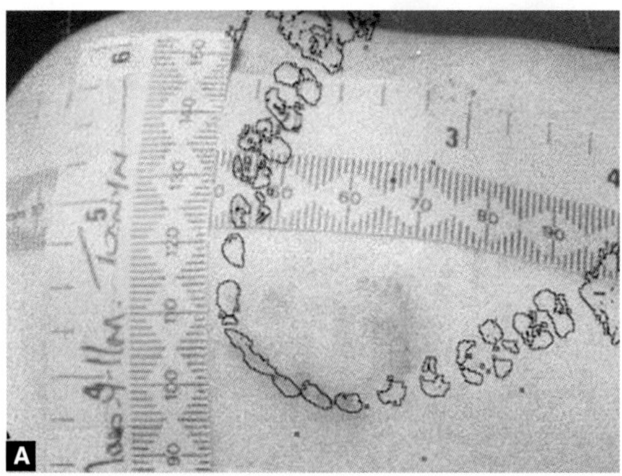

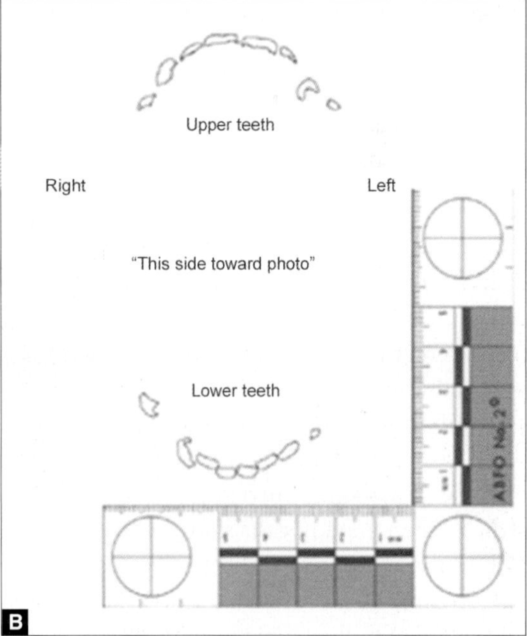

Figs 6.22A and B: The overlay technique for transferring the indented bite marks from the victim or from the cast of the suspect and its subsequent comparison with those of actual left bite marks

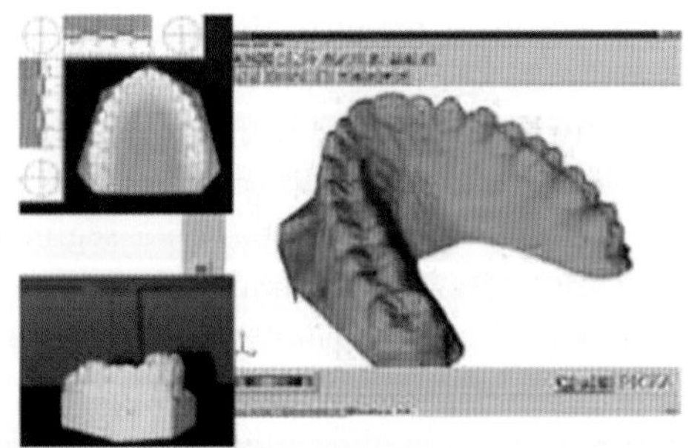

Fig. 6.23: The more sophisticated technique of using computers in case of bite mark cases

Using this premise, the article then stated that the probability of finding two sets of dentition with all six teeth in the same position was 1.4×10^{13}. With an assumed world population of 4 billion (4×10^9) Rawson stated that a match at five teeth on a bite mark would be sufficient evidence to positively identify an individual as the biter to the exclusion of all others.

Forensic Physical Comparison of Exhibits

It is simply the comparison of bite evidence to the suspect evidence to determine if a correlation exists. The most common methods to determine if the suspect's teeth caused the bite mark include techniques to compare the pattern of the teeth (shape, size, position of teeth, individually and collectively) with similar traits and characteristics present in life-sized photographs of the injury using transparent overlays. These overlays have been produced using various techniques.

The most accurate technique has been found to be a method using a computer. Other comparison methods include the direct comparison of the suspect's study casts with photographs of the bite mark, comparison of test bites produced from the suspect's teeth with the actual bite mark, and the use of radiographic imaging and scanning electron microscopy. A 1994 survey of Diplomates of the American Board of Forensic Odontology indicated that they presently use the following analytic methods in the comparison of Bite mark evidence.

The purpose of bite mark analysis is to compare the bite evidence with the suspect evidence and to determine if correlation exists. Analysis usually involves visualization and comparison, formation of an opinion and often court testimony.

The responsibility of comparing the photographs of the bite pattern injury with the dentition of the suspect rests with the forensic dentist.

The foundation of bite mark analysis lies in the following premises:

1. Each individual's dentition is presumed to be unique.
2. This presumed uniqueness is accurately recorded in the characteristics of the injury on the skin or object. Consequently, bite mark evidence has become legally accepted and admissible in courts of law.
3. Numerous cases have involved bite mark evidence in criminal proceedings
4. Criticism of bite mark evidence as a reliable scientific tool has been expressed due to the subjective nature of comparative analysis.

The dynamics of biting make analysis of the bite mark and its comparison to the suspect's teeth challenging. In addition to jaw movements, one needs to consider movement on part of the victim, the flexibility of the bitten tissue, as well as distortion introduced during photography. Bearing this in mind, one may proceed with the analysis. It is important to consider uncommon characteristics of the bite mark such as presence or absence of a particular tooth, mesiodistal dimension, rotation, fracture, diastema, and other unusual features of the teeth as these may help in implicating a suspect.

Ideally, bite mark analysis should begin with a qualitative and quantitative analysis in situ. This should be followed by the analysis of life sized or enlarged photographs. Models and impressions of bite marks add to the evaluation. A separate qualitative and quantitative analysis of the models and occlusal registrations from the suspect's dentition should be performed at this stage; only after these steps should one proceed towards comparison, as it avoids bias.

The protocol for bite mark comparison is made up of two broad categories:

i. The measurement of specific features of the bite mark and suspect's dentition, called "metric analysis"

ii. Matching the pattern of injury to the configuration of teeth on the suspect's dental cast, called "pattern association".

Metric Analysis

The following features captured in the bite mark should be measured and recorded:

- The length, width, and depth of the tooth
- Overall size of the mark
- Intercanine distance
- Spacing between tooth marks
- Rotation from normal arch form

A similar procedure is employed with the suspect's casts. The measurements thus obtained are compared to one another. Simple instruments such as a vernier caliper may be used for obtaining the measurements. More recently, computer based analysis such as Adobe Photoshop has also been used. Metric analysis however, should not be used alone, but rather in conjunction with pattern association.

Pattern Association

Pattern association involves direct methods and indirect methods of comparison. Direct method is where the suspect's models are placed directly over the photograph of the bite mark or the bite mark itself, i.e. in situ. Bite registrations obtained from the suspect may also be compared with the actual bite mark.

Indirect method uses the following:

1. Superimposing transparent overlays of the suspect's bite edges and the bite mark photograph
2. Computer software programmes such as Adobe Photoshop
3. CAT scans.

The newer trends are moving towards the use of computer software programs suggested by Johansen and Bowers. A 3-D/CAD supported photogrammetry approach developed by Thali and coworkers holds promise for the future.

Based upon the 3D detailed representation of the cast with the 3D topographic characteristics of the teeth, the interaction with the 3D documented skin can be visualized and analyzed on the computer screen. It is possible to demonstrate the progression of the biting action and the development of the subsequent injury pattern.

Bite mark identification is based on the individuality of a dentition, which is used to match a bite mark to a suspected perpetrator. This matching is based on a tooth-by-tooth and arch-to-arch comparison utilizing parameters of size, shape and alignment. The most common method used to analyze bite mark is carried out in 2D space. That means that the 3D information is preserved only two dimensionally with distortions.

Biological Techniques for Bite Mark Comparisons

The biological basis of bite mark analysis has centered on the recovery of salivary DNA and Sweet has pioneered much of this work. While such techniques offer an objective, scientifically validated method of bite mark, analysis by the systems employed are expensive and require extensive laboratory equipment and expertise.

A new technique that has attracted attention is the genotyping of oral bacteria, mostly oral streptococci. With over 2000 species in an individual's mouth it is possible to develop a bacterial 'fingerprint' due to the diversity of such populations.

Comparison Techniques

Bite mark comparison protocols include measurement and analysis of the pattern, size and shape of teeth against similar characteristics observed in an injury on skin or a mark on an object.

The comparison involves not only the use of superimposition techniques but also, more importantly; the collection of all the evidence, including the physical features as well as the dynamics of the bite and the compatibility of the features with the suspect's teeth.

Whatever the techniques used the odontologist must have confidence in the findings and be prepared to demonstrate them clearly and simply to the jury in the courtroom.

The comparison techniques have been divided into two categories life size and assisted comparisons. Comparisons are made between life-size 1:1 photographs and a variety of tracings and overlays or reproduction of the biting surfaces of the suspect's teeth. Assisted comparisons involve the use of microscopes of varying types, electronic, histological, radiographic and specialized techniques including the use of experimental bite marks.

Life-size Comparisons

Life-size comparison is the most common type undertaken by the odontologist using the life-size 1:1 photographs with the models of the teeth.

Direct method

The models are placed directly over the photographs and the concordant points demonstrated, e.g. the fit of the incisal edges (**Fig. 6.24**). It is worth remembering that the comparison is of a three-dimensional model with a two-dimensional photograph. An advantage of this method is that the model can be moved to illustrate the dynamics of the bite by showing slippage and scraping.

West and Friar used direct model-to-victim comparisons to demonstrate marks caused by slippage of the teeth, by placing the model directly over the breast of a deceased victim and dragging the model across the skin to demonstrate how the marks were produced in vivo. The entire procedure was photographed, videotaped and produced as evidence.

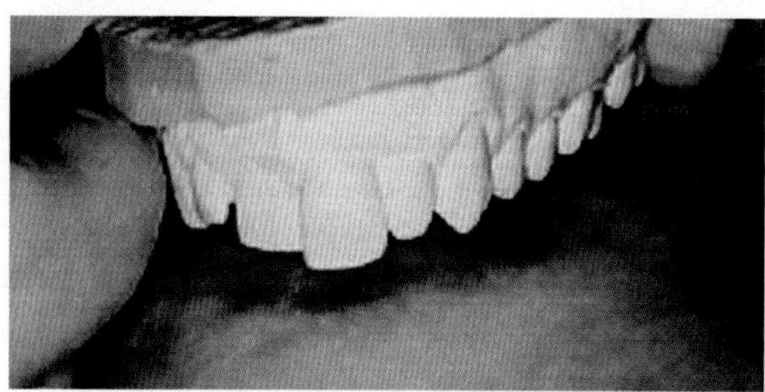

Fig. 6.24: Picture showing the comparison of the cast of the suspect to those of photograph of actual bite marks left on the victim

Furness described a method similar to that used by fingerprint officers, where lines are used linking various points of correspondence between the models and the teeth. The advantage of this technique is that fine detail such as cervical margin indentations can be seen and compared.

The disadvantage is that the technique cannot be used on grossly distorted marks, as the lines will not tally and could require lengthy court explanations.

Indirect methods

Indirect comparison is made using transparent overlays on which the biting surfaces of the teeth are recorded; these are then placed directly over the marks on the photograph. This method was first used by Sorup in 1924 and cited by Strom. The most common methods used to compare a suspected biter's dentition with a bite mark injury involve some form of overlay technique. Morgen used photographs of the models to produce overlays. The photographic production of overlays by various methods is the most reliable way of producing true reproduction of the dentition.

Camerson and Sims in 1974 described a method of using a closely adapted acetate film on the model and tracing the biting surfaces of the teeth on it.

The use of photographic tracings can be enhanced by using oblique lighting on the model to highlight specific features.

Other methods such as pressing the teeth into wax and photographing the indentations can produce accurate overlays. The indentations can be enhanced if sprinkled with radiopaque powder and radio graphed.

Overlays of the chewing surfaces of teeth can be obtained by:

1. Tracing these surfaces on a sheet of transparent acetate.
2. A glass of photocopier machine and duplicating on transparencies or special paper
3. Utilizing the computer, scanner, Adobe Photoshop
4. Radiographic technique using metal fillings painted into test bite indentations created in plaster or wax wafers
5. Inking the incisal edges of anterior teeth on stone models of suspect's teeth and imprinting the inked edges on various materials.

Use of hand tracings has been discontinued largely in favor of less subjective methods.

Overlays created using a computer; scanner and Adobe Photoshop were found to be more accurate and less subjective **(Fig. 6.25).** Computer-based technique for the production of life sized bite mark comparison overlays allows accurate and objective selection of the biting surfaces of a suspect's teeth from dental study casts. Images of the teeth of interest can then be exported to transparent acetate film. Comparison overlays produced by this method are referred to as hollow volume overlays since they record the perimeter of each tooth's biting edge, leaving the inner aspect of the tooth blank.

In a study of comparison between five commonly used methods of overlay production (computer based method, hand-traced from stone casts, hand traced from wax impressions, xerographic method and radiopaque impression method) from dental casts, it was found that the computer based method was the most accurate followed by xerographic method. The radiopaque impression method was found to be the least accurate followed by the hand tracing from the dental casts.

Farrell et al used computerized axial tomography scanning to produce overlays of the dentition at varying depths, so that the teeth not involved initially in the bite were shown at the precise depth at which they began to be involved in the mark. Despite this overabundance of methods a recent survey of 72 odontologists found that over 90 percent used some form of overlay as their sole method of pattern analysis.

Assisted Comparisons

This approach to the comparison of bite mark and dentition encompasses simple procedures such as measurements of inter-canine distances as well as complex electronic methods. These can be used where the mark is either distorted or not clearly defined. Jacobsen and Keiser-Nielsen point out that any measurements taken should be from within the arch and not between the arches. If overlay method fails to produce a clear result then other methods may be tried. It should be noted that these methods

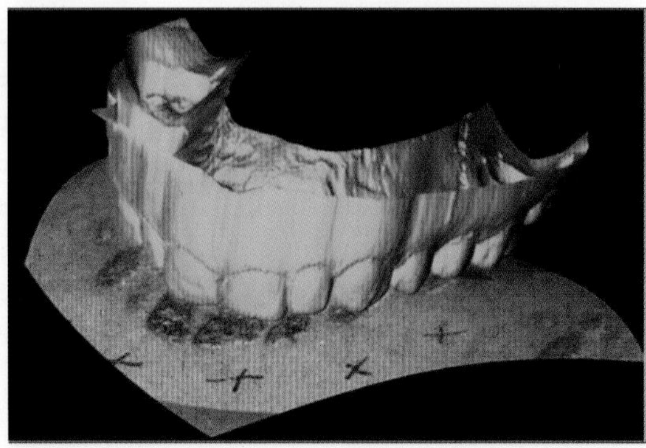

Fig. 6.25: Another picture showing the similar comparisons with the help of computers

are best used as confirmation of result rather than a sole assessment.

Tsutsumi and Furukawa described the use of a measuring instrument called a Vectron, which is similar to a dental surveyor and measures distances between fixed points, angles and radii.

Bang used stereo metric graphic analysis in mark investigation and produced a contour map of features of the mark and suspect dentition. A visual representation is then available which is compared electronically with the mark in terms of longitudinal contours and topographical features.

Light, electron and split image microscopy can be used. Bang and David both described the use of the scanning electron microscope (SEM) to good effect.

Ligthelm et al have added the reflex microscope to range of microscopes in use.

SEM is capable of detecting individual characteristics due to its high level of resolution. Using SEM it has been demonstrated that a single class characteristic contains individual charac-teristics. SEM may help to create an opinion that contains a higher degree of certainty that a specific set of teeth made a certain set of marks. Various electronic techniques such as splitting the image, image stacking, bite edge enhancement etc can be used.

Specialized Techniques

Xeroradiography and transillumination, as described by Rawson et al and Dorion respectively are specialized techniques that have been used in bite mark analysis. Both these techniques require the removal of the bitten tissue. In case of the xeroradiographic technique a layer of iodine contrast material is used and radiographs of the mark are taken. Xeroradiography is only applicable when indentations are present.

Transillumination utilizes the changed hemorrhagic structure of the tissue, which is viewed under a light source that enhances the areas of varying hemorrhagic density. This is a useful technique when the mark is very diffuse. Removal of the tissue does involve some distortion, and steps must be taken to minimize it.

Biopsy and histological examination of bitemarks is confined to the deceased. Whittaker refers to methods of staining for iron, other blood products, elastic fibers and collagen. He also describes the use of histological techniques to establish whether the mark was inflicted ante or postmortem.

Glass et al used histology to demonstrate the presence of microorganisms and calculus within the lesion, thereby confirming that the mark was caused by teeth.

The use of reflected, or direct, ultra violet photography can be of great value for three reasons.

- They provide greatly enhanced surface detail because a greater proportion of radiation of the wavelength used is reflected from the epidermis than is the spectrum of visible light.
- They may enhance the clarity of outlines of injuries due to their ability to record subtle and even invisible pigmentary changes that are known to occur after injury
- They may be taken, sometimes to great effect, many weeks and, some claim, even months after injury and still provide useful evidence, since the pigmentary changes referred to above take some time to occur.

Although acceptance of bite mark evidence has progressed, there is still a constant search for new methods, which improve on the shortcomings of traditional techniques. Recent methods described include infrared and ultra violet photography, scanning electron microscopy, computerized image enhancement, radiographic techniques, stereo metric graphic plotting and the use of three-dimensional measuring instruments. Shortcomings of these methods include inaccurate visual, photographic or graphic matching and damage to the bite mark due to certain procedures such as the making of impression.

Experimental Marks

The use of experimental marks to analyze a bite mark has been used as an aid to comparisons. They stipulate that three criteria should be met before undertaking experimental bite marks:

- The mark has been established as having made by teeth
- A reliable reproduction, example: A photograph
- The circumstances under which the bite was inflicted are known.

Vale et al made a rubber model of the part that was bitten, in this case a nose, and produced similar marks using the suspect's dentition on the model. Many other materials have been used in attempts to produce a skin like substance, such as baker's dough or pig-skin.

Bite Marks in Inanimate Objects

There are numerous examples in the literature of criminals who have left impressions of their teeth at the scene of a crime. The materials which are best able to record such marks are cheese, chocolate and metal tapes, where as those which present considerable difficulties are softer materials such as fruits, apples, cooked foodstuffs **(Figs 6.26A and B).** The same recording procedures are used as have been described in the case of human flesh so that the mark should be photographed under standardized conditions and a description produced of the type of dentition resulting in the mark.

If the services of a forensic dentist are not immediately available, it may be necessary to preserve the material in which the mark was made. If it is foodstuff, the simplest and most effective method is to wrap the object in slightly dampened tissues and to then place in a sealed jar in the main body of a refrigerator at about +2°C. The interpretation of the marks will differ from those seen in skin because during the biting of hard objects the teeth slide through the foodstuff and produce not only marks relating to the incisal edges but also gouges as the teeth travel through the material. In addition, brittle materials may fracture through the point of biting. A very useful technique may be to take silicone rubber impressions of the marks in some of these materials, and these may be retained not only for analysis but for final presentation in court.

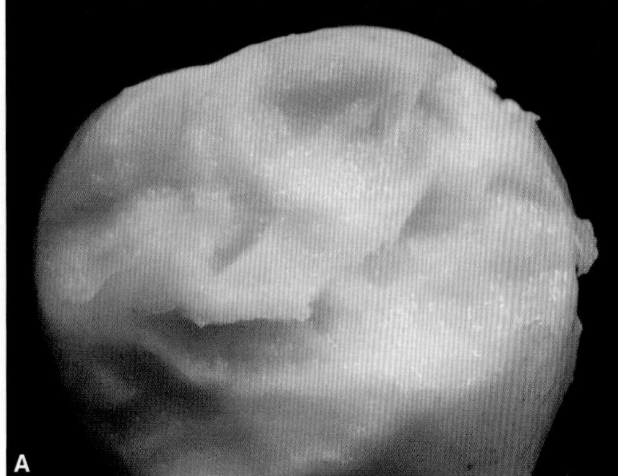

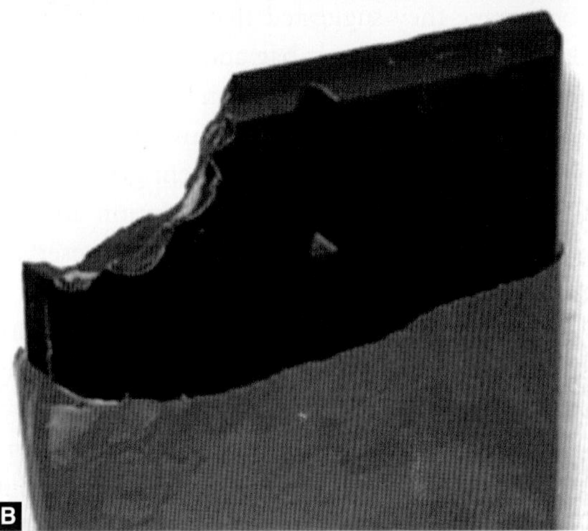

Figs 6.26A and B: Bite marks left in inanimate subjects at the scene of crime like those on food stuffs, like apple and chocolates as shown here

Inanimate objects like cheese, fruits, bread, chewing gum in which tooth mark fall into three broad categories.

- Edible substances
- Objects that are habitually chewed

- Substances making contact with teeth during fall or skirmishes.

Preservation and Collection of Inanimate Evidence

Saliva swabbing should be carried out and the object should be examined for fingerprints, as it must have been handled to reach the mouth. The preservation of foodstuffs is an urgent priority as all food deteriorates once exposed to air. Criminals are known to take bites out of apples or cheese, and to leave chewing gum at the scene of the crime. For storage they suggested that the specimen be placed in a sealed plastic bag and kept refrigerated until impressions and models can be taken from it. For long term storage Rudland found that immersion in a medium of 5 percent glacial acetic acid, 40 percent formaldehyde solution and 70 percent ethanol in the ratio of 5:5:90 preserved apples for 10 years.

It should be noted that the best marks are produced on the skin of fruit and not in the fleshly parts.

According to Webster and Mac Donald, cheese will undergo a nine percent weight loss and eight percent shrinkage after exposure for 72 hours. This can be considerably reduced if the cheese is refrigerated within this period. Layton describes a procedure for reproducing cheese bites in plaster of Paris. Chocolate is stable if refrigerated for up to one year.

Non-perishable substances: Non-perishable objects may reproduce marks well and dimensionally stable. Some of the objects are include a bullet, pipe stems and soap. Care must be taken to store and handle these objects carefully; any careless handling could introduce additional marks that might invalidate the analysis.

Long-Term Preservation

Long-term preservation can be achieved by two methods, photography or making models.

a. Photography

Marks should be photographed from various directions to show not only the point of tooth entry but also the exposed parts. Photographic principles for bite marks should be followed.

b. Models

Stoddart described a method for making models of perishable substances. For other inanimate objects, modern two-stage crown and bridge impression materials give satisfactory results. Depending on the type of analysis required, models can be made using plaster, acrylic or composite restorative materials.

Analysis and Comparison in Inanimate Objects

Analysis and comparison should follow the same format as that for skin, i.e. a quantitative and qualitative analysis of the marked object and the subject's dentition prior to a comparison being made.

Having a life-size model of the teeth and model of the object will enable a direct comparison to be made. Alternatively, if no suspect is available, acrylic teeth can be shaped to fit the marks and set up in. wax so that some idea of the dentition responsible can be obtained. Comparison can also be made using overlays, photographs or any of the specialized techniques. Jonason et al used a stereomicroscope to analyze the marks on a pipe stem. Mills placed a bullet directly onto articulated models of the suspect's teeth to demonstrate how the marks were produced.

Bite marks in cheese, butter and chewing gum are often difficult and sometimes impossible to identify due to shortcomings in the present techniques. The reflex microscope can be used to evaluate and identify bite marks in inanimate objects. Positive identification using the reflex microscope has become possible with a high level of accuracy.

One of the most important features of the reflex microscope is that non-contact measurements in three dimensions can be made directly of bite marks otherwise not suitable for taking measurements or impressions, such as butter.

Habitual Chewing Marks

Usually found on pipe stems, pencil and key bows. Very often in harder substances only cusp marks are present, and if the object has been bitten repeatedly, isolating and differentiating these marks can prove difficult. Cusp marks made by human canines, premolars and molars can be similar to those produced by the dentition of dogs and cats.

Bite Mark Pattern in 3-dimensional Settings

Foundation lies in the fact of overall relationship of bite mark to the teeth that caused injury. We know that photos give 2-D architecture of 3-D substances. Also it has been shown that one or more teeth may imprint on skin before an adjacent tooth begins to touch tissues, thus it is important to understand that absence of an individual mark in injury pattern does not mean associated tooth is missing, as the tooth may be below the occlusal plane. In such a scenario study casts may provide a substitute for the process.

Some effort has been made to standardize the comparison procedures but, unfortunately, the conclusions are often based on the expert's level of personal experience and judgement. The American Board of Forensic Odontology has worked hard to establish guidelines for independent examination of the same evidence by second and third odontologists before the primary expert submits a final report. Regardless, many cases have been disputed because of differing expert opinions, attacks on the scientific basis of physical comparisons because of the elasticity of skin and the question of uniqueness of the human dentition.

Human Bites as Forensic Biological Evidence

During the process of biting and also during kissing and sucking, saliva is deposited on the skin's surface. It has been shown that this trace evidence is present in sufficient quantity and quality to enable PCR-based typing of the DNA that is present in saliva from white blood cells and possibly from sloughed epithelial cells. Significantly, since high-intensity alternative light sources and lasers are now widely used by the police to locate stains from bodily fluids at the crime scene, saliva stains deposited on skin—even in the absence of marks from teeth—can be found and recovered. After analyzing the salivary DNA and establishing the depositor's DNA profile, this result can be compared with the DNA profile of any suspects obtained from buccal swabs containing saliva or whole blood taken using a lancet.

Terms Indicating Degree of Confidence that an Injury is a Bite mark

Possible bite mark: An injury showing a pattern that may or may not be caused by teeth; could be caused by other factors but biting cannot be ruled out.

Criteria: General shape and size are present but distinctive features such as tooth marks are missing, incomplete or distorted or a few marks resembling tooth marks are present but the arch configuration is missing.

Probable bite mark: The pattern strongly suggests or supports origin from teeth but could conceivably be caused by something else.

Criteria: pattern shows some, basic, general characteristics of teeth arranged around arches.

Definite bite mark: There is no reasonable doubt that teeth created the pattern; other possibilities were considered and excluded.

Criteria: Pattern conclusively illustrates (classic features) all the characteristics of dental arches and human teeth in proper arrangement so that it is recognizable as an impression of the human dentition.

Descriptions and Terms Used to Relate Bite Mark to the Suspected Biter

Reasonable dental/Medical certainty: Beyond a reasonable doubt.

Probable: More likely than not.

Exclusion: Ruled out.

Inconclusive: Insufficient evidence to relate the bite mark to the suspected biter.

Terminologies Used in Analysis of Bite Mark Cases

Point

- A singular unit or feature available for comparison or evaluation
- An area attributable to a tooth
- A way of counting features

This term is used as a convenience in reports to address specific components of the bite mark which are being compared to teeth. A point does not imply any degree of specificity and not a characteristic.

Concordant point:

- Point seen in both the bite mark and the suspect's exemplars.
- Corresponding feature.
- Comparable element.
- Unit of similarity.
- Matching point.

Area of comparison:

- A dynamic or specific region to be compared.
- A complex or pattern made up of a conglomerate of several points or a group of features.

Match:

- Nonspecific term indicating some degree of concordance between a single feature.
- Combination of features or a whole case.
- An expression of similarity without stating degree of probability or specificity.

This term "match" or "positive match" should not be used as a definitive expression of an opinion in a Bite mark case.

Consistent (compatible) with:

Synonymous to "match", a similarity is present but specificity is unstated.

If used to represent the odontologist's conclusion, the term "consistent with" should be explained in the report or testimony as indicating similarity but implying no degree of specificity to the match.

Possible biter:

Could have done it; may or may not have. Teeth like the suspect's could be expected to create a mark like the one examined but so could other dentitions.

Criteria: There is a nonspecific similarity or a similarity of class characteristics; match points are general and/or few, and there are no incompatible inconsistencies that would serve to exclude.

Probable biter:

Suspect most likely made the bite; most people in the population could not leave such a mark.

Criteria: Bite mark shows some degree of specificity to the individual suspect's teeth by virtue of a sufficient number of concordant points including some corresponding individual characteristics. There is an absence of any unexplainable discrepancies.

Reasonable medical certainty:

Highest order of certainty that suspect made the bite. The investigator is confident that the suspect made the mark. Perpetrator is identified for all practical and reasonable purposes by the bite mark. Any expert with similar training and experience, evaluating the same evidence should come to the same conclusion of certainty. Any other opinion would be unreasonable.

Criteria: There is a concordance of sufficient distinctive, individual characteristics to confer (virtual) uniqueness within the population under consideration. There is absence of any unexplainable discrepancies.

The term reasonable medical certainty conveys the connotation of virtual certainty or beyond reasonable doubt. The term deliberately avoids the message of unconditional certainty only in deference to the scientific maxim that one can never be absolutely positive unless everyone in the world was examined or the expert was an eye witness. The Board (ABFO), considers that a statement of absolute certainty such as "indeed, without a doubt", is un-provable and reckless. Reasonable medical certainty represents the highest order of confidence in a comparison. It is, however, acceptable to state that there is "no doubt in my mind" **(Table 6.1).**

The following list of Bite mark terminology standards has been accepted by the American Board of Forensic Odontology.

1. Terms assuring unconditional identification of a perpetrator, without doubt, on the basis of an epidermal bite mark and an open population is not sanctioned as a final conclusion.
2. Terms used in a different manner from the recommended guidelines should be explained in the body of a report or in testimony.
3. Certain terms have been used in a non-uniform manner by odontologists. To prevent mis-communication, the following terms, if used as a conclusion in a report or in testimony, should be explained:
   - Match; positive match.
   - Consistent with.
   - Compatible with.
   - Unique.
4. The following terms should not be used to describe bite marks:
   - Suck mark.
   - Incised wound.

Table 6.1: Showing ABFO scoring criterion

	Features	*No. of Points*
Gross	All teeth present	One/arch
	Size of arch consistent	One/arch
	Shape of arch consistent	One/arch
Tooth position	Same labio-lingual position	One/tooth
	Same rotational position	One/tooth
	Vertical position	One/tooth
	Spacing	One/space
Inter-dental Features	M- D width	One/tooth
	L-L width	Three/tooth
	Incisal edge curvature	Three/tooth
	Other distinctive features	Three/tooth
Miscellaneous	edentulous arch	Three

Using the following guide for scoring:

0- Excluded/no match
1- Possible match/some similar features
2- Probable match/several similar features
3- Definite match

Differences in Bite Patterns of Child and Adults

The relationship of biter to victim is also complex. This relationship may be seen amongst adult to adult, adult to child, child to adult or child to child. Both adults and children may self inflict bites in a surprisingly aggressive manner.

Adults biting other adults or children will almost inevitably constitute criminal activity and may be associated with actual or grievous bodily harm, rape, and murder or child abuse. Common areas include head, neck, limbs and trunk.

Most common age groups for these bite marks appears to be for;

- Male victims: 4 to 10 years
- Female victims: 11 to 14 years.

Non-accidental Injury to Children

It is now almost 30 years since the first description of the battered child syndrome and it is important that dentists are aware of the possibility of child abuse and have a knowledge of the key factors in its diagnosis. Police surgeons may also be involved at an early stage of an investigation and if there are marks present on the child which have the appearance of human bites, they may wish to call in the services of a forensic dentist.

Human bites, be they from a child or an adult, are usually oval or circular in shape. It may be possible to distinguish between the halves of the circle, having been produced by upper or lower arches of the dentition, and it may ideally be possible to distinguish marks made by individual teeth and even to pick up irregularities in those teeth. There may, in addition, be evidence of petechial haemorrhage in the centre of the circular bite. This is due to tongue pressure or suction at the time of the injury. It is essential that high quality photographs are taken of the bites and these must be accompanied by standard centimetre scales. The bite should be photographed as soon as possible and it may be necessary to re-photograph at 12 or 24-hour intervals.

Although it may be difficult to determine, in some instances, whether a child has suffered non-accidental injury (NAI), the presence of a human bite mark is indicative of NAI. However, it must be remembered that siblings may inflict an injury and indeed the child may self-inflict a bite mark providing the part of the body is accessible. The importance of the human adult bite in a non-accidental injury case is obvious. If it is present, non accidental injury by definition has occurred and the injury is one of the very few that may be related to the assailant, providing the image of the bite contains sufficient characteristics. It is difficult to determine whether the incidence of NAI to children is increasing but the forensic dentist is certainly called to see more cases than in the past. In addition to human bites there may be extra-oral injuries, such as bruising of the facial tissues, cigarette burns, lacerations and also intraoral injuries, including fractures of the teeth and/or jaw bones. It has been said in the past that the ruptured labial frenum is indicative of non-accidental child injury but it is now recognised that there may be other causes.

Animal Bites

When investigating bite marks it is important to remember that they may not always be produced by humans. Animals are capable of biting both the living and the dead. Bites from animals are rarely the object of bite mark analysis. About one percent of causalities in USA clinics are of bite marks (human or animal) **(Fig. 6.27A)**. The teeth of animals leave patterned injuries that appear quite different from those created by human teeth. This is especially true with dogs **(Fig. 6.27B)**, which are predominant culprits in bites to humans who bite at a rate eight times more frequently than humans bite each other. However, such bites may need to be analyzed in order to distinguish what species of animal may have been the attacker, or exclude one or more animals when there is more than one possible offender.

Carnivorous animals, like dogs or tigers, use their teeth in two distinct ways. They kill their prey primarily using their canines and they tear and slice the flesh to produce digestible fragments. Human teeth are designed principally to cut and grind food which is usually previously prepared. Some people appear to revert to more primitive instincts and use their canines and incisors to inflict bites on victims.

The size and distribution of the animal's teeth are likely to be very different to those of the human. For example, the bite of a dog consists, in principle, of four puncture wounds representing the perforation of the skin by the four large canines **(Fig. 6.27C)**. The incisors are small and rarely leave a mark. The bite may be complicated by tearing of tissue. Smaller animals, such as rodents may produce small, horizontal puncture wounds from their razor sharp incisors but may also produce long lacerations of any length produced by swinging their sharp incisors across the surface of the skin.

Cases have arisen where it has been necessary to demonstrate that more than one dog has been involved in a particular biting incident, and this may be possible by careful measurement of inter-canine widths. Distinguishing between animal bites requires a knowledge of comparative dental anatomy but it

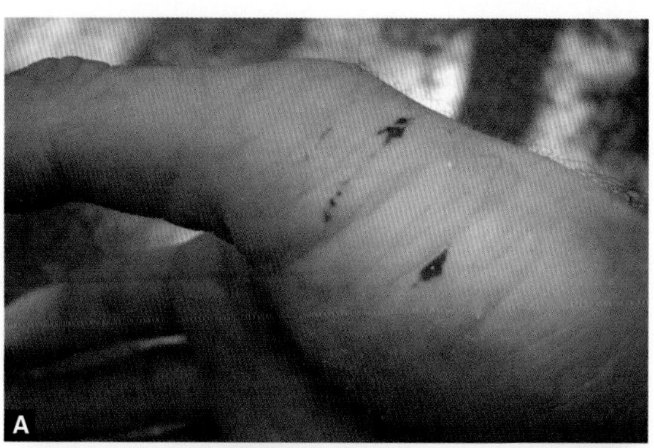

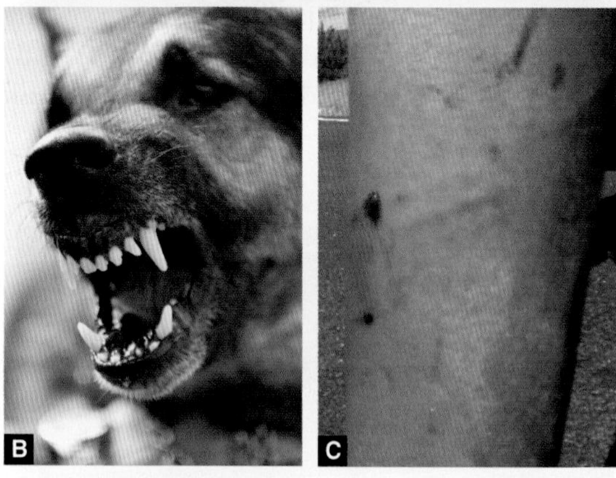

Figs 6.27A to C: Bite marks resulting because of animal bites most notably, dogs, cats, and reptiles. Shown here in the first picture is the bite marks because of a rattle snake and in the third picture, because of a dog bite. Note the two puncture wound resulting because of sharper canines of the dog

may be important, medicolegally, to determine the type of animal concerned **(Table 6.2)**.

Table 6.2: Showing characteristic differences in bite patterns between human and animals

Characteristics	*Human*	*Animal*
Basic outline	U shaped	V shaped
Area bitten	Broad	Elongated
Overall shape	Somewhat circular/oval	Narrow in anterior aspect
Morphology of anteriors	Broad centrals, relatively narrow lateral incisors	Broad laterals, narrow centrals
Canines	Blunt	Sharper and deeper canine marks

Bites, Bite Wound Infections, Prevention and Management

Prevalence of Bites

Bite wounds are among the commonest types of trauma to which a man is subjected. In urban areas dogs, cats and humans cause the majority of such wounds. A large percentage of dog and human bites are located on the face. Children often being the victims of family pets and to a lesser extent to human bites. Biting of one human by another is the third most common bite injury followed by dogs and cats and was first reported in the literature by Hultzen in 1910, who described an infective sequel to a human bite. About one half of the people in united states will be bitten by an animal or human during their lifetime, and these injuries account for one percent of all emergency department admissions and cost more than 25 million dollars in health care expenses per year. Studies found that the incidence in children is close to one human bite/600 pediatric emergency department visits. Bite wounds contaminated by animal and human oral flora are relatively common. These may be infected by the organisms causing virulent infections, including rabies.

Nature of Bites

Depending on the ferocity and anatomical characteristics of the biter, the bite may either be perforating, laceration, crushing, avulsive or combinations of any of these. Bites can be described in an ascending scale of severity; petechial, hemorrhage, contusion, abrasion, laceration and avulsion.

Animal Bites

Dog bites

Dogs are responsible for the vast majority of animal bite wounds. Dog bite related mortality is a well recognized aspect of this problem, amounting to at least 15 deaths per year in the United States. Dog bites account for 80 to 90 percent of all animal bites requiring medical care. The incidence rates are significantly higher among children aged 0 to 9 years especially among boys.

The peak incidence of dog bites occur in young children, most documented injuries have been to the head, face or neck region, whereas in older children and adults dog bites most commonly involve the limbs. Dogs are more likely to inflict superficial abrasions and lacerations. Dog bites wounds are frequently complicated with crush injury as a result of high masticatory forces that can be delivered by large breeds. Dog bites involve a combination of penetrating and avulsive injuries. They may be very disfiguring **(Figs 6.28 and 6.29)**, and may also cause serious damage to the eye and its adnexae. Injury in the region of the medial canthus is common with damage to the lacrimal system found in 15 of 16-periorbital dog bites. A snap provoked pet dog may inflict a deep perforation, even through a child's skull; however, the dog will often withdraw at once, and not tear as a wild carnivore might.

Cat bites

Tend to occur on the arms, commonly affecting women older than 20 years of age. Because of their slender, sharp teeth, more often cause deep puncture **(Fig. 6.30)** wounds. Cats inflict punctures without tearing or avulsing, and like other Felines may scratch as well as bite. Large carnivores may inflict gross mutilations on their victims, and treatment is often complicated by delay in seeking expert management.

Bear bites

Govilla et al reported a case in which a bear bit off 8 cm of jaw from the mandible of an Indian woman; the avulsed jaw was brought to a surgeon, but too late for implantation. Davis states that the North American bear typically bite the face or scalp. Illukol has described her own experience as a small girl in the Karimojong tribe of Uganda. A hyena attacked her, and her lips, nose and right maxillary region were avulsed, with loss of scalp. A crocodile on the other hand may seize and crush, being eager to drag its whole victim under water rather than to bite off a portion.

Human bites

Most common human bites occur during fights whereas a substantial percentage is related to sexual activities. Human bites have been described to occur in a number of situations, including overtly aggressive behavior, accidents and sexual activity. The site of bite is an important variable in the risk of infection.

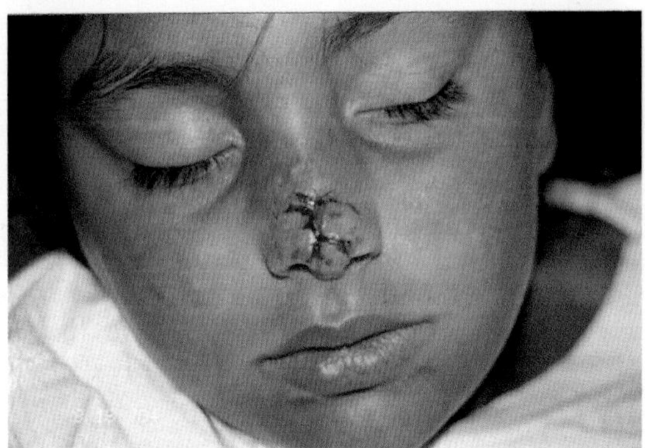

Fig. 6.28: An injured victim with his treatment done following an episode of a dog bite

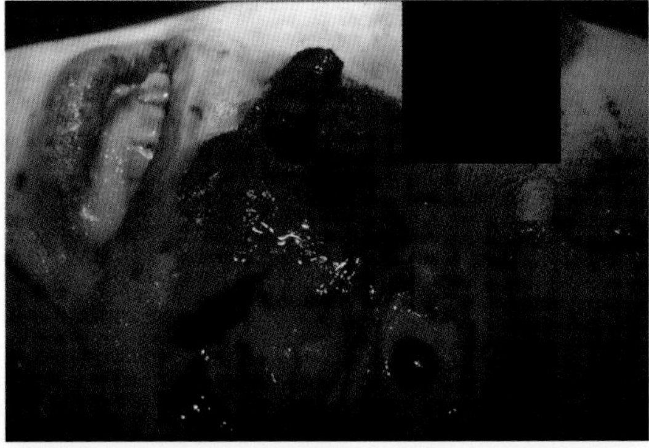

Fig. 6.29: A very severely disfiguring bite mark with a severity of grade 6, carrying no forensic significance, left after a traumatic bite by an animal

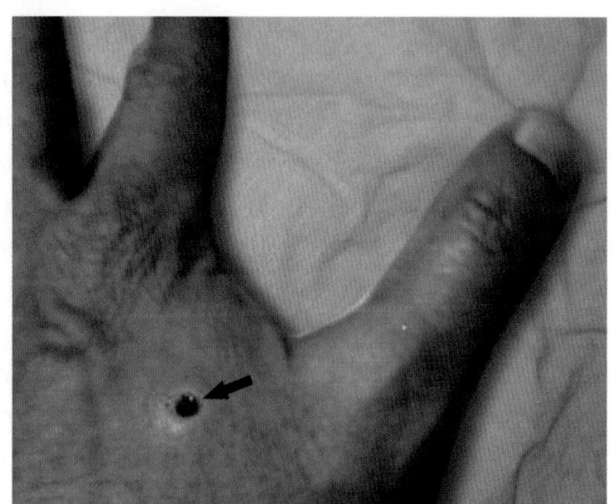

Fig. 6.30: A puncture wound reflecting a bite mark by an animal on the hand of a young victim

The prominent parts of the face are usually bitten; the lips, nose and ears are often attacked and loss of tissue is common. The amount of tissue removed is limited by the size of the human mouth and the anatomy of the dentition

Human bites include a specific type of wound, the clenched fist injury, which is sustained by the attacker, most commonly to the third metacarpophalangeal joint of the dominant hand, as a result of a clenched fist against the teeth of the opponent. In the clenched fist injury, a laceration of roughly 5mm occurs, typically in the third metacarpophalangeal joint. Some authors believe that a clenched fist injury is a separate entity from that of the bite mark and should be separated in bite classifications. The reported infection rate of a human bite varies. The infection rate for a bite to hand was 28 percent in one study, compared with only 4 percent for bites to the facial area.

Human bites are thought to be more serious than animal bites because of a higher incidence of infectious complications. Human saliva is considered a more virulent inoculum, with bacterial loads at the order of 10^8 per milliliter, which significantly increase in cases of periodontal disease and oral sepsis. Transmission of several systemic bacterial and viral infections has been reported to occur with human bites including hepatitis B and C, tuberculosis, syphilis and tetanus.

Transmission of human immunodeficiency virus following an accidental human bite has been documented. A bite injury that transmits HIV to the recipient could be classified as assault with a deadly weapon. The risk of HIV transmission following a bite injury is important to many groups of people. The first are those who are likely to be bitten as an occupational risk, such as police officers, medical personnel and institutional staff. The other group is represented by victims and perpetrators of crimes involving biting, both in attack and defense situations.

The severity of the bite injury is one factor that is likely to increase the chance of HIV transmission. To access the victim's blood, a bite must break the skin: thus an abrasion or more severe injury is required. Consideration must also be given to skin that is already broken. Studies show that the viral quantity in saliva is low or is supplemented by the presence of blood contamination. The source of this may be from undetectable micro lesions, trauma or periodontal disease.

It is possible that a bite from an HIV infected individual may transmit HIV. The likely risk of transmission is increased if; blood is present in the oral cavity, the bite breaks the skin, the bite is associated with a previous injury and the biter has a deficiency of anti HIV salivary elements (IgA deficient).

The recommendations for such bites are as follows: If an individual is bitten, treatment should be sought immediately and a risk analysis performed. The use of prophylactic antiretroviral agents may be appropriate in such situations. Health care workers, caregivers, police officers and others at risk of bites should be aware of this potential transmission route and use preventive measures such as hand and arm protection.

Physicians and other health care workers who care for patients who have sustained human bite marks need a working protocol to ensure that these patients receive proper care. The earliest report of a human bite in medical literature is by Burnett in 1898, numerous authors have described their successes and failures in treating human bites.

Diagnosis of Infection

Infected bite wounds are usually manifested by pain, edema localized at the site of the injury frequently associated with a purulent discharge and possibly regional lymphadenitis. The latency period between the bite and the appearance of the first symptoms of infection appears to be significantly shorter for cat bites than for human and dog bites.

Radiological Assessment

Teeth can penetrate the skull, and the associated scalp wound may be alarming. It is therefore necessary to obtain X-ray pictures of the skull or facial skeleton in case of facial or calvarial bites. Computed tomographic scans with appropriate window settings visualize small calvarial punctures well, and show the depth of cerebral penetration and the presence of in driven bone.

Microbiological Assessment

Once the guidelines for bite mark analysis have been addressed, all wounds should be smeared for gram stain analysis and cultured both aerobically and anaerobically. High-risk individuals should be tested for hepatitis antigens and HIV.

The microbiology of bite wounds is polymicrobial. Anaerobes usually account for the largest proportion and include species such as Prevotella and Porphyromonas. Many of the anaerobes isolated are beta lactamase producers.

A 22-month-old boy who, subsequent to a dog bite over the left maxilla, suffered infection of the dental follicle of the primary canine with Pasteurella multocida and this was the first case of an infected dental follicle secondary to an animal bite.

Various microbes have been implicated in infection from dog bites, including staphylococcus aureus, Pasteurella multocida and anaerobic cocci, pseudomonas aeruginosa, staph epidermidis and various streptococci. Pasteurella multocida may cause acute local cellulitis and lymphangitis and also has the capacity to cause meningitis and cerebral abscess. *Capnocytophaga canimorsus,* a common isolate from the dog's mouth, may produce fulminant septicemia in patients who are immuno suppressed. Staphylococci and streptococci have been isolated more frequently from nonpurlent infections, whereas anaerobic organisms are more commonly associated with abscesses both in dog and cat bite infections and in human infections.

The bacteriology of dog and cat bite wounds generally reflects, the oropharyngeal flora of the biting animal, as it is the animal saliva rather than the victim's skin flora that seems to be the major source of bacteria isolated from bite wound cultures. Various bacteriae have been isolated from human bite wounds; staphylococcus aureus is found in 25 percent and anaerobic bacteria, especially the bacteroides species, are found in greater than 50 percent of bite wounds.

Cultures are frequently recommended as standard procedures for all infected bite wounds. As the bacteriology of bite wound infection has been so extensively studied, cultures are probably helpful only in cases of treatment failure or severe or high-risk infections.

Complications

Bacteria in the wound will also hinder normal wound healing by enlarging the wound and competing for vital nutrients such as oxygen and glucose needed for wound healing. This causes further tissue anoxia, the production of lactic acid, and further breakdown of the wound.

Bite wounds may look innocuous initially; they frequently lead to infection that can progress to more serious complications like cellulitis, osteomyelitis, septicemia and death.

Biting of buccal mucosa is a very frequent injury; emphysema causing puffing of the cheek through a self-inflicted bite of the buccal mucosa has been reported.

Management

Many individuals do not seek treatment for human bites because of embarrassment and possible legal repercussions.

General

The management of human bite injuries is separated into two categories:

a) The care of adults with human bites and

b) The care of children with human bites

The treatment of bite wounds is two-fold: adequate surgical debridement and appropriate antibiotic treatment where indicated.

All bite injuries should undergo early wound decontamination unless there are obvious signs that infection is already present. The single most important step in prevention of infection is decontamination by forced irrigation using at least 200 ml of normal saline through a 19 gauge needle. This has been shown to reduce wound infections very substantially. Lavage with dilute povidone-iodine or chlorhexidine solution may also be used. If rabies is suspected, a viricide should be used. Antimicrobial prophylaxis for all bite wounds is controversial, and depends on the age of the wound and the extent and presence of patient risk factors such as asplenism, immunosuppression and immunocompromization. There has been a diversity of opinion with regard to the management of human bite wounds of the orofacial region.

Tomasetti et al. while reporting 25 cases of human bite wounds of the face, stated that surgical treatment should be dependent upon the presence or absence of infection, the length of time from initial trauma, and the size of the wound. His recommendation was that all recent, non-infected wounds should be evaluated for primary closure. It is this recommendation that appears to be the generally accepted concept of treatment now, but many authors have added a restricted period ranging from 12 to 84 hours after injury, beyond which primary closure should not be considered.

In 1976, one author reported the use of hyaluronidase injections around the wound site, in conjunction with conventional soft tissue wound repair, to successfully manage immediate primary closure, grossly contaminated and/or locally infected wounds of the orofacial region. According to McCarthy, when the patient is seen at a later stage with extensive tissue edema, crushed wound edges and with contused devitalized tissue, the purpose is to delay primary closure conditions for primary healing are more preferable. The technique he recommends consists of limited debridement to remove nonvital tissue, the application of wet dressings and antibiotic therapy until there is resolution of edema and a cleaner appearance of the wound. It is at this time that one could expect that a closure would be successful. Ordinarily, this process takes three to five days.

Surgical repair should be undertaken using the standard soft tissue repair techniques. In the past, fear of infection often led to a policy of delayed wound closure, with poor aesthetic results. If the bite has amputated a piece of tissue, replantation is sometimes possible; the amputated fragment should be washed in warm sterile saline and taken as soon as possible for consideration by the micro surgeon. If there is any delay, the tissue should be kept cool but not frozen.

Facial Bites (Table 6.3)

Peri-orbital bites

Standard ocular techniques are used to repair eyelid wounds if less than six to eight hour. If there is marked tissue edema, hemorrhage or suspected of infection, operation must be postponed for two to three days. Spinelli et al reported five cases in which large pieces of eyelid had been bitten off in passion or combat; the morsels were replaced and survived though loss of cilia was seen when there was delay in replantation. When the surgery was done within 14 hours, the cilia survived.

Bites of the lips

The lips were the leading sites of dog bites in reported series, being lacerated or amputated in 63/148 bites. It is sometimes possible to replant an amputated lip. Jeng et al replaced the vermillion area of a lower lip after eight hours by reanastomosing one inferior labial artery and joining the other to the vein.

Bites of the nose

These are very disfiguringand in some communities carry cruel implications of punishment for domestic or political crime.

Bites of the ear

These are relatively less disfiguring and indeed may be a source of mild pride when sustained in a combat. When a large piece of an ear has been bitten off, microvascular repair may be warranted. But for a majority of the people, covering the area with the by hair may be sufficient aesthetic management.

Bites on knuckles/fingers

The recognition of human bites on the body is generally easy for, there are usually abrasions, contusions, petechiae and tooth marks present. Those on the nose, finger or knuckle may be more difficult to recognize. Bites on the fingers are generally on the distal phalanx. They vary from simple abrasion to compound fractures. These are potentially dangerous and should be kept under observation for the development of felon or tendon sheath invasion. The incidence of wound contamination by mouth organisms is undoubtedly great due to the frequency of thumb sucking, hand nail biting, and other habits which bring saliva contact with wound.

The impact of the tooth produces a laceration over the knuckles of the index or middle fingers. It is tiny but deep, frequently penetrating the extensor tendon and usually entering the joint. Pain on movement of the finger indicates the progression of a septic arthritis. The joint mobility is restricted. Lymphangitis may be present. In favorable cases surgical intervention brings relief and decrease the temperature.

Massive avulsive bites

In the case of bear bite reported by Govilla et al the lower jaw was successfully reconstructed with a pectoralis major island flap containing a length of the rib.

Craniocerebral bites

The sharp teeth of a dog may perforate the infant's calvarial bone and pierce the underlying cerebral cortex. Klein and Cohen reported a case where failure to explore the wound led to the development of a brain abscess, the organism responsible being Pasteurella multocida.

Table 6.3: Classification of facial bite injuries (modified from Lackmann et al.)

Type	*Clinical Findings*
I	Superficial injury without muscle involvement
IIA	Deep injury with muscle involvement
IIB	Full thickness injury of the cheek or lip with oral mucosal involvement (through and through)
IIIA	Deep injury with tissue defect (complete avulsion)
IIIB	Deep avulsive injury exposing nasal or auricular cartilage
IVA	Deep injury with severed facial nerve and or parotid duct
IVB	Deep injury with concomitant bone fracture

In general, superficial injuries can be treated in the outpatient setting, whereas for type III and IV injuries hospitalization is required for special surgical care.

Prophylaxis

The first line antimicrobial is coamoxiclav when allergic to pencillin the options include a combination of both metronidazole and azithromycin.

When bite is the cause of a facial injury it is important to determine the immune status of the patient including the record of tetanus immunization. Tetanus antitoxin should be given to all patients.

Rabies is endemic in most parts of world, except the United Kingdom, Ireland, Sweden, Taiwan, Japan and Australia, which are at present supposedly free. The virus is commonly transmitted by dog bites. A rabid animal may be unbelievably ferocious and can attack the head or face. The incubation period for rabies is typically 2 to 8 weeks, but much longer periods have been reported. A person bitten by a rabid animal will obviously be under prolonged emotional strain, and should be counseled and reassured. In some developed countries, domestic dogs and cats are routinely vaccinated.

If a criminal act has been committed, it is the treating physician's responsibility to notify the proper authorities. Patients who are sexually abused require proper legal counseling, and the physician must report the incident to the law enforcement agency. If a child is found to be accidentally biting other children, the parents must be informed and proper counseling offered.

Sex Determination in Bite Marks

The possibility of obtaining exfoliated buccal epithelial cells in saliva on bite marks has increased the possibility of sex determination of the perpetrator. The duration of this line of inquiry is apparently possible for several weeks post deposition, depending on the materials containing the impressions and environmental factors. Two parameters have been proposed, both based on successful efforts to sex bloodstains:

1. The presence and detection of sex chromatin (Barr bodies in females, and F bodies in males); and
2. Sex hormone level determinations based on detectable quantities and ratios of testosterone and 17B-estradiol by radioimmunoassay (RIA).

The former parameter has been demonstrated successfully in saliva stains; this author is unaware of any successful attempt to identify sex in saliva by means of hormonal ratios.

Interpretation of such investigatory efforts must be dependent on an understanding of the possible variations that might be encountered. Discrepancies noted in tests for sex chromatin include:

1. Chromatin negative females, e.g. Turner's Syndrome and testicular feminization,
2. Chromatin positive males, e.g. Klinefelter's Syndrome, and
3. Genetic mosaics.

In each case, a sufficient number of nucleated cells must be obtained, fixed, and stained. Alcohol fixation and H and E stains have been used successfully for detection of Barr bodies or "drumsticks" in materials containing at least 100 nucleated cells. An aceto-orcein staining process was described by Sanderson and Stewart in 1961. Determination of sex by DNA analysis according to Sensabaugh and Blake is possible by using PCR based on the characteristics of the mammalian sex chromosomes, X and Y. Normal females have two X chromosomes and males have an X and Y chromosome. The development of a mammalian embryo as male is determined by genes on the Y chromosome and the phenotypic sex of individuals with an abnormal complement of sex chromosomes depends only on the presence or absence of the Y chromosome. According to various authors, a number of X and Y chromo-some-specific sequences have been identified and serve as potential markers for sex determination.

Several PCR-based approaches have been used. The simplest is the amplification of a Y specific sequence; the presence of a PCR product indicates the sample contains male cells. With this assay, the absence of a product cannot be interpreted unless there is an amplification control. An assay using the DYZ1 repeat sequence for the Y marker and either an Alu repeat or DQA sequences as amplification controls is an example of such testing.

Witt and Erikson described an assay using both X and Y specific centromeric alphoid repeat sequences as the chromosome markers. Amplification of these two sequences employ different primer sets but can be co-amplified. Male DNA shows both X and Y PCR products, whereas female DNA shows only the X product. Gaensslen et al. reported this application in 1992 on forensic specimens.

A third method, described by Aasen and Medrano amplifies both the X and Y specific sequences using a single primer set. The human ZFY and ZFX genes possess regions of conserved sequence permitting the design of primers capable of amplifying both. The two sequences are then distinguished by a sequence-specific restriction assay using Hae III. The ZFX gene is marked by a characteristic 400-base-pair fragment and the ZFY gene by a 317-base-pair fragment. Because both sequences are amplified from the same set of primers, the assay has a built-in control for the amplification reaction from both sexes. The gene sequences are also species-specific according to Aasen and Medrano.

Psychological Aspects of Bite Marks

Infliction of bite mark wounds represents highly complex thoughts and emotions expressed through a screen of fantasy, the mortal state of the victim, location of wound sites, and stigmatic destructiveness (tool marks). Suckling marks, tearing and abrasion pattern are all important factors in identifying the psychological dynamics and behavioral tracts of the biter.

Due to a pattern of psychologically expressed ritualism, the perpetrator will often inadvertently leave important psychological clues at the crime scene. After reviewing cases reported in the literature and after conducting psychological interviews with perpetrators, three major groups of perpetrators seem to be apparent. The first group is motivated out of an anger track, the second group is motivated out of sadistic biting, and the third is out of the more traditional "cannibal complex" motif.

Based upon the physiological and psychological materials, there emerge three major motivational categories in which bite mark evidence can be classified

1. Anger — impulsive biting
2. Sadistic biting
3. Ego — cannibalistic biting

Anger—impulsive Biting

This is consistent with the overaggressive and under controlled display of impulsive anger. This type of biter is often nettled by frustration and incompetence while dealing with any conflict situation.

When the biter reaches an apex of emotional excitation, the situational loss of self-control allows for an impulsive act of revenge by inflicting a tool mark bite on the victim.

Although biter may not derive specialized satisfaction from inflicting the tool mark wound, his pleasure is derived from the ability to effectively hurt and humiliate the victim by his "Wolf – like" ferocity.

Sadistic Biting

In the continuum of sexual sadistic biting, the themes of blood, flesh, and object symbolization become important to the cultivated sensualization of power of ripping, tearing, and utilizing the ability to render the victim helpless and incapacitated. By a protracted and ritualistic biting of the victim, the aggressor can satisfy not only the cultivated power symbols, but satiate his increasing lust for domination, control and omniscience.

Bite marks found in the most advanced forms of sadism can range from an early fetishism for blood to the bite marks found on the internal organs from an eviscerated body.

Ego — cannibalistic Biting

The most vicious and destructive type of biting is within this complex. In this category of biting, the assailant's major thrust is to satiate ego demands by annihilating, consuming and absorbing life essences from their victims.

Signature Implicants

In bite mark cases, when the wound indicant is linked with the overall crime scene evidence, the signature theme of biting motivations can be examined for signs and symbols revealing stylized intents. Since the assailants often use central themes of aggression with personalized adaptations, a psychology cannot make a "fingerprint" of the crime, it can give signature importance to bite mark evidence in relationship to the crime. It is recognized that psychology cannot "Solve" cases, but it can yield valuable information about the crime through examining the underlying structures and themes. To this goal, the psychological understanding of bite mark evidence can and should be used as a clarifying tool.

The Pitfalls of Bite Mark Analysis Systems in Forensic Settings

Human bites on skin are difficult to interpret because skin is not a good 'impression' material, moreover, victims may struggle and movement will distort the image of the bite. Skin surfaces are not flat and visual distortion may be present, often heightened by photographic distortion caused by inadequate imaging techniques.

Human dentitions, whilst possibly being unique in the sense of small nuances of tooth size, shape, angulations and texture may not inflict unique bite marks which can only record gross and not fine detail. If the victim survives, the injury may change due to infection or subsequent healing and if the victim is deceased, putrefaction may introduce distortion.

The forensic dentist will be asked to determine whether or not the injury is, in fact a human bite mark? Is it compatible with an adult dentition and can the perpetrator be identified from the information present in the injury? What is the optimum protocol available when an odontologists compares a suspect to a possible bite mark when the DNA results are still pending?

The purists would say the two fields—physical matching and DNA analysis — are independent, this is despite the fact that physical matching of bite marks is a non-science which was developed with little testing and no published error rate. Alternatively, the statistical justification for DNA has been scrutinized and approved. The frequencies in the population of polymorphic loci are also known.

What the, should a prudent odontologists do in this situation?

The temptation to create an opinion early in an investigation is normal. Who wants to say that odontology cannot conclusively establish a bite mark as unique? The greater experience of one expert over another has been argued as a guarantee of a "better" result. This is unproven conjecture and serves as the single support for proponents of the non-science approach. How does one weigh the importance of a single rotated tooth in a bite mark when the suspect has a similar tooth?

The value judgments range widely on the value of this feature. This is not science. Instead, statistical levels of confidence must be included in this process. Until then, the DNA results are far superior to the odontologist's position. There is no honest way to deny this. The majority of cases will be proven conclusively by the biological tests, if they are performed. If the two independent tests do not correlate, I hope odontologists will not rely on the theory that there were two assailants involved in the same case-one biting and the other spitting.

Summary

1. Bite marks can be useful physical evidence.
2. The effect of skin variability has not yet been determined and further research is required in this area. The distortion of various anatomical locations is subject to curvature, bone and adipose deposits.
3. Currently, digitally created overlays can be regarded as best practice although no official recommendation has been made by either US or UK bodies.
4. Care must be taken when expressing certainty, especially with regard to the product rule.
5. Forensic dentistry requires more research to investigate bite mark accuracy and reliability.

Bibliography

1. Arhearta KL, Pretty IA. Results of the 4th ABFO Bite mark Workshop—1999. Forensic Science International 2001;124:104-11.
2. American Board of Forensic Odontology. ABFO Guidelines and Standards. In Bowers C M, Bell G L (ed) Manual of Forensic Odontology. 3rd ed. pp299, 334-353. Colorado Springs: American Society of Forensic Odontology, 1995.
3. Dr. Shwetha Aacharya. Bite marks. Library dissertation submitted to Rajive Gandhi university of health sciences in partial fulfillment for the degree of masters of dental surgery in the speciality of Oral pathology at Bangalore, Karnatka, India 2005-2008.
4. Guidelines for bite-mark analysis, American Board of Forensic Odontology, J Am Dent Assoc 1986; 112:383-6.
5. John D. McDowell. A commentary on the current status of bite marks. Dental abstracts. Volume 54, Issue 1, 2009.
6. Michael BC. Problem-based analysis of bite mark misidentifications: The role of DNA. Forensic Science International 2006;159S:S104-S109.
7. Pretty IA, Sweet D. Digital bite mark overlays—an analysis of effectiveness, J For Sci 2001;46:1385-9.
8. Pretty IA, Sweet D. Anatomical locations of bite marks and associated findings in 101 cases from the United States. J Forensic Sci 2000;45:812-4.
9. Sweet D, Pretty IA. A look at forensic dentistry—Part 2: Teeth as weapons of violence—identification of bite mark perpetrators BDJ, Volume 190, no. 8, April 28, 2001.
10. Sweet D, Lorente J A, Lorente M, Valenzuela A, Villanueva E. PCR–based typing of DNA from saliva recovered from human skin. J Forensic Sci. 1997;42:447-51.
11. Vale G L, Noguchi TT. Anatomical distribution of human bite-marks in a series of 67 cases. J Forensic Sci. 1983;28:61-9.

Chapter 7

Cheiloscopy and Palatoscopy

Gaurav Atreja

Chapter Overview

- Cheiloscopy
- Anatomical Aspects
- Palatoscopy
- Historical aspects
- Anatomical aspects
- Classification
- Analyzing and recording palatal rugae
- Problems with palatoscopy
- Future prospects

INTRODUCTION

In some particular circumstances, often related to a criminal investigation, there can be other data, which are important to the process of human identification. Some of those data result from soft oral and perioral tissue prints **(Fig. 7.1)**.

In fact, lips, as well as the hard palate, are known to have features that can lead to a person's identification. The study of lip prints is known as Cheiloscopy; the study of hard palate anatomy to establish someone's identity is called Palatoscopy

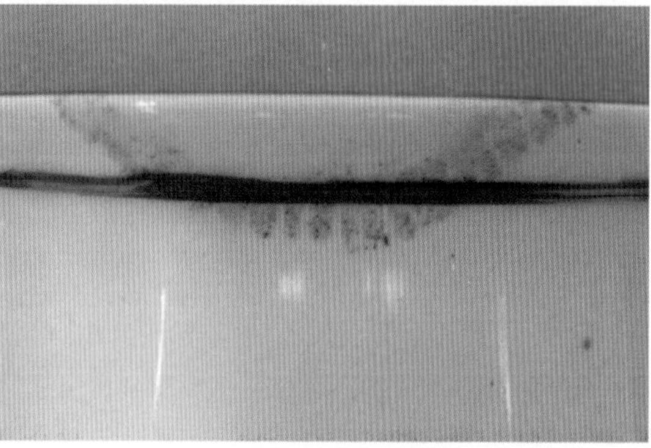

Fig. 7.1: A lip print formed on the glass plate by oral and perioral soft tissues

CHEILOSCOPY

Cheiloscopy, (from the Greek words cheilos, lips) is the name given to the lip print studies. The importance is linked to the fact that lip prints are unique to one person, except in monozygotic twins. Like fingerprints and palatal rugae, lip grooves are permanent and unchangeable. It is possible to identify lip patterns as early as the 6th week of intrauterine life.

From that moment on, lip groove patterns rarely change, resisting many afflictions, such as herpetic lesions. In fact, only those pathologies that damage the lip substance like burns, seem to rule out cheiloscopic study.

Historical Review of Cheiloscopy

1902 First described by Fisher

1930 Diou de Lille developed some studies which led to lip print use in criminology

1932 Edmond Locard, one of France's greatest criminologists, acknowledged the importance of cheiloscopy

1950 Le Moyer Snyder, in his book "Homicide Investigation" mentioned the possibility of using lip prints in the matter of human identification

1960 Santos, suggested that the fissures and the criss-cross lines in the lips could be divided into different groups

1972 Renaud, studied 4000 lip prints and confirmed the singularity of each one, supporting the idea of lip print singularity

Suzuki and Tsuchihashi in their study, over a long period of time, confirmed not only lip print singularity, but also lip response to trauma; in fact, these authors observed that after healing, the lip pattern was equal to that before the injury occurred.

Anatomical Aspects

Lips are highly sensitive mobile folds, composed of skin, muscle, glands and mucous membrane **(Fig. 7.2)**. Anatomically, whether covered with skin or mucosa, the surface that forms the oral sphincter is the lip area. There are two different kinds of lip covering—skin or mucosa. When the two meet, a white wavy line is formed – the labial cord – which is quite prominent in Negroes.

Where identification is concerned, the mucosal area holds the most interest. This area, also called Klein's zone, is covered with wrinkles and grooves that form a characteristic pattern— the lip print. However, this is not the only area that deserves careful study. In fact, in cheiloscopy, one should also analyze lip anatomy, considering their thickness and the position.

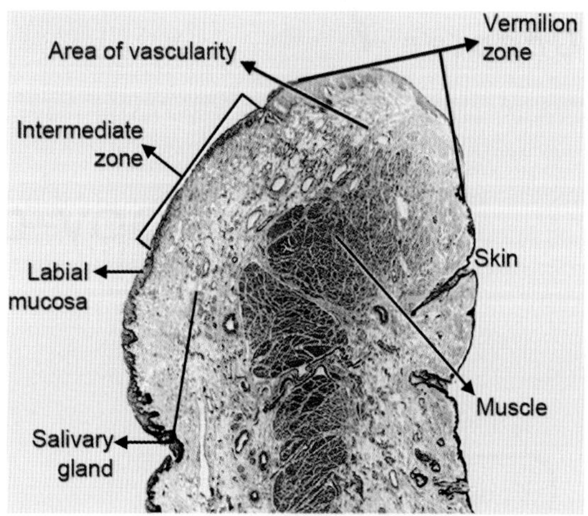

Fig. 7.2: Vermillion border histology

The lips can be horizontal, elevated or depressed and, according to their thickness, it is possible to identify the following four groups: also, illustrated in the diagram below is the pictorial representation of the same **(Fig. 7.3).**

1. Thin lips (common in the European, Caucasian)
2. Medium lips (from 8 to 10 mm, are the most common type)
3. Thick or very thick lips (usually having an inversion of the lip cord and are usually seen in Negroes)
4. Mix lips (usually seen in Orientals)

Various classification system proposed for the cheiloscopy study are:

A. Suzuki and Tsuchihashi classification
B. Renaud classification.
C. Martin Santos classification.
D Afchar-Bayat classification.
E. Jose Maria Dominguez classification.

A. Suzuki and Tsuchihashi Classification (Table 7.1)

These authors considered six **(Fig. 7.4)** different types of grooves, as seen in the following table.

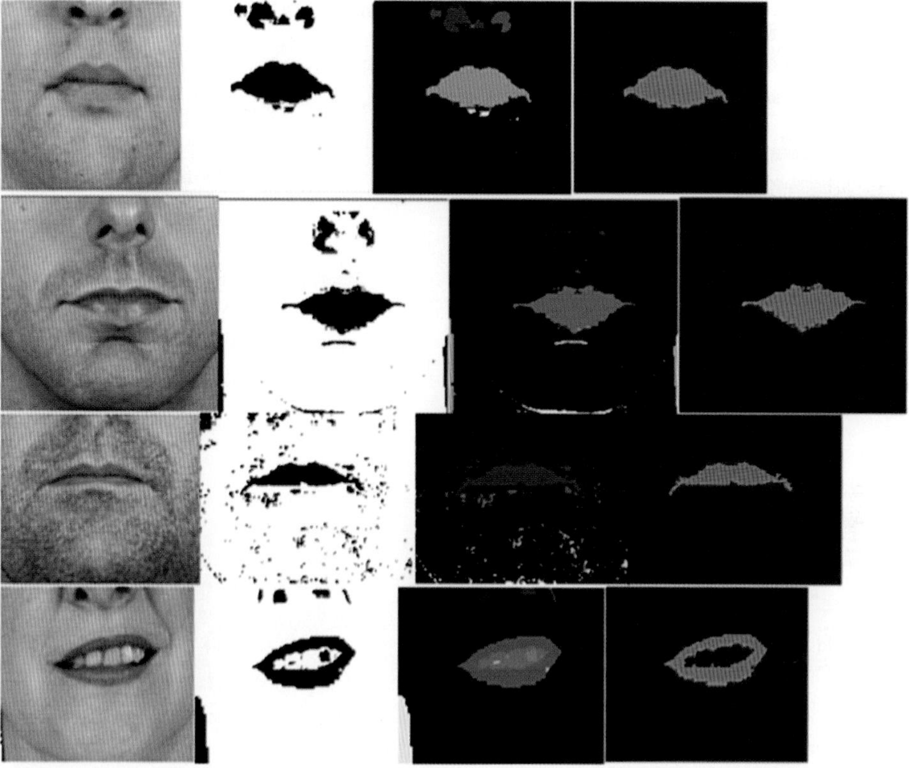

Fig. 7.3: Chief types of lip pattern in world population

Table 7.1: Suzuki and Tsuchihashi classification

Classification	*Groove type*
Type I	Complete vertical
Type I'	Incomplete vertical
Type II	Bracnched
Type III	Intersected
Type IV	Reticular pattern
Type V	Irregular

B. Renaud Classification

This is, probably, the most complete classification. The lips are studied in halves (left and right), and every groove, according to its form, has a number. A formula is then elaborated using capital letters to describe the upper lip left (L) and right (R) sides, and small letters to classify each groove **(Table 7.2)**.

In the lower lip, it is done the other way around, using capital letters to classify the grooves, and small letters to separate left from right sides.

C. Afchar-Bayat Lip Prints Classification

This classification, dated from 1979, is based on a six-type groove organization, as seen in the table below **(Table 7.3)**.

D. Jose´ Maria Dominguez Classification

This is a classification based on the one made by Suzuki and T. suchihashi. In the grooves classified as Type II of Suzuki and Tsuchihashi, the author and his co-workers observed, with some frequency, a slight variation: they observed that branched grooves often divided upwards in the upper lip, and downwards in the lower, as reported by Suzuki

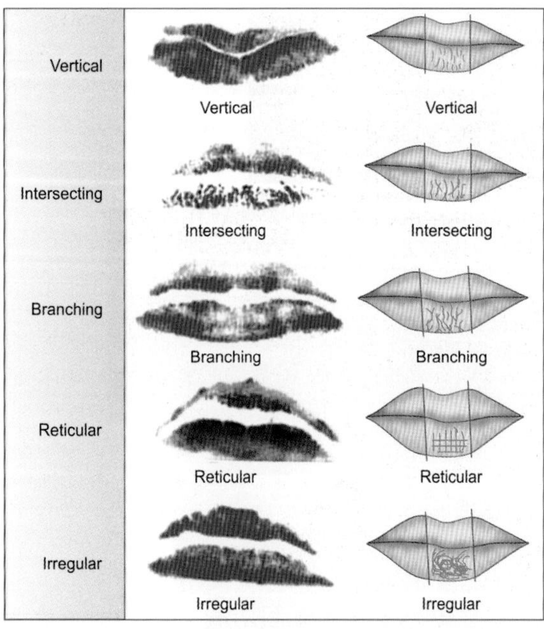

Fig. 7.4: Suzuki and Tsushihashi classification of various lip types

Table 7.2: Renaud classification

Classification	*Groove type*
A	Complete vertical
B	Incomplete vertical
C	Complete Bifurcated
D	Incomplete Bifurcated
E	Complete branched
F	Incomplete branched
G	Reticular pattern
H	X or Coma form
I	Horizontal
J	Other forms (ellipse, triangle)

and Tsuchihashi; but they also realise that some grooves, the so called II0 type branched the other way around.

Analyzing and Recording Lip Prints

Lip prints can link a subject to a specific location if found on clothes or other objects, such as glasses, cups (**Fig. 7.5**) or even cigarette buts. Sometimes lip prints will be seen as lipstick smears. Lipsticks are complex substances, which have in their constitution, several compounds, oils or waxes; color of the lipsticks is due to organic inks and inorganic pigments.

However, all lip prints are important, even the ones that are not visible. In fact, this complex process is not restricted to studying visible prints, but also the latent ones. The vermillion border of the lips has minor salivary and sebaceous glands which, together with the moisturizing done by the tongue, leads to the possibility of the existence of latent lip prints.

When searching for lip prints, one must always consider that not all lipstick smears are colored; in fact, in recent years the cosmetic industry has been developing new lipsticks which do not leave a

Table 7.3: Afchar-Bayat lip prints classification

Classification	*Groove type*
A1	Vertical and straight grooves covering whole lips
A2	Like the former, but not covering the whole lip
B1	Straight branched grooves
B2	Angulated branched grooves
C	Converging grooves
D	Reticular pattern grooves
E	Other grooves

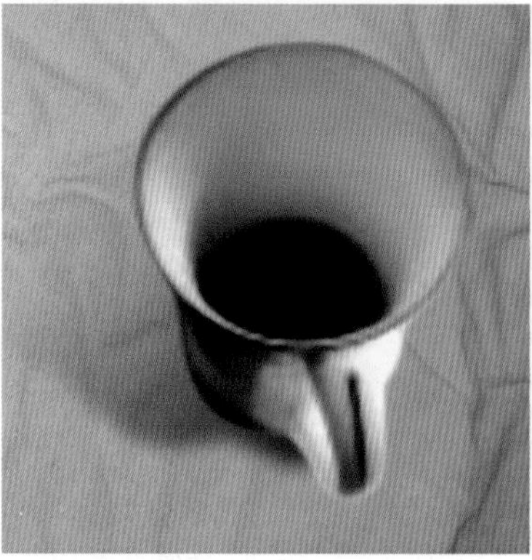

Fig. 7.5: Lip print on a coffee mug

visible smear or mark when they come in contact with different items—these are called persistent lipsticks.

A group of Spanish investigators has studied latent lip prints and concluded that they could be studied in a similar way to fingerprints, using similar techniques. In fact, even when located on "difficult" surfaces (such as porous or multicolored ones), latent prints can be easily seen using fluorescent dyes **(Fig. 7.6)**.

When dealing with lip prints from persistent lipsticks, one must always remember that persistent lipsticks have minimal oil content and therefore, their development using conventional powders (developers) might not be effective. Lysochromes should then be used since they have the ability to dye fatty acids and are very effective when used on long-lasting lipstick prints, even on porous surfaces. In this manner, latent lip prints should always be considered when processing a crime scene, even if there are no traces of lipstick.

Processing lip prints depends on the anatomical, morphological and histological tissue features of lips. Observation should be the first step using white and ultraviolet light. Photographs should be made prior to any processing in order to protect the evidence.

According to FBI guidelines latent prints should be photographed individually with an identification label and a scale; each step in the sequence must be photographed. If lipstick is present, it should be analyzed in order to determine its constitution. About 65 percent of lipsticks share the same ingredients, however some are different and this difference can provide the identification of the lipstick manufacturer.

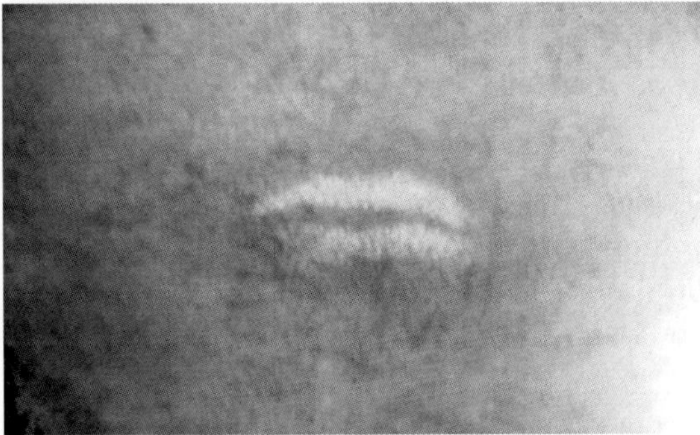

Fig. 7.6: Lip print visualized after fluorescent examination

Lip Prints can be Recorded in a Number of Ways

If located on a non-porous surface, lip prints can be photographed and enlarged. Using transparent overlays, it is possible to make an overlay tracing. As previously referred to, the development of lip prints can be made using several substances known as developers, such as aluminium powder, silver metallic powder, silver nitrate powder, plumb carbonate powder, fat black aniline dyer or cobalt oxide.

All lip prints contain lipids which make their development possible by using lysochromes dyes (Sudan III, Oil Red O, Sudan Black) **(Figs 7.7A to D)**. Sometimes, the use of fluorescent reagents is necessary, especially when the color of the developer and the color of the surface on which the lip print lies are the same, or when the lip print is an old brand.

Developers Commonly Used are–

Plumb carbonate: Over smooth, polished, metallic or plastic surfaces. Its only limitation is its use over white surfaces, use black marphill powder in such cases

Silver nitrate: Non ideal surfaces, such as untreated wood or cardboard

DFO and Ninhydrin: Porous surfaces

Cyanoacrylate dye: On plastic or waxed surfaces, or on vinyl gloves

Cyanoacrilate dye or an iodine spray reagent: In photographs, latent prints can be developed

Lips may also be studied and recorded in order to allow a proper comparative analysis. Although

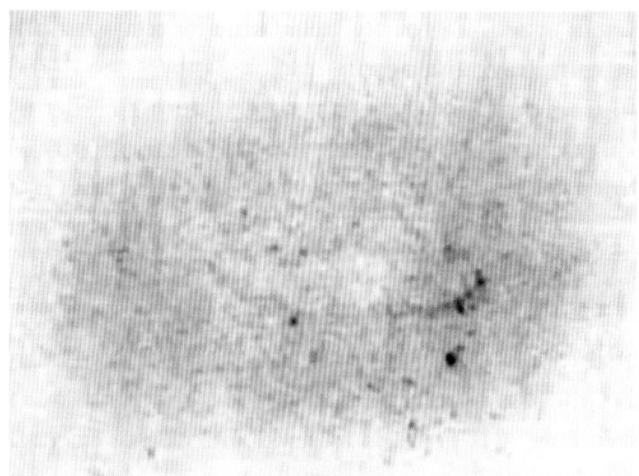

Fig. 7.7A: Latent lip print visualized after using a developer black powder on a cotton fabric after 30 days

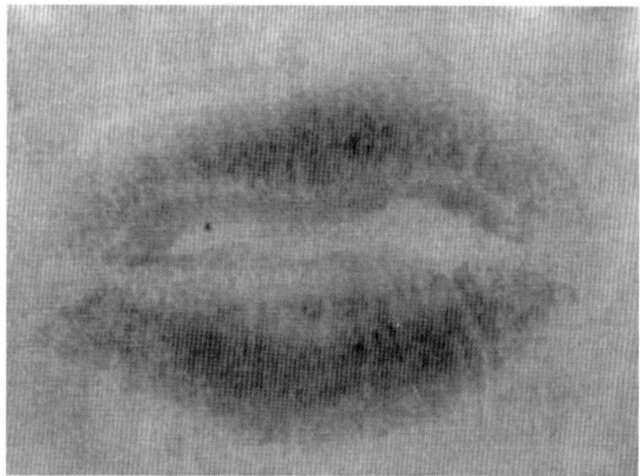

Fig. 7.7B: Latent lip print visualized after using a developer oil red O

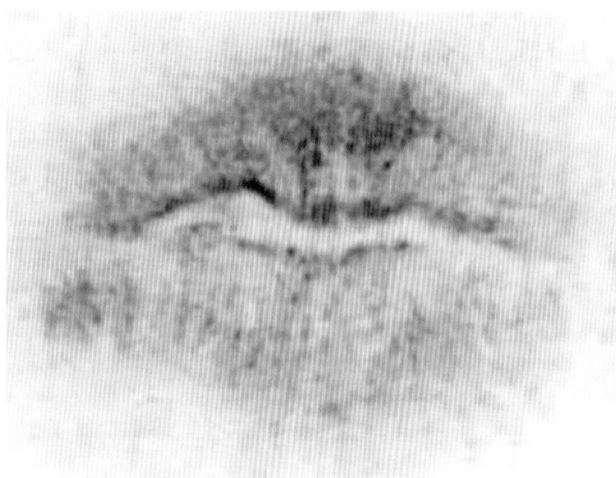

Fig. 7.7C: Another lip print visualized after using a developer oil red O

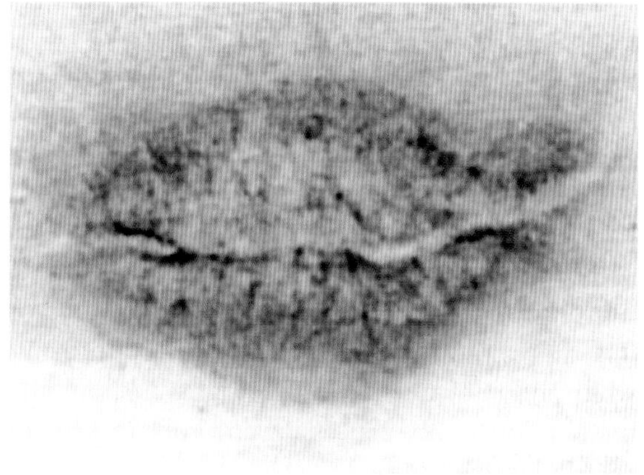

Fig. 7.7D: Lip print obtained after using Sudan black dye

lips can be photographed directly, covering them with lipstick allows better groove visualization. The lip prints should be recorded, making several recordings until all transfer mediums are exhausted. Then, prints are covered with transparent overlays and, when using a magnifying lens, a trace can be successfully done

Problems with Cheiloscopy

Lip print is produced by a substantially mobile portion of the lip. This fact alone explains the reason why the same person can produce different lip prints, according to the pressure, direction and method used in taking the print. If lipstick is used, the amount can also affect the print. This problem however, can be solved if recordings are made until all of the substance is used.

Manual register of the overlay is another problem, due to the possibility of some subjectivity. Another factor to be considered is the existence of some pathological conditions (lymphangioma, congenital lip fistula, lip seleroderma, Merkelson-Rosenthal syndrome, syphilis, angular cheilitis, among others), which can invalidate the cheiloscopic study.

One must also consider the possibility of post-mortem changes of lip prints from cadavers with various causes of death. It should also be pointed out that only in very limited circumstances, is there antemortem data referring to lip prints, which obviously impairs a comparative study where necro identification is concerned. The main feature for dental identification is the existence of ante mortem data, which cannot be expected in cheiloscopy. Therefore, the only use of cheiloscopy will be to relate lip prints to the lips that produced them

Future Prospects of Cheiloscopy

Cheiloscopy is interesting mostly in identifying the living, since it can be the only way to link somebody to someone or to a specific location. However, although lip prints have previously been used in a court of law, its use is not consensual and some authors believe further evidence is needed to confirm their uniqueness. In fact, lip print use is controversial and rare.

The FBI has used this kind of evidence only in a single case in order to obtain a positive identification. Nowadays, new research allows for cheiloscopy use in a court of law in the USA. Recent studies also point out other possibilities namely, DNA detection in latent lip prints where some researchers are trying to relate characteristic lip patterns with a person's gender. Another aspect that might be interesting to study is the possibility of using identifiable lip prints obtained from the skin of assault and murder victims, in a similar way to what has already been done with latent finger prints.

Palatoscopy

Identifying live or dead people is often a difficult and time consuming process. Identifying living people is sometimes difficult because people do not normally wish to be identified. Therefore, in order to achieve this goal, people disguise their presence in various ways. Identifying the dead raises a whole different set of problems, which relate to;

The natural process of decomposition;

Scavenger animal actions;

The circumstances in which death occurred.

Palatoscopy, or palatal rugoscopy, is the name given to the study of palatal rugae in order to establish a person's identity.

Due to anatomical position, it is unlikely that the study of palatal rugae could be used in the process of linking a suspect to a crime scene. On the other hand, palatoscopy may be used as a necro-identification technique. As previously mentioned, it will be in these particular circumstances that palatoscopy is most valuable. The possibility of finding antemortem data supports this idea. Nowadays, palatal rugae patterns are considered a viable alternative for identification purposes. Some investigators aim to assess its feasibility with the aid of a computer and a software program. The results so far are good, but expected to be better.

In fact, the Brazilian Aeronautic Minister demands palatal rugoscopy of all its pilots, in order to ensure their identification in case of accident.

Historical Review

1897 Kuppler was the first person to study palatal anatomy to identify racial anatomic features.

1932 Palatal rugoscopy was first proposed in 1932, by a Spanish investigator called Trobo Hermosa.

1937 Carrea developed a detailed study and established a way to classify palatal rugae One year later, Da Silva proposed another classification.

1946 Martins dos Santos presented a practical classification based on rugae location.

1983 Brinon, following the studies of Carrea, divided palatal rugae into two groups (fundamental and specific) in a similar way to that done with fingerprints.

In this manner, dactiloscopy and Palatoscopy were united as similar methods based on the same scientific principles and are sometimes complementary: For instance, Palatoscopy can be of special interest in those cases where there are no fingers to be studied (burned bodies or bodies in severe decomposition).

Anatomical Aspects

The surface of the oral mucosa is mostly flat and smooth without grooves or **(Figs 7.8A to C)** crests, this happens in order to achieve the best performance in oral functions. Nevertheless, there are some exceptions, like back of the tongue, which is covered with papillae; the anterior portion of the palatal mucosa, having a dense system of rugae, firmly attached to the underling bone. Palatal rugae are irregular, asymmetric ridges of mucous membrane extending lateral from the incisive papilla and the anterior part of the median palatal raphe whose purpose is to facilitate food transportation through the oral cavity, prevent loss of food from the mouth and participate in the chewing process. Due to the presence of gustatory and tactile receptors, they contribute to the perception of taste, the texture of food qualities and tongue position. Generally, there is no bilateral symmetry in the number of primary rugae or in their distribution from the midline. It has been found that there are slightly more rugae in males and on the left side in both genders.

Their role in human oral function seems to be increasingly less important, which might explain why their development time is retarded. Palatal rugae are formed in the 3rd month in utero from the hard connective tissue covering the bone. Once formed, they do not undergo any changes except in length, due to normal growth, remaining in the same position through out an entire person's life. Not even diseases, chemical aggression or trauma seem to be able to change palatal rugae form.

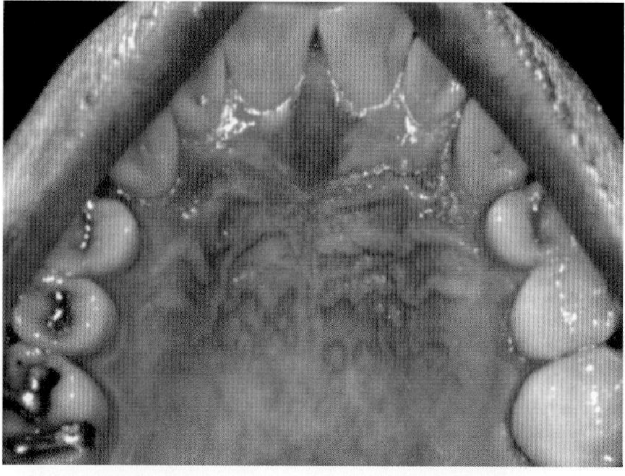

Fig. 7.8A: A clinical picture of palatal rugae

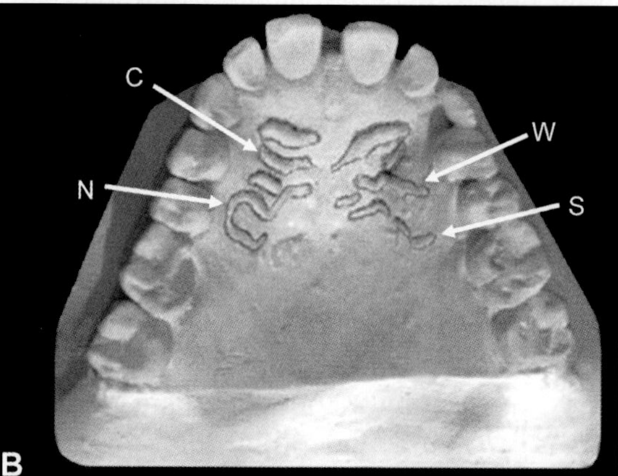

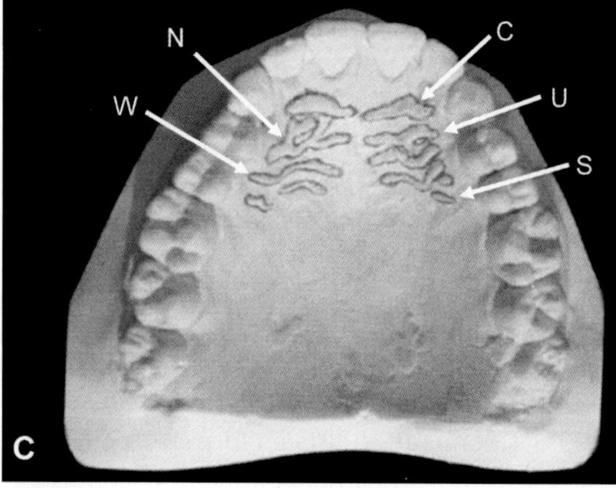

Figs 7.8B and C: Cast showing the palatine rugae

Investigations have been carried out to study the thermal effects and the decomposition changes on the palatal rugae of burn victims with pan facial third degree burns, and have concluded that most victims did not sustain any palatal rugae pattern changes, and when changes were noted, they were less pronounced than in the generalized body state.

Furthermore, the ability of palatal rugae to resist decomposition changes for up to seven days after death was also noted. However, some events can contribute to changes in rugae pattern, including extreme finger sucking in infancy and persistent pressure due to orthodontic treatment.

Nevertheless, in most cases, one must account for palatal rugae persistency. Camargo et al have referred that, in gingival graft surgery, the selection of the palatal donor site should avoid the rugae areas because they may persist in the grafted tissue. However, extractions may produce a local effect on the direction of the rugae. In fact, palatal rugae stability is considered an important factor when teeth are extracted as has been demonstrated in several studies, which point out the stability of the rugae medial points over the lateral points. These features where first noticed in 1967, by Peavy and Kendrick, who said, the closer the rugae are to the teeth, the more prone they are to stretch in the direction that their associated teeth move. In addition to these findings of the importance of using medial points, it has been said that the more posterior rugae are less susceptible to changes with tooth movement, being the third palatal rugae pair in particular the most stable reference. Other studies however, point out that the first rugae is the most stable. Many authors however believe that further studies are needed in order to define which rugae is the most stable. The occurrence, number and arrangement of palatal rugae in mammals are species-specific. In humans they are asymmetrical, which is an exclusive feature of human beings. According to English's studies, palatal rugae patterns are sufficiently characteristic to discriminate between individuals. In fact, these authors found it legitimate to base identification upon their comparison, allowing for human identification even in extreme circumstances.

Palatal Rugae Classifications

The supposed uniqueness and overall stability of palatal rugae suggest their use for forensic identification. Palatal rugae are used in human identification not only due to their singularity and unchangeable nature, but also due to other advantages, namely their low utilization costs. Researchers have found the task of classification a difficult aspect of rugae studies. The subjective nature of observation and interpretation within and between observers poses a problem. Nowadays, there are several known palatal rugae classifications. However, according to several authors, Lysell, in 1955, developed the first classification system for palatal rugae pairs:

Various classification system proposed for Palatoscopy are as outlined below:

A. Carrea classification
B. Martins dos Santos classification
C. Lo´pez de Le´on classification
D. Da Silva classification
E. Trobo classification
F. Basauri classification

Carrea Palatal Rugae Classification

This author divides palatal rugae into four different types, as shown in below **(Table 7.4)**. Palatal rugae are classified only according to their form and no formula (rugogram) is developed.

Martins Dos Santos Classification

Based on the form and position of each palatal rugae, this classification indicates and characterizes the following **(Table 7.5)**:

Table 7.4: Carrea palatal rugae classification

Classification	*Rugae type*
Type I	Posterior- anterior directed rugae
Type II	Rugae perpendicular to the raphe
Type III	Anterior- posterior directed rugae
Type IV	Rugae directed in several directions

Table 7.5: Martins dos Santos classification

Rugae type	*Anterior position*	*Other positions*
Point	P	0
Line	L	1
Curve	C	2
Angle	A	3
Circle	C	4
Sinuous	S	5
Bifurcated	B	6
Trifurcated	T	7
Interrupt	I	8
Anomaly	An	9

One initial rugae; the most anterior one on the right side is represented by a capital letter.

Several complementary rugae; the other right rugae are represented by numbers; One subinitial rugae; the most anterior one on the left side is represented by a capital letter; Several sub-complementary rugae; the other left rugae are represented by numbers. The numbers and letters given to each rugae, relate to its form and can be seen in **Table 7.5**.

Lo´Pez De Le´On Classification

Dating from 1924, this classification has only historic relevance. The author proposed the existence of a link between a person's personality and palatal rugae morphology. In this manner, there were four known types of palatal rugae:
B—Bilious personality rugae;
N—Nervous personality rugae;
S—Sanguinary personality rugae;
L—Lymphatic personality rugae.
The letters B, N, L, and S, stand for the different personalities. The letters l and r stand for the left and right side of the palate, and are followed by a number, which specifies the palatal rugae number on each side. For instances, a possible rugogram would be Br6; Bl8.

Table 7.6: Da Silva palatal rugae classification

Classification	*Rugae type*
1.	Line
2.	Curve
3.	Angle
4.	Circle
5.	Wavy
6.	Point

Table 7.7: Trobo classification

Classification	*Rugae type*
Type-A	Point
Type-B	Line
Type-C	Curve
Type-D	Angle
Type-E	Sinuous
Type-F	Circle

Da Silva Palatal Rugae Classification

In this classification, palatal rugae are divided into two groups: simple, from 1 to 6 and composed, resulting from two or more simple rugae. They are named according to each rugae number. It is possible to classify each ruga individually (describing its form), but also to describe all the palatal rugae system (describing each ruga type number), making this a difficult classification to use **(Table 7.6)**.

Trobo Classification

This classification also divides rugae into two groups: Simple ruga, classified from A to F and composed rugae, classified with the letter X. Composed rugae result from two or more simple rugae unions. The rugogram is made from right to left, beginning with the principal ruga (the one closest to the raphae), which is classified with a capital letter. The following rugae are classified with small letters. Finally, the left side of the palate is described using the same criteria **(Table 7.7)**.

Basauri Classification

Like the Trobo classification, this is a very easy classification to use. It distinguishes between the principal rugae, which is the more anterior one (labeled with letters) and the accessory rugae, which concerns all the remaining rugae (labeled with numbers), as seen in Table. The rugogram is elaborated beginning from the right side of the palate **(Table 7.8)**.

Cormoy System

This system classifies palatal rugae according to their size, in:

1. Principal rugae (over 5 mm);
2. Accessory rugae (ranging from 3 to 4 mm);
3. Fragmental rugae (with less than 3 mm length).

The form (line, curve, and angle), origin (medial extremity) and direction of each ruga are also described. Possible ramifications are also pointed out. Rugae that share the same origin, interrupted rugae and the incisive papilla are described as well. It is a very complete system. However, its use does not lead to rugogram elaboration, which makes the managing and processing of data difficult.

Correia Classification

Rugae are labeled with numbers or letters, according to their form. The rugogram is formed like a fractional equation. The right side is the numerator and the left side is the denominator. The first right and the first left palatal rugae (initial and subinitial rugae) are classified by a letter and the other right and left (complementar and subcomplementar rugae) are assigned numbers.

Table 7.8: Basauri classification

Principal rugae classification	*Accessory rugae classification*	*Rugae anatomy*
A	1	Point
B	2	Line
C	3	Angle
D	4	Sinuous
E	5	Curve
F	6	Circle
X	7	Polymorphic

Palatoscopy in Edentulous Cases

When a victim has no teeth, information for use in personal identification based on methods available in forensic odontology is much more limited than in the case of dentate victims. For edentulous victims, **(Fig. 7.9)** some identification methods are available, such as comparing the anatomy of the Paranasal sinuses and comparing bony patterns seen on radiographs.

Furthermore, the victims' dentures themselves, can provide us with more personal information with regard to denture making, denture materials, and their unique shapes, for use as antemortem data or postmortem evidence **(Fig. 7.10).** Among the evidence taken from an edentulous victim, a palatal rugae pattern is one of the unique and relatively obtainable morphological features, and the pattern can be taken not only directly from the hard palate, but also from the mucosal surface of the dentures.

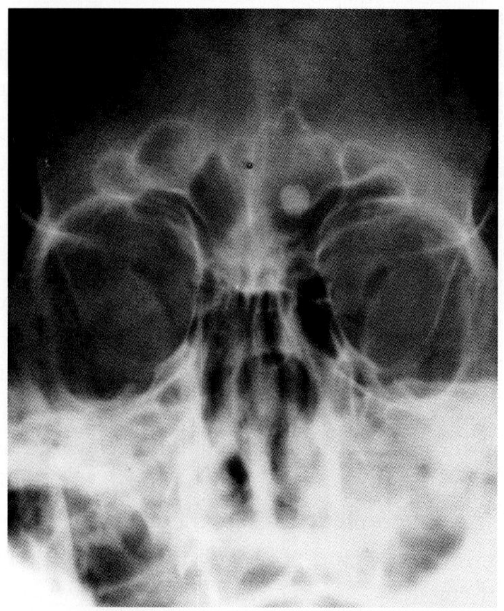

Fig. 7.9: Radiograph of an edentulous patient showing paranasal sinuses

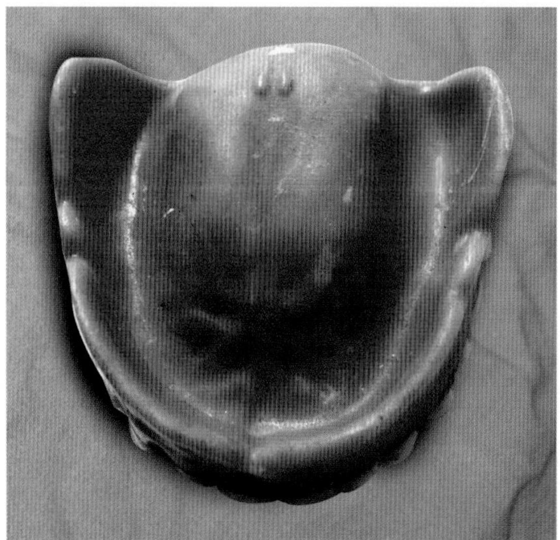

Fig. 7.10: Mucosal surface of maxillary denture showing palatine rugae

Application of palatal rugae patterns to personal ID was 1st suggested by Allen in 1889. Subsequently, its usefulness has mainly been established in dentate cases. In contrast, the usefulness of this method for edentulous victims has not yet been fully established.

Thomas and Wyk proposed the usefulness of rugae pattern for personal identification by comparing its morphological features with the victim's dentures. They successfully identified a severely burnt edentulous body by comparing the rugae to those on the victim's old denture indicating, among other things, that rugae are stable in adult life. However, Jacob and Shalla doubted its usefulness because the accuracy of identification based on palatal rugae tracings was only 79 percent in their trials.

M Ohtani et al in their study analyzed the incidence of obtaining a correct match in such edentulous case, revealed that there were three major misleading shapes that could give rise to a low rate of correct matches; these are:

1. Severely low and poorly demarcated eminences of rugae,
2. Change of palatal height, and
3. Non-complex rugae pattern.

These features are mainly due to the shape of the edentulous palate itself and rarely due to the dentures, and could lead to difficulties in finding unique points for use in matching rugae patterns. These findings as notified by the authors suggest that an appropriate selection of cases, taking into consideration the above misleading shapes, may establish an increased rate of accuracy for identification with this method, thereby bringing the percentage of correct matches closer to 100 in edentulous cases, which is also the percentage of correct matches previously reported in dentate cases.

The use of teeth in postmortem identification has gained prominence over the last half-century; the rugae are well protected by the lips, buccal pad of fat and teeth and hence, survive postmortem insults. Postmortem dental identification is, however, not possible in the edentulous and palatal rugae can be used as a supplement in such instances.

Thus, palatal rugae appear to possess the features of an ideal forensic identification parameter because of their:

1. Uniqueness,
2. Postmortem resistance and
3. Stability

In addition, rugae pattern may be specific to racial groups facilitating population identification (which may be required post-disasters).

Analyzing and Recording Palatal Rugae

There are several ways to analyse palatal rugae. Intraoral inspection is probably the most used and also the easiest and the cheapest. However, it can create difficulties if a future comparative exam is required. A more detailed and exact study, as well as the need to preserve evidence may justify oral photography or oral impressions. Calcorrugoscopy, or the overlay print of palatal rugae in a maxillary cast, can be used in order to perform comparative analysis. Other more complex techniques are also available. By using stereoscopy, for example, one can obtain a three dimensional image of palatal rugae anatomy. It is based on the analysis of two pictures taken with the same camera, from two different points, using special equipment. Another technique is the sterophotogrammetry which, by using a special device called Traster Marker, allows for an accurate determination of the length and position of every single palatal rugae. However, due to its simplicity, price and reliability, the study of maxillary dental casts is the most used technique.

Genetic Influence on Palatal Rugae

Population differences pose the question as to how much is attributable to genetic differences and how much is the result of environmental affects. While intraoral environmental influences such as denture wearing, tooth malposition and palatal pathology are considered to affect rugae pattern, some consider it "very unlikely" that they affect formation of rugae and believe rugae pattern is genetically controlled. Furthermore, twin studies show that rugae pattern has an underlying genetic basis. According to Luke, the rugae develop as localised regions of epithelial proliferation and thickening. Fibroblasts and collagen fibres then accumulate in the connective tissue beneath the thickened epithelium and assume distinct orientation. "The fibres running anteroposteriorly within the core and in concentric curves across the base of each ruga" determine their orientation. It is plausible that certain, as yet unidentified, genes influence orientation of the collagen fibres during embryogenesis and post-natal growth and govern rugae pattern in different populations. Hence, rugae shape may be used as genetic markers for further research on population groups.

Problems with Palatoscopy

Palatoscopy is a technique that can be of great interest in human identification. In fact, contrary to lip prints, it is possible to have antemortem data established such as records found in dental practice in different forms (dental casts, old prosthetic maxillary devices and intraoral photographs). However, palatoscopy might not be so useful in crime scene investigations in the linking of suspects to crime scenes. In fact, this kind of evidence is not expected to be found in such circumstances.

Another aspect of palatoscopy that one must consider is the possibility of rugae pattern forgery. In a case report, Gitto et al. described a method where palatal rugae were added to a complete denture in order to improve speech patterns in some patients. This process can lead to false identity exclusion due to misleading antemortem data.

Future Prospects

As with cheiloscopy, other aspects of palatoscopy have been studied. For instances, Thomas et al. have worked on the possible use of palatal ruga patterns in paternity determination. This possibility was first suggested by Lysell. However, there were no findings to link the two aspects. Kratzsch and Opitz developed a study in cleft patients whose results suggest that palatal rugae, in combination with measuring points of the cleft palate, can serve to depict changes occurring in the anterior palate during various stages of therapy and growth. These findings suggest that some facial changes can be expected when studying specific rugae patterns. Few studies using palatal rugae as a means of forensic identification are found in literature. However, the idea of rugae being unique to an individual is promising and deserves further investigation.

Bibliography

1. Burris BG, Harris EF. Identification of race and sex from palate dimensions, J Forensic Sci. 1998;43(5):959-63.
2. Ehara Y, Marumo Y. Identification of lipstick smears by fluorescence observation and purge-and-trap gas chromatography, Forensic Sci Int. 1998;96:1-10.

3. English WR, Robinson SF, Summitt JB, et al. Individuality of human palatal rugae, J Forensic Sci. 1988;33:718-26.
4. Gitto CA, Exposito SJ, Draper JM. A simple method of adding palatal rugae to a complete denture, J Prosthet Dent. 1999;81;237-9.
5. Ine's Morais Caldas. Review Establishing identity using cheiloscopy and palatoscopy. Forensic Science International. 2007;165:1-9
6. Kaur R, Garg RK. Personal identification from lip prints. Abstracts/Forensic Science International. 2007;169S:S47-S49.
7. Latent Prints Examinations, http://www.fbi.gov/hq/lab/handbook/intro9. html.
8. Lip prints could help forensic science, The Indian Express, http://www. indianexpress.com.
9. Maki Ohtani, et al. Indication and limitations of using palatal rugae for personal identification in edentulous cases. Forensic Science International 2008;176:178-82.
10. Sivapathasundharam B, Prakash PA, Sivakumar G, Lip prints (Cheiloscopy), Ind J Dent Res. 2001;12(4):234-7.
11. Thomas CJ, Rossouw RJ, The early development of palatal rugae in the rat, Aust Dent J 1991;36(5):342-8.
12. Thomas CJ, The role of the denture in identification: a review, J Forensic. Odontostomatol. 1984;2:13-6.
13. Thomas CJ, Van Wyk CW The palatal rugae in an identification, J Forensic Odontostomatol. 1988;6:21-7.

Chapter 8

Forensic Facial Reconstruction

Nitul Jain, Sohail Lattoo, Vishwas Bhatia

Chapter Overview

- Daubert standard
- Theoretic foundations
- Types of identification
- Types of reconstructions
- History
- Technique for creating a three-dimensional clay reconstruction
- Currently used methods
- Problems with facial reconstruction
- Facial reconstruction and the media

INTRODUCTION

Whenever human remains are found, attempts are made to assign these to a definite person. Current methods of identification include odontostomatology (comparison of teeth), DNA analysis, dactyloscopy, and analysis by x-ray comparison. No method of identification offers 100 percent certainty that the parts definitely belong to that person; it cannot be excluded that somewhere in the world there is or was another person who has the same features. At the end of the examination the probability that the identity is correct should always approach 100 percent. When the probability exceeds 99.8 percent, this is referred to as a "probability bordering on certainty".

Forensic facial reconstruction (or forensic facial approximation) is the process of recreating the face of an unidentified individual from their skeletal remains through an amalgamation of artistry, forensic science, anthropology, osteology, and anatomy. It is easily the most subjective—as well as one of the most controversial—techniques in the field of forensic anthropology. Despite this controversy, facial reconstruction has proved successful frequently enough that research and methodological developments continue to be advanced.

All identification methods require comparative data and materials from the person concerned. For DNA analysis and fingerprints, databases exist whose data can be compared against the collected data. If a targeted person's data are, however, not in a file or they have not visited a dentist in the preceding years, then inquiry approaches and morphological investigations have to be used to identify a comparable person. Depending on the extent of decomposition and completeness of the human remains, forensic autopsy or forensic-osteological examination may offer information regarding sex, age, size, proportions, ethnic origin, and habits or diseases.

The face, which has an excess of a hundred individual features, is of great value in recognizing/identifying a person. In unknown dead bodies, a facial photograph is taken, which is sometimes digitally processed, so that it becomes suitable as a portrait image for witnesses to study or for newspapers to publish. For the purposes of legal identification of a dead body—which requires a person to take a look at it, for example, a family member—the face is often the only body part to be uncovered. In many unidentified dead bodies, the face has been rendered unrecognizable to the point of complete skeletization through autolysis, decay, by animals, or other destruction. If the listed methods do not succeed in identifying the body, facial reconstruction may be used as a method of last resort. Here in this chapter, I have tried out to sketch out the historic development of forensic facial reconstruction and critically discuss the different methods and current developments.

In addition to remains involved in criminal investigations, facial reconstructions are created for remains believed to be of historical value and for remains of prehistoric hominids and humans. For example, recently all of us had seen recreation of the face of King Tut's Mummy, **(Fig. 8.1)** the young ruler of Ancient Egypt. Based on an earlier CT Scan of the boy king's mummy, Paris-based forensic sculptor Elisabeth Daynès created a silicon-skinned bust using the previously acquired data and combined it with average traits of today's Egyptians. The CT data was then sent to a US forensic team, who worked to verify the findings, without knowledge of who their subject was. The reconstruction was featured in the June, 2005 issue of National Geographic magazine **(Fig. 8.2)**, in the touring exhibit Tutankhamun and the Golden Age of the Pharaohs, and on the National Geographic Channel's special documentary named King Tut's Final Secrets.

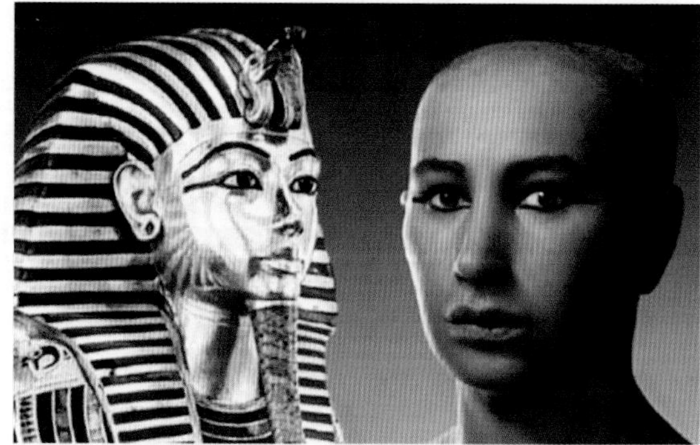

Fig. 8.1: The famous reconstruction of king Tut's face from the ancient recovered mummy

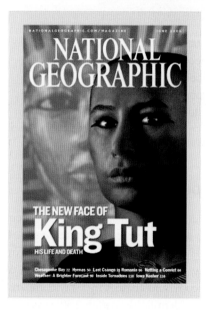

Fig. 8.2: National Geographic magazine, which had first reported the existence of king Tut's mummy

Daubert Standard

In the US, the Daubert Standard is a legal precedent set in 1993 by the Supreme Court regarding the admissibility of expert witness testimony during legal proceedings. This standard was set in place to ensure that expert witness testimony is based upon sufficient facts or data, is the product of reliable principles and/or methods (including peer review), as well as ensuring that the witness has applied the principles and methods reliably to the facts of the case.

When multiple forensic artists produce approximations for the same set of skeletal remains, no two reconstructions are ever the same and the data from which approximations are created are largely incomplete. Because of this, forensic facial reconstruction does not uphold the Daubert Standard, is not included as one of the legally recognized techniques for positive identification, and is not admissible as expert witness testimony. Currently, reconstructions are only produced to aid the process of positive identification in conjunction with verified methods.

Theoretic Foundations

In forensic facial reconstruction, or rather, forensic reconstruction of soft facial parts, the basic premise is that in certain anatomical points of the skull there are definable soft tissue thicknesses. In several studies, these were measured, and the mean thickness for the respective point (so called landmarks) **(Fig. 8.3)** was calculated. The measurements used to be taken on dead bodies, with needles, MRI, or CT.

The imaging methods provided an opportunity to perform measurements in living subjects, to be able to exclude postmortem changes and artifacts.

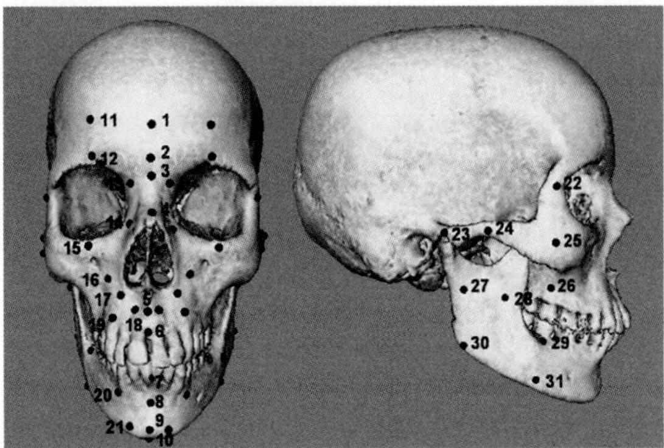

Fig. 8.3: Some of the most important anatomic landmarks used on the skull for facial reconstruction

In living subjects, however, substantial differences in the measurement results were noted depending on the bodily position of the subject. Measurements taken in an upright position on the head and in a seated position are most meaningful, **(Figs 8.4 A and B)**, because they correspond best with the usual position of the head in living persons. Measurements taken in a seated position are possible only by using ultrasonography, whose resolution, however, is limited.

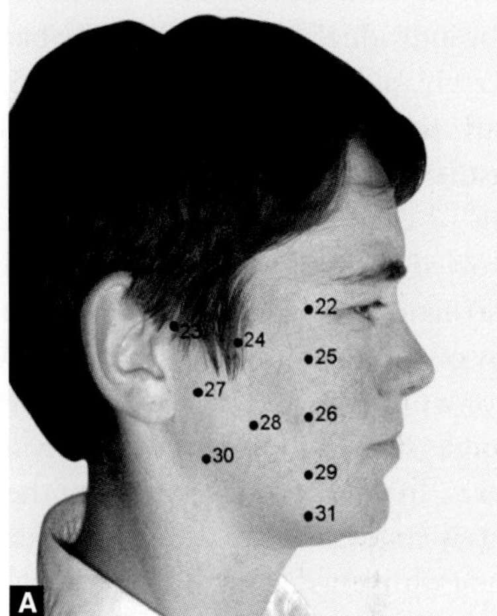

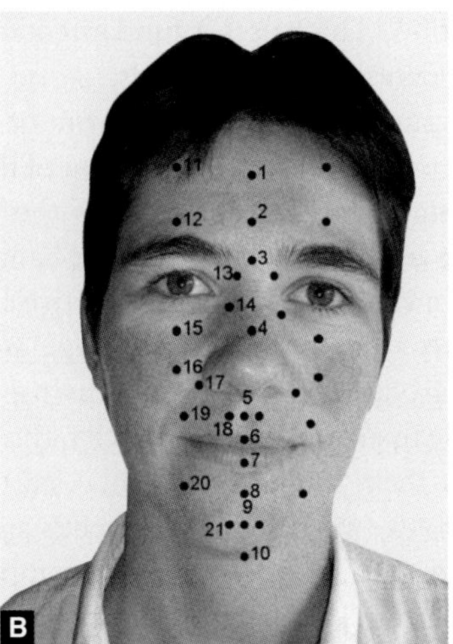

Figs 8.4 A and B: The various soft tissue thickness at specific location used for facial reconstruction

For the training in facial reconstruction, skulls should be used for whom a portrait photograph is available to enable a comparison after the reconstruction has been completed. But an exact reconstruction does not necessarily mean that the model will be recognized as the missing person. If a missing person is identified after the publication of a police search photograph that is based on a facial reconstruction, then the question is what has led to this. If a conspicuous beard or hairstyle, combined with unusual clothing, have been faithfully reproduced in a police search photograph, then the individual face fades into the background. Conversely, a face that has been reconstructed perfectly, to the last detail, but is surrounded by an unsuitable hairstyle, can make recognition difficult or even impossible. Gerasimov is said to have solved nearly 100 percent of cases in 140 reconstructions. The Two dimensional reconstruction of the French national police, which was based on a phantom image, however, did not result in a single successful identification in more than 100 cases. In critical consideration of these results, then it is impossible in the individual case to conclude with any degree of certainty whether the facial reconstruction or other elements of the inquiry have provided the decisive clues for the identification. This poses a fundamental problem in the validation of the methods.

More crucial than technical errors or measurement errors related to the positioning of the subject during data collection, however, is the extent to which the actual value in the case at hand deviates from the mean value for the respective landmark. Further to a person's sex, their age is a highly influential variable. With increasing age, the connective tissues lose their elasticity, the soft facial parts lose their firmness, and they start hanging down in folds/wrinkles. The subject's age is to be taken into consideration in most samples to be investigated. The largest individual influence for the thickness of the soft tissues on the landmarks, however, is due to by the individual's nutritional condition. The problem is, on the one hand, that this has not been taken into consideration during data collection and therefore, this variable cannot be captured statistically. On the other hand, it is difficult in a decomposed or skeletized corpse to determine the dead person's nutritional condition before death.

Types of Identification

There are two types of identification in forensic anthropology: circumstantial and positive.

Circumstantial identification is established when an individual fits the biological profile of a set of skeletal remains. This type of identification does not prove or verify identity because any number of individuals may fit the same biological description.

Positive identification is one of the foremost goals of forensic science, is established when a unique set of biological characteristics of an individual are matched with a set of skeletal remains. This type of identification requires the skeletal remains to correspond with medical or dental records, unique antemortem wounds or pathologies, DNA analysis, and still other means.

Facial reconstruction presents investigators and family members involved in criminal cases concerning unidentified remains with a unique alternative when all other identification techniques have failed. Facial approximations often provide the stimuli that eventually lead to the positive identification of remains.

Types of Reconstructions

Two-dimensional Reconstructions

Two-dimensional facial reconstructions are hand-drawn facial images based on antemortem photographs, and the skull. Occasionally skull radiographs are used but this is not ideal since many cranial structures are not visible or at the correct scale. This method usually requires the collaboration of an artist and a forensic anthropologist. A commonly used method of two-dimensional facial reconstruction was pioneered by Karen T Taylor of Austin, Texas during the 1980s. Taylor's method involves adhering tissue depth markers on an unidentified skull at various anthropological landmarks, then photographing the skull. Life-size or one-to-one frontal and lateral photographic prints are then used as a foundation for facial drawings done on transparent vellum. Recently developed, the FACE and CARES computer software programs quickly produce two-dimensional facial approximations that can be edited and manipulated with relative ease. These programs may help speed the reconstruction process and allow subtle variations to be applied to the drawing, though they may produce more generic images than hand-drawn artwork.

Three-dimensional Reconstructions

Three-dimensional facial reconstructions are either:

A. Sculptures (made from casts of cranial remains) created with modeling clay and other materials.
   or
B. High-resolution, three-dimensional computer images.

Like two-dimensional reconstructions, three-dimensional reconstructions usually require both an artist and a forensic anthropologist. Computer programs create three-dimensional reconstructions by manipulating scanned photographs of the unidentified cranial remains, stock photographs of facial features, and other available reconstructions. These computer approximations are usually most effective in victim identification because they do not appear too picturesque or too artificial.

Superimposition

Superimposition is a technique that is sometimes included among the methods of forensic facial reconstruction. It is not always included as a technique because investigators must already have some kind of knowledge about the identity of the skeletal remains with which they are dealing (as opposed to 2D and 3D reconstructions, when the identity of the skeletal remains is generally completely unknown). Forensic superimpositions are created by superimposing a photograph of an individual suspected of belonging to the unidentified skeletal remains over an X-ray of the unidentified skull. If the skull and the photograph are of the same individual, then the anatomical features of the face should align accurately.

History

It was Mr M Gerasimov (1965), Soviet archeologist and anthropologist who developed the first technique of forensic sculpture.

The article by Grüner offers a good historic overview. Facial reconstruction was preceded by the comparison of skulls with portrait images, for the purposes of identification. In the 19th century, attempts were already made to reconcile found skulls with portrait paintings, albeit in an unsystematic fashion and by using outline sketches.

Welcker (1883) and His (1895) were the first to reproduce three-dimensional facial approximations from cranial remains. Most sources, however, acknowledge His as the forerunner in advancing the technique. His also produced the first data on average facial tissue thickness followed by Kollmann and Buchly who later collected additional data and compiled tables that are still referenced in most laboratories working on facial reproductions today. Facial reconstruction originated in two of the four major subfields of anthropology. In biological anthropology, they were used to approximate the appearance of early hominid forms, while in archaeology they were used to validate the remains of historic figures. In 1964, Gerasimov was probably the first to attempt paleoanthropological facial reconstruction to estimate the appearance of ancient peoples.

Initially, forensic reconstruction of soft facial parts aimed to reconstruct a face for historic skulls. This was also the case for the work of Gerasimov, who used clay to sculpt his faces. He was the first to apply his techniques to forensic investigations. The authorities asked his help in solving the cases of unknown dead bodies whose aspect had been changed beyond any recognition. The facial reconstructions of Gerasimov are reputed to have facilitated recognition and later identification of many victims among the population.

Although students of Gerasimov later used his techniques to aid in criminal investigations, it was Wilton M Krogman who popularized facial reconstruction's application to the forensic field. Krogman presented his method for facial reconstruction in his 1962 book, detailing his method for approximation. Others who helped popularize three-dimensional facial reconstruction include Cherry (1977), Angel (1977), Gatliff (1984), Snow (1979), and Iscan (1986).

The "super projection procedure" was the first purely photographic method: the portrait photograph, a pane of acrylic glass, and the skull marked with landmarks were lined up on an optic bench. The landmarks from the photograph and the lines emanating resulting from this were transferred to the acrylic glass. After removal of the photograph, the skull was adjusted according to the drawings on the acrylic pane. Finally, skull and photograph were photographed in the calculated position on the optic bench. This method was simplified with the help of a procedure whereby two television cameras recorded photograph and skull simultaneously; the images were then projected with a video image mixer. Nowadays, digital image processing is available for the super-projection/superimposition of skulls and portrait photograph.

In 2004, it was noted by Dr Andrew Nelson of the University of Western Ontario, Department of Anthropology that noted Canadian artist Christian Corbet created the first forensic facial reconstruction of an approximate 2,200 year old mummy based on CT and laser scans. This reconstruction is known as the Sulman Mummy project.

Technique for Creating a Three-Dimensional Clay Reconstruction

Note: Because a standard method for creating three-dimensional forensic facial reconstructions has not been widely agreed upon, multiple methods and techniques are used. The process detailed below reflects the method presented by Taylor and Angel from their chapter in Craniofacial Identification in Forensic Medicine, pages 177-185. This method assumes that the sex, age, and race of the remains to undergo facial reconstruction have already been determined through traditional forensic anthropological techniques.

The skull is the basis of facial reconstruction; however, other physical remains that are sometimes available often prove to be valuable. Occasionally, remnants of soft tissue are found on a set of remains. Through close inspection, the forensic artist can easily approximate the thickness of the soft tissue over the remaining areas of the skull based on the presence of these tissues. This eliminates one of the most difficult aspects of reconstruction, the estimation of tissue thickness. Additionally, any other bodily or physical evidence found in association with remains (e.g. jewelry, hair, glasses, etc.) are vital to the final stages of reconstruction because they directly reflect the appearance of the individual in question.

Most commonly, however, only the bony skull and minimal or no other soft tissues are present on the remains presented to forensic artists. In this case, a thorough examination of the skull is completed. This examination focuses on, but is not limited to, the identification of any bony pathologies or unusual landmarks, ruggedness of muscle attachments, profile of the mandible, symmetry of the nasal bones, dentition, and wear of the occlusal surfaces.

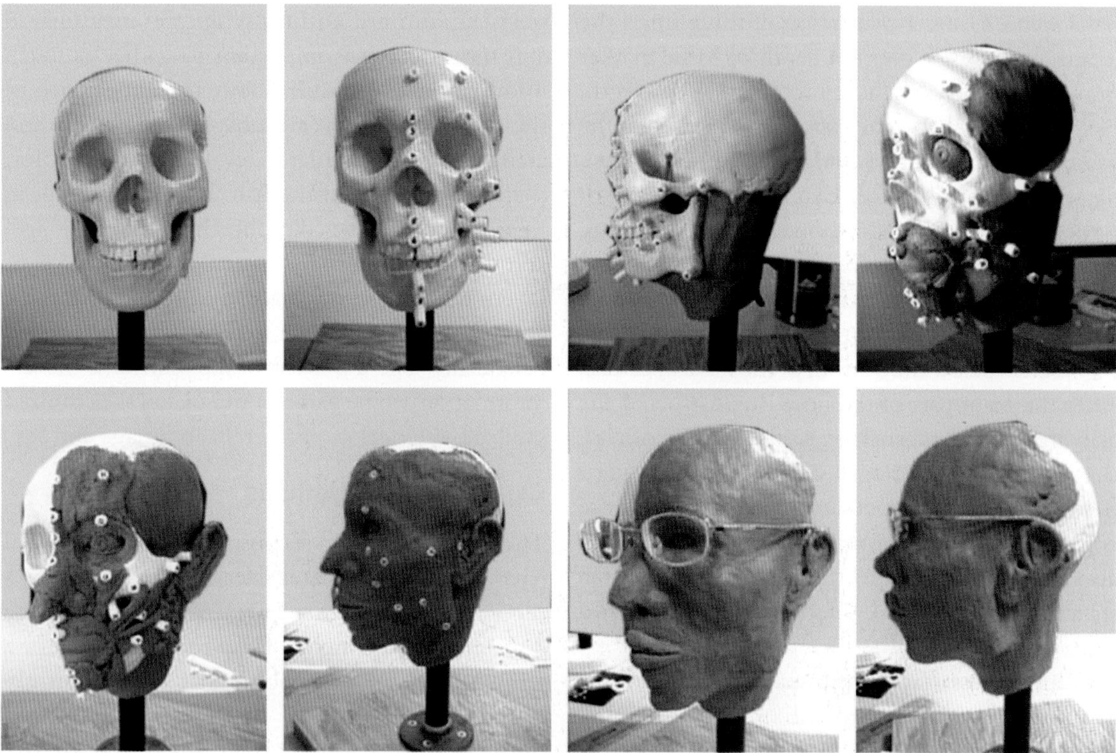

Fig. 8.5: The sequence of events depicting facial reconstruction using clay technique

All of these features have an effect on the appearance of an individual's face.

Once the examination is complete, the skull is cleaned and any damaged or fragmented areas are repaired with wax. The mandible is then reattached, again with wax, according to the alignment of teeth, or, if no teeth are present, by averaging the vertical dimensions between the mandible and maxilla. Undercuts (like the nasal openings) are filled in with modeling clay and prosthetic eyes are inserted into the orbits centered between the superior and inferior orbital rims. At this point, a plaster cast of the skull is prepared. Extensive detail of the preparation of such a cast is presented in the article from which these methods are presented.

After the cast is set, colored plastics or the colored ends of safety matches are attached at twenty-one specific "landmark" areas that correspond to the reference data. These sites represent the average facial tissue thickness for persons of the same sex, race, and age as that of the remains. From this point on, all features are added using modeling clay **(Fig. 8.5)**.

First, the facial muscles are layered onto the cast in the following order: temporalis, masseter, buccinator and occipitofrontals, and finally the soft tissues of the neck. Next, the nose and lips are reconstructed before any of the other muscles are formed. The lips are approximately as wide as the interpupillary distance. However, this distance varies significantly with age, sex, race, and occlusion. The nose is one of the most difficult facial features to reconstruct because the underlying bone is limited and the possibility of variation is expansive. The nasal profile is constructed by first measuring the width of the nasal aperture and the nasal spine. Using a calculation of three times the length of the spine plus the depth of tissue marker number five will yield the approximate nose length. Next, the pitch of the nose is determined by examining the direction of the nasal spine—down, flat, or up. A block of clay, that is the proper length is then placed on the nasal spine and the remaining nasal tissue is filled in using tissue markers two and three as a guide for the bridge of the nose. The alae are created by first marking a point, five millimeters below the bottom of the nasal aperture. After the main part of the nose is constructed the alae are created as small egg-shaped balls of clay, that are five millimeters in diameter at the widest point, these are positioned on the sides of the nose corresponding with the mark made previously. The alae are then blended to the nose and the overall structure of the nose is rounded out and shaped appropriately.

The muscles of facial expression and the soft tissue around the eyes are added next. Additional measurements are made according to race (especially for those with eye folds characteristic of Asian descent) during this stage. Next, tissues are built up to within one millimeter of the tissue thickness markers and the ears (noted as being extremely complicated to reproduce) are added. Finally, the face is "fleshed," meaning clay is added until the tissue thickness markers are covered, and any specific characterization is added (for example, hair, wrinkles in the skin, noted racial traits, glasses, etc.).

Currently Used Methods

Requirements for a Forensic Reconstruction of Soft Facial Parts

The prerequisite for every method used for facial reconstruction is a mostly intact skull, preferably with the lower jaw bone present. If bone injuries or destruction are present, then the skull will have to be reconstructed before the facial reconstruction can take place. Before the reconstruction work can start, the skull and remaining parts of the post-cranium are anthropologically investigated and measured. It is important to gather as much information as possible about the appearance of the deceased from the available human remains and artifacts. Of particular relevance are the color, shape, and length of the hair, beard/facial hair in men, skin color, eye color, height and weight, age, and ethnicity.

For the later model, traces of clothing or hats are also useful. They provide vital clues to the person's personality. The less is left of the individual the less information can be gained. An isolated skeletonized skull allows conclusions merely about age and sex.

Classic Manual Methods

The aim of forensic reconstruction of soft facial parts can be formulated clearly: it is to create a recognizable image of a missing person. The assessment of a concrete facial reconstruction or a whole method is problematic. A seemingly objective method is the comparison of a photograph of the person with that of the reconstruction, after successful identification has taken place. For the classic manual techniques, several studies exist that have shown a good consistency between the reconstruction, their reproduceability, and the actual looks of the person. Such results are so far lacking for computer aided methods. Basically, the classic manual methods allow application of the soft facial parts that are to be reconstructed directly on to the skull in the form of clay, wax, or synthetic substances. Such an approach, however, has to be rejected from an ethics perspective if a funeral is planned after successful identification. In all cultures and belief systems, the head is a central element of the body.

The standard procedure is therefore to cast the skull as a first step. Silicone is most suitable for this. Using the templates produced in this manner, the skull is cast in synthetic material or plaster. The resulting skull model then forms the basis for the reconstruction of the soft facial parts. The skull model is then marked with landmarks and the distance holders fixed on to these, whose lengths reflect the average soft tissue thickness above the respective landmark **(Figs 8.4A and B).**

In the so called *Manchester method*, the face is reconstructed from the musculature step by step with clay **(Figs 8.6A to E)**. The muscular tracks on the bone indicate whether the musculature was more or less strongly developed. Glass eye models are inserted into the eye sockets. After the musculature has been completed, the epidermis, glands, and skin are applied according to their anatomic position. For this step, the nutritional condition and the biological age of the person are essential for deciding the thickness of the layer. This information, combined with the extent to which the facial muscles were developed, helps the person doing the reconstruction to decide whether to intentionally exceed or undercut the soft tissue thickness that are indicated on the landmarks with distance holders. After subsequent smoothing and sculpting of the skin, a sculpture-like face has been created.

In the "*American method*" the soft parts are applied at first in the shape of ribbons in the area of the spacer device. The spaces in between are filled in subsequently. This method also offers flexibility with regard to the shaping of the nutritional condition, but the influences of the facial muscles cannot be taken into consideration as in the Manchester method.

The sculpture-like head model (crude model) has to be furnished with a skin color and hair, and maybe a beard. The head thus constructed can be photographed on its own or on a body model wearing the clothes of the deceased. The result: a photograph that can be used in the police search. Using the reconstructed head, several variations of hair and clothing may be undertaken and documented by photography.

Classic manual forensic reconstruction of soft facial parts is labor intensive and therefore cost intensive for the client. Even a practiced craftsman will take a minimum of 40 hours.

Graphic Methods

To undertake facial reconstruction in the sense of a phantom drawing, detailed anatomic knowledge of the head will have to be combined with artistic skills. The three dimensional reconstruction of the soft facial parts occurs in the mind of the investigator, who puts on paper the image of the person he is reconstructing. This method is fast but can hardly be checked and largely depends on the individual skill of the investigator.

Computer Aided Reconstruction of the Soft Facial Parts

With regard to the enormous expenditure in terms of time for manual forensic reconstruction of the

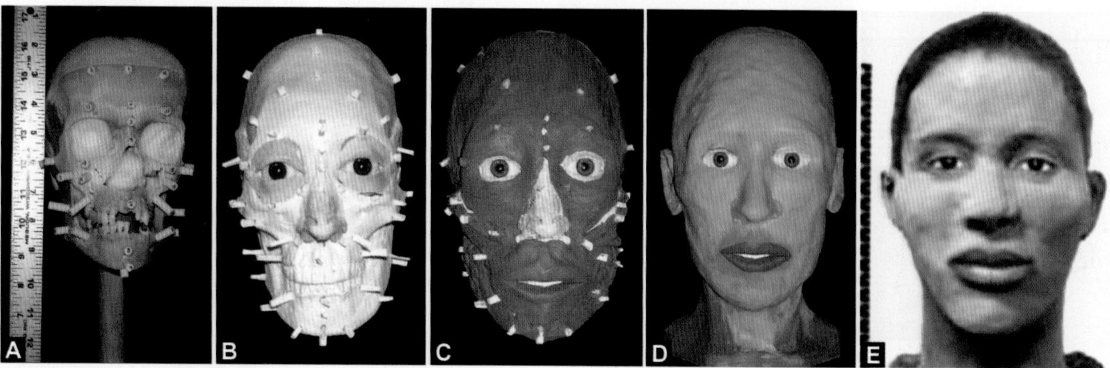

Fig. 8.6A to E: Pictures showing step-wise process in developing a face from the skull

soft facial parts on the one hand and the ever increasing capabilities of computers on the other hand, it is understandable that there is a desire to develop a fast, efficient, and cost effective computer aided forensic facial reconstruction tool. Improved objectivity is another desirable effect that is hoped for.

The three dimensional digital capture of the skull is the first step. Mostly, a surface scanner or a CT scan is used for this (**Fig. 8.7**). This step is faster than making a real copy of the skull. The soft facial parts have to be applied to the virtual skull copy. Most methodological approaches are based on the experiences of classic forensic reconstruction of the soft facial parts. Usually, the same landmarks with their respective soft tissue thickness are used.

Programs have already been developed that place the landmarks automatically, but this often leads to gross mistakes. Therefore, such programs have the capability to manually correct the landmarks or place them primarily manually. These steps are much more labor intensive than fixing the spacer to the landmarks of the real skull copy.

After the virtual anchoring of the landmarks and their spacers, the ends of the landmarks are joined together and the spaces in the resulting lattice pattern filled in and the edges smoothed over. Depending on how powerful the computer is, digital reconstruction of the soft facial parts can

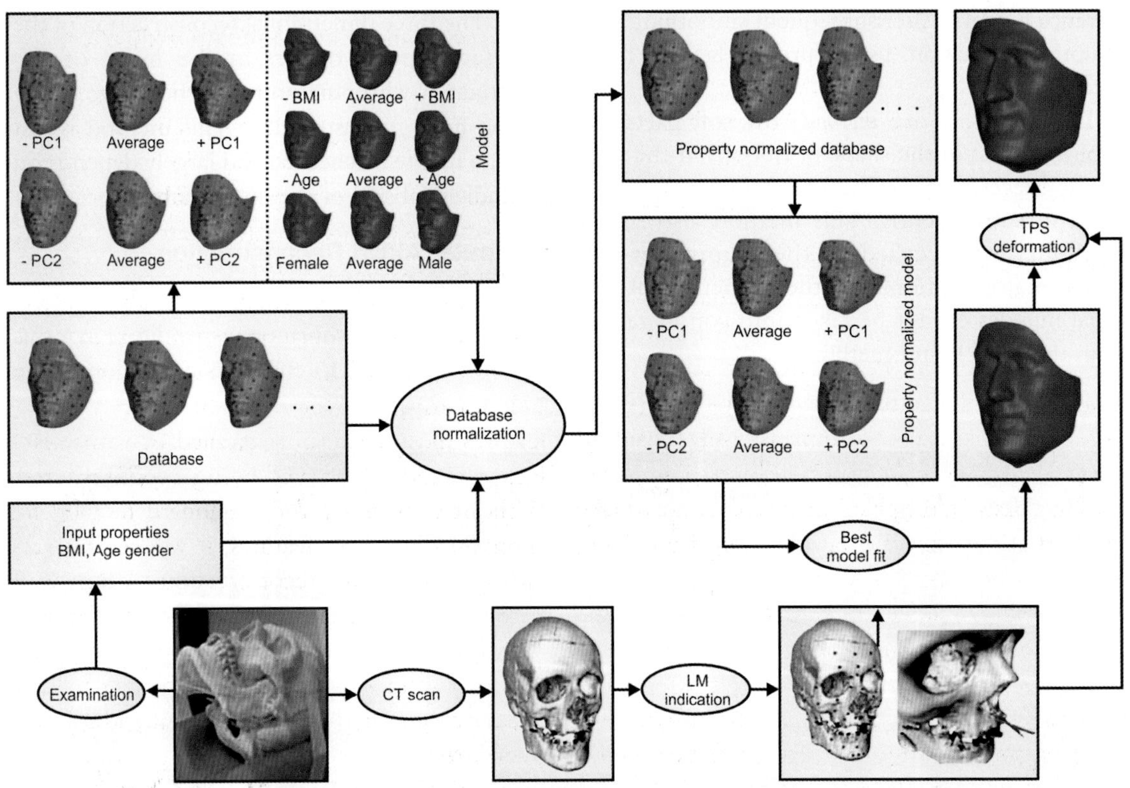

Fig. 8.7: The computerized technique using MRI, CT Scan and computer database to visualize the face from skull

be achieved in seconds. The problem is that the resulting faces do not have any individual features and are reminiscent of an adversary in a computer game rather than a real person. On this background, attempts are currently being made to establish methods that enable the investigator to use several methods for the reconstruction. For example, it is being attempted to undertake the virtual facial reconstruction on screen step by step, just as in the classic manual methods. This takes more time, but the advantage is that as many intermediate steps can be saved as desired, and steps can be repeated or used in a different variation.

Another approach that several working groups have trialed entails correlating morphometric and morphological skull variables with existing phantom images (for example, from the German federal criminal office or the French national police), in order to produce an automatic phantom image of the unknown skull. Such a file then contains a certain number of portrait photographs (frontal aspect), whose individual facial components (for example, the nose, ears, or mouth) can be used in isolation and combined into new faces. This way, phantom images can be put together according to witness statements.

The use of such phantom image data for facial reconstruction has, however, fundamental weaknesses. A three dimensional structure (face) based on another three dimensional entity (skull) is being reconstructed two dimensionally (phantom image) without an intermediate step. The image data as a basis for the phantom image file are usually (at least at the time of data collection) from living persons, whose skull shape is unknown.

Critically, in some cases, the phantom image method is being aggressively promoted with the argument that it is faster and more cost effective than the conventional method. For the prosecution or the police, the lure of having a facial reconstruction at a fraction of the usual cost and achieving a result within very few days is quite understandable.

Problems with Facial Reconstruction

Insufficient Tissue Thickness Data

There are multiple outstanding problems associated with forensic facial reconstruction. The most pressing issue relates to the data used to average facial tissue thickness. The data available to forensic artists are still very limited in ranges of ages, sexes, and body builds. This disparity greatly affects the accuracy of reconstructions. Until this data is expanded, the likelihood of producing the most accurate reconstruction possible is largely limited.

Lack of Methodological Standardization

A second problem is the lack of a methodological standardization in approximating facial features and individuating characteristics. Forensic anthropologists and artists have published individual techniques used in their own practices. However, a single, official method for reconstructing the face has yet to be recognized. This also presents major setback in facial approximation because facial features like the eyes and nose and individuating characteristics like hairstyle—the features most likely to be recalled by witnesses—lack a standard way of being reconstructed. Without consistency and a standard method for approximating these features, it will remain very difficult for forensic reconstruction to earn wide recognition as a legitimate form of forensic identification. Recent research on computer-assisted methods, which take advantage of digital image processing, pattern recognition, promises to overcome current limitations in facial reconstruction and linkage.

Subjectivity

Reconstructions only reveal the type of face a person may have exhibited because of artistic subjectivity. The position and general shape of the main facial features are mostly accurate because they are greatly determined by the skull, but subtle details like certain wrinkles, birthmarks, skin folds, the shape of the nose and ears, etc. are unavoidably speculative **(Fig. 8.8)** because skeletal remains leave no evidence of their appearance. The success of reconstruction depends as much upon the circumstances pertaining to the subject under investigation as it does upon the accuracy of the technique.

Facial Reconstruction and the Media

In historic skulls, the idea of being able to look into a face from a long gone past and thus into another world, is particularly attractive. In addition to the necessary authenticity, the most important target variable is presumably in the field of esthetics.

For example, the facial reconstruction of Tutankhamun as shown on the cover of National

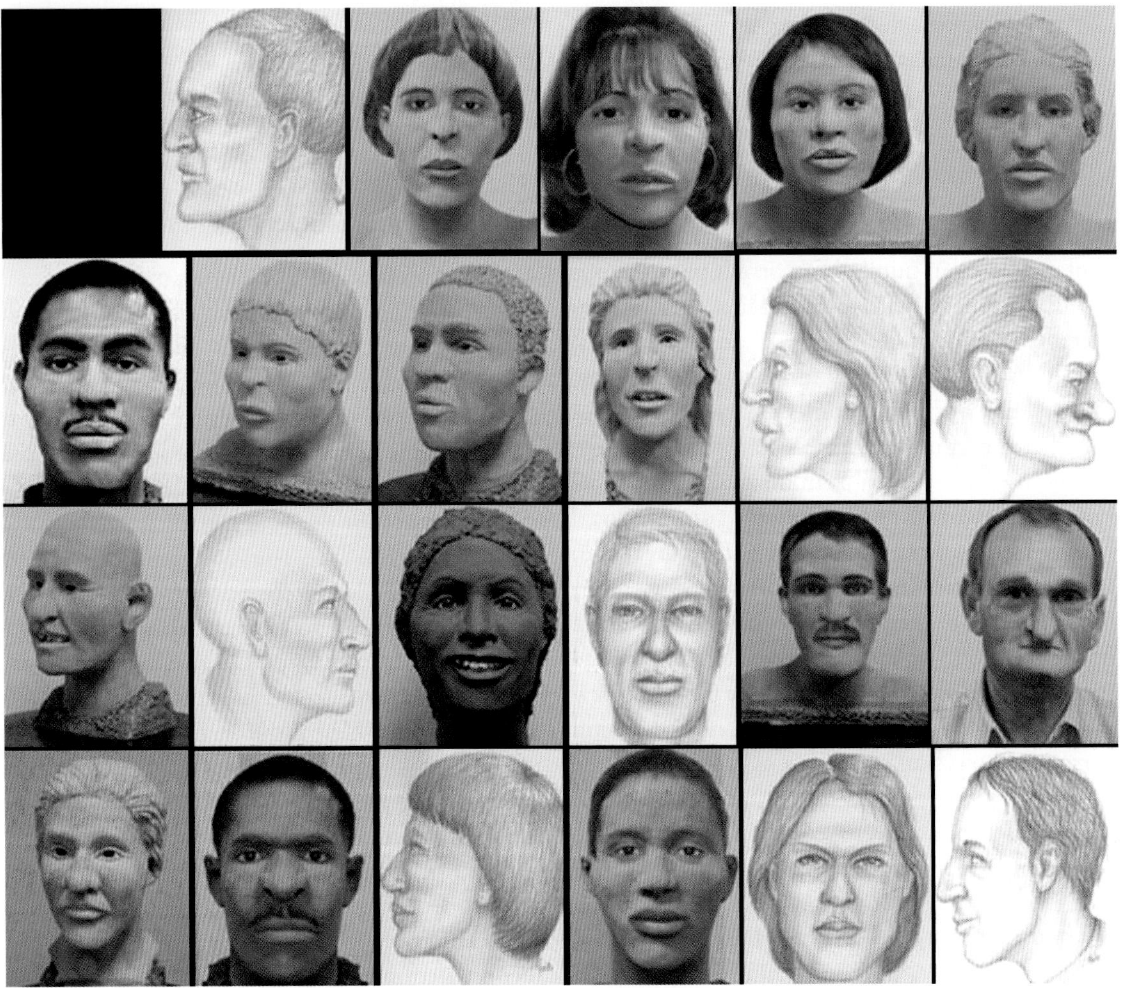

Fig. 8.8: The composite picture showing the facial subjectivity in process of facial reconstruction

Geographic in 2005 has gained an excessive media attention.

Due to the recent rise in popularity of television shows (e.g. CSI: Crime Scene Investigation, CSI: Miami, CSI: NY, NCIS, Bones, and the UK programme Meet the Ancestors) and feature films concerned with criminal investigations, forensics, and law enforcement, the presence of forensic facial reconstructions in the entertainment industry and the media has also increased. The way the fictional criminal investigators and forensic anthropologists utilize forensics and facial reconstructions are, however, often misrepresented, an influence known as the "CSI effect". For example, the fictional forensic investigators will often call for the creation of a facial reconstruction as soon as a set of skeletal remains is discovered. In reality, facial reconstructions are widely used as a last resort to stimulate the possibility of identifying a victim.

In conclusion, the classic methods of forensic reconstruction on the facial soft parts—if done carefully—offer an opportunity to recreate the missing face to a skull. For the appearance of the face, other components play a part in addition to the soft parts: hairstyle and beard, skin color, and clothing. The manual, computer aided methods provide a chance to alleviate the workload and improve speed for the future. However, they need to be used by morphologically versed investigators if not interdisciplinary teams. Practicing the manual methods will be indispensable in learning the morphologic fundamentals/basics now and for the future.

Bibliography

1. Kreutz K, Marcel A Verhoff. Review article: Forensic facial reconstruction – Identification based on skeletal findings. Dtsch Arztebl. 2007;104(17): A1160-5
2. S De Greef, et al. Large-scale in-vivo Caucasian facial soft tissue thickness database for craniofacial reconstruction/Forensic Science International. 2006;159S:S126-S146

Chapter 9

Mass Disaster Victim Identification and Dentist's Role

Ajay Telang, Anil Pandey

Chapter Overview

- What is a disaster and a mass fatality incident?
- Kinds of disaster
- Need for the preparedness
- The ways a dentist can be of help in case need arises in disaster management
- Preparation for unfortunate disasters and protocols
- Role of dentists in mass disaster forensics
- Phases of response
- The standard operating procedures
- Chain of custody
- Evidence collection and preservation
- Dental records and mass disasters
- Man made disasters
- Dental radiography in mass disasters

What is a Disaster and a Mass Fatality Incident?

A disaster is a sudden occurrence that exceeds the resources available in a community to deal with it. A mass fatality incident is an occurrence that causes loss of life that exceeds death investigation resources in a community. A disaster contingency plan identifies and develops plans to use such resources should the need arise.

In India, we come across such kind of disasters very often, which may take any shape and can cause loss of life in any proportion, be it the terrorist evoked bombings, natural flood/earthquakes or train mishaps/accidents. These horrifying incidences cause a great loss of life leaving behind many of the family members grieving and economically unstable. This chapter particularly draws attention of dentist to the various events and happening, where they can provide some sort of help to the various authorities in resolution of the aftermath effects.

Kinds of Disaster

Basically they can be divided into three broader categories **(Figs 9.1 A to E).** The initial response as well as the management of each kind of disaster is slightly different, in terms of various protocols and rules to be followed. These are:

Natural: Tsunami, volcanic eruptions, floods, cyclones, earthquakes

Accidental: Mine explosion, plane/train crashes, fires, unusual calamities

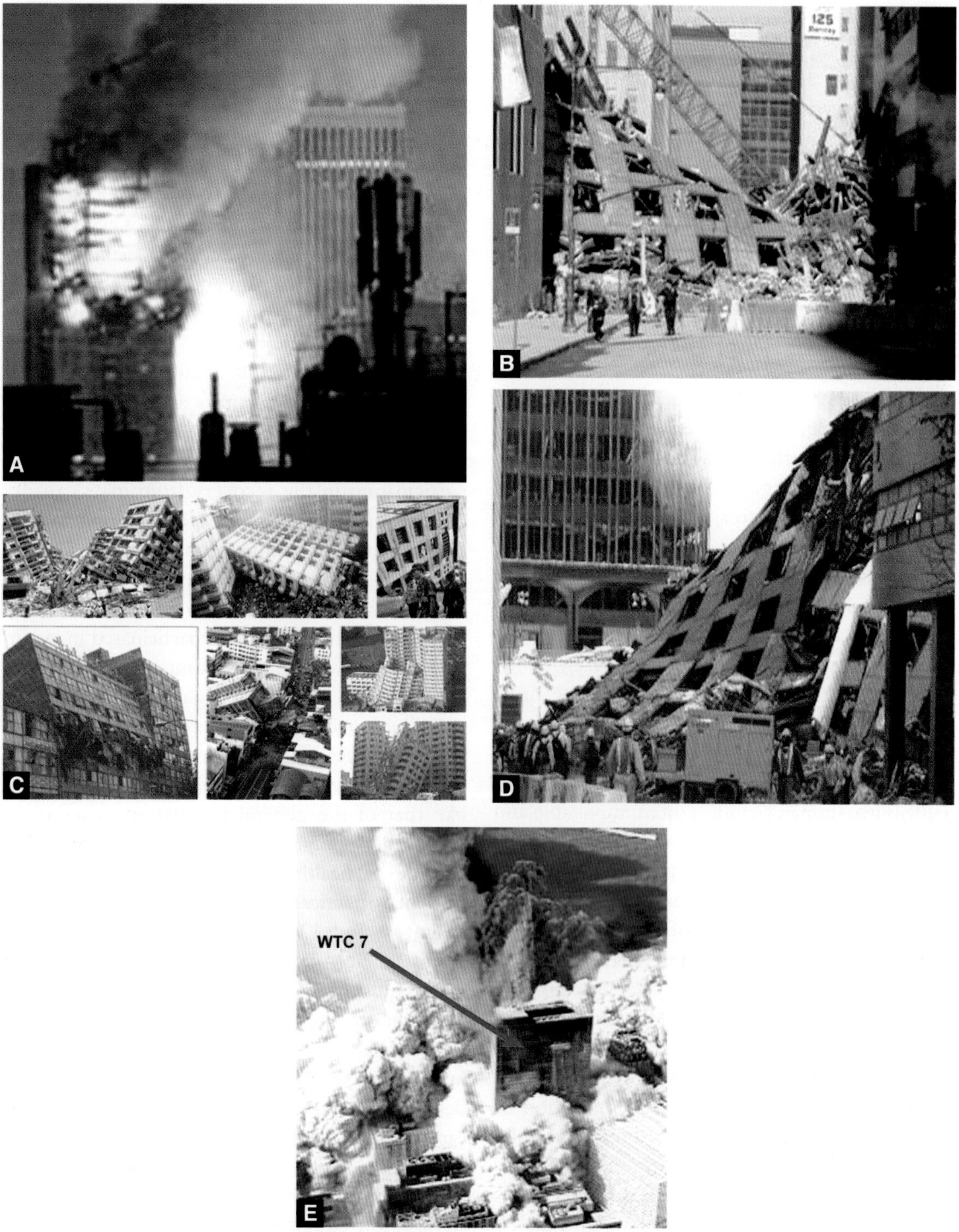

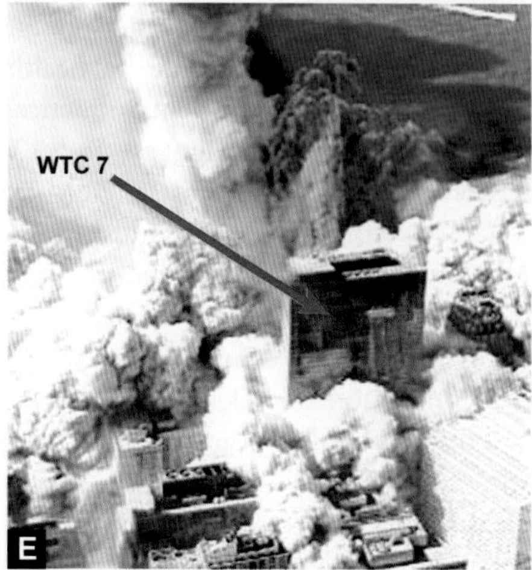

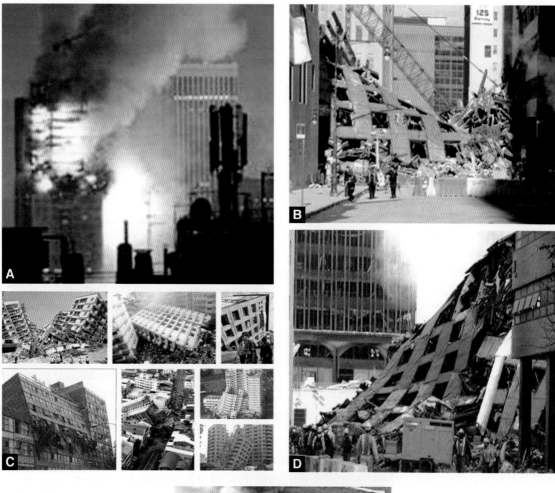

Figs 9.1A to E: Various kinds of disasters; man made, natural and terrorist evoked

Terrorism and military evoked: Bomb explosions, military attacks, serial killings.

Teamwork and planning are two overlying principles crucial to disaster management. Dental team preplanning includes training, formal agreements with medical examiner, supply sources and immunizations. Dental teams are generally included in the operations sections under the mortuary services branch in the identification group in the identification processing unit.

Need for the Preparedness

Mass disasters represent a significant challenge for dental personnel who are frequently called upon to provide identifications. Recently-published materials have highlighted the need to prepare such groups for the disaster challenge and report inadequacies in existing preparation methods with an emphasis on team integration, organization and the psychological and emotional effects of such work.

In the last few decades, identification by dental means has been described as one of the most reliable methods for identification of victims in mass disasters and when one individual must be identified. Visual recognition of facial features in badly burnt human victims is often impossible and identification by fingerprints may not be possible due to the degree of destruction of the bodies. Dental identification may be based on pathological conditions, disturbances of tooth eruption, malocclusions and on dental treatment. The identity of an individual may be established on the basis of the uniqueness of concordant ante and postmortem dental features. A comparison between antemortem records and postmortem findings may thus often lead to identification or provide convincing proof to rule out a particular identity.

Also, it is evident from recent catastrophic events that the traditional medical care system may be overwhelmed because many medical centers operate close to capacity on a daily basis. Add the generation of mass casualties by a major incident or a significant bioterrorism attack into the equation, and a basic life-saving response by the existing medical care system becomes nearly impossible. There is a need to marshal all available resources in response to a disaster of great magnitude if losses and disruption of everyday life are to be minimized and recovery facilitated.

Professionals who plan and manage emergency responses must reach out to groups that have assets to contribute to the response effort but are not intrinsically tied to the medical response (e.g. hospital personnel). Dentists and dental staff are examples of such groups. For a long time, dentistry has played a well-acknowledged role in participating in the recovery from mass casualty events, such as natural disasters, bombings, and transportation accidents, primarily in the forensic identification of victims when identities can not be established by conventional means. Some individual dentists also have participated in victim rescue and treatment. For the most part, the dental profession is a loosely organized network of individual practitioners. There are approximately 175,000 professionally active dentists in the United States, and they are distributed in a manner much like that of the general population. They own, equip, and supply the office facilities in which they provide oral health care. Approximately 85 percent of dental practices in the United States are solo practices, and 11 percent are made up of two dentists. The consolidation that has characterized many industries and businesses in the United States, including medicine has not occurred in dentistry. Only a small proportion of dental care is provided in a hospital setting. In contrast to medicine, most dental care is provided to patients by one primary care dentist in one facility. The average dental office is essentially a mini-hospital or an outpatient clinic. It is equipped with radiographic capability, sterilization equipment, central suction, medical gasses and various anesthesia capabilities, suites with surgical lighting, some surgical equipment and supplies, laboratory space, and administrative areas for records and patient reception. Trained and experienced office staff are present to operate in these areas. Dental offices are dispersed throughout the community.

Dentists are exposed to information in many general medical areas during their predoctoral education that can be useful in disaster response situations. They also routinely perform many tasks that emergency responders may be required to do, such as perform minor surgery, dispense drugs, give injections, and administer anesthesia. It should be apparent from this description that dentistry has much to contribute to the response to a major disaster in terms of personnel and facilities when the traditional medical care system in an area is overwhelmed.

After the seminal events that occurred in the fall 2001, particularly the deliberate attempts to spread weapons-grade *Bacillus anthracis* spores **(Figs 9.2A and B)** through the US mail system, the American Dental Association convened two workshops to determine how dentistry could contribute to the response to mass casualty disasters and how dentistry could become better prepared to respond.

It is generally thought that dentistry can be of greatest assistance immediately after the occurrence of a mass disaster before the full force of federal assistance can be mobilized effectively. During recent disasters, this mobilization time varied from a few days to a week. Many victims of disasters cannot wait that long for help. When local medical resources are unable to cope adequately with a huge number of victims, dentists can be recruited to provide certain services that will allow physicians to do things only they can do. Dentists can enhance the surge capacity of the local medical system until additional physicians arrive or the demand for immediate care decreases.

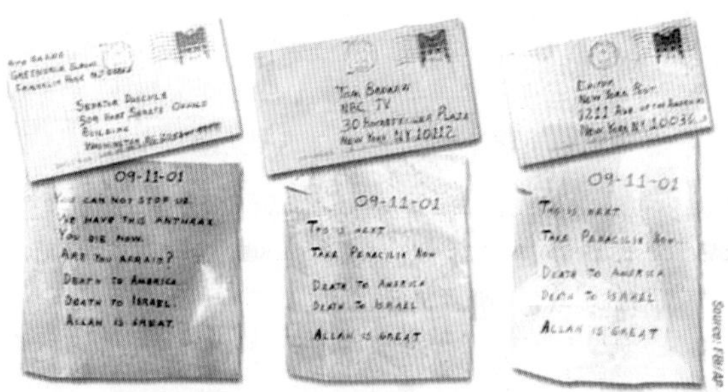

Fig. 9.2A: Postal letters containing anthrax spores which created havoc in United States postal departments

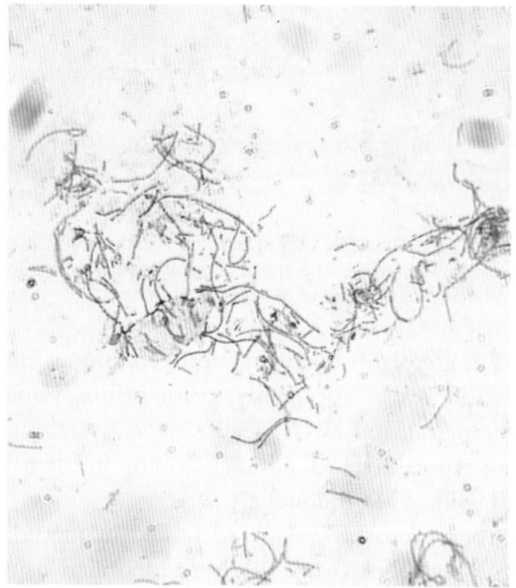

Fig. 9.2B: Microscopic picture of anthrax spores recovered from the postal letters in United States

The Historical Perspective

Case report 1: "The Alfred P Murrah Federal Building bomb blast, **(Fig. 9.3)** Oklahoma City on April 19, 1995".

It has always been considered as the Gold Standard of disaster response. The forensic teams worked for 16 days × 12 hours shifts daily, because of whom 168 confirmed victims and 168 positive identifications were made. Out of these cases, 45 cases were identified on the basis of Dental identifications, 77 cases by a combined Dental ID

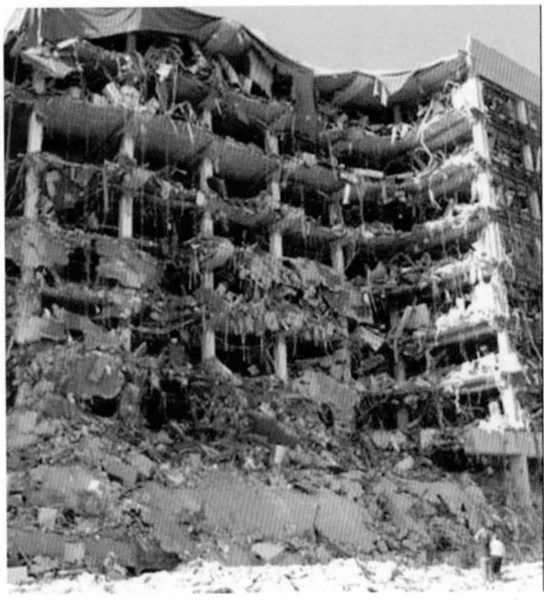

Fig. 9.3: The Alfred P Murrah building explosion in City of IOWA, United States. This mass disaster is referred to Gold standard in mass disaster management

and fingerprints identification techniques and Remainders by footprints, palm prints, visual, radiological, and DNA means.

Case report 2: Horrendous bombing incident in Bali, **(Fig. 9.4)** Indonesia.

There were 115 people identified by methods including DNA, while 12 were identified using fingerprints. About 100 were identified by methods including dental records, and 7 identified by methods including medical records. Searches were made, using the DNA profile, for varying levels of kinship such as parents, children or siblings.

Case report 3, Asian tsunami December 2004 **(Figs 9.5 A and B).**

In the Asian tsunami of 2004, dental records contributed to nearly 85 percent of the identifications. The tsunami provides an example of the problems that can arise in a forensic response to a mass disaster. This case involved over 200,000 dead and injured persons. Nearly 60 nations were represented in the victims, and ten nations were affected by the disaster. Disaster relief came from

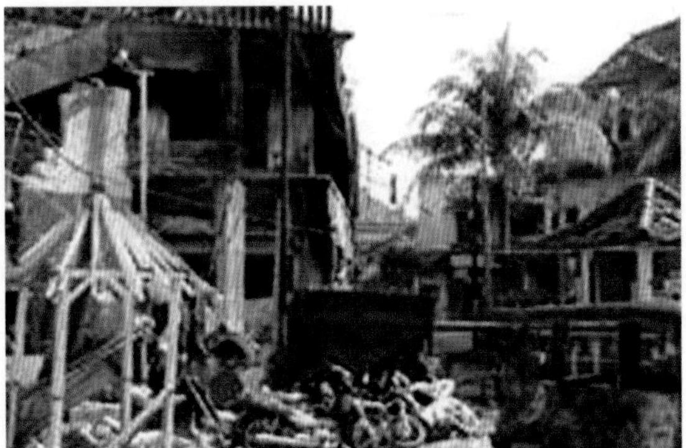

Fig. 9.4: Pictures showing the incidence of bomb explosions in Bali, Indonesia.

around the world, and victim identification teams were sent from more than 20 countries, necessitating the adoption of universal protocols before evidence collection and analysis.

In another example, the USS Iowa explosion, 45 of 47 victims were identified through dental comparison either alone or in conjunction with fingerprint matching. Because the victims were active duty military personnel, high quality, up-to-date dental records were easily available, providing optimum circumstances for dental comparisons to be completed.

The crash of Arrow Airways Flight 950 near Gander Airport in Newfoundland, Canada provides a contrast to the ideal operational conditions in the USS Iowa investigation. As in the previous case, forensic odontology contributed to a significant number of the nearly 250 US Army personnel identifications; however, unlike in the USS Iowa explosion, the servicemen were carrying their medical and dental records during the flight. The Armed Forces Institute of Pathology was charged with the identification of the victims. The team consisted of 23 armed forces dental officers and 16 support staff. One subgroup of these personnel, the dental registrar, was charged with the receipt, inventory, and custody of all obtained medical records. Because the primary dental records were mostly fragmented or destroyed in the crash, records were obtained from civilian sources.

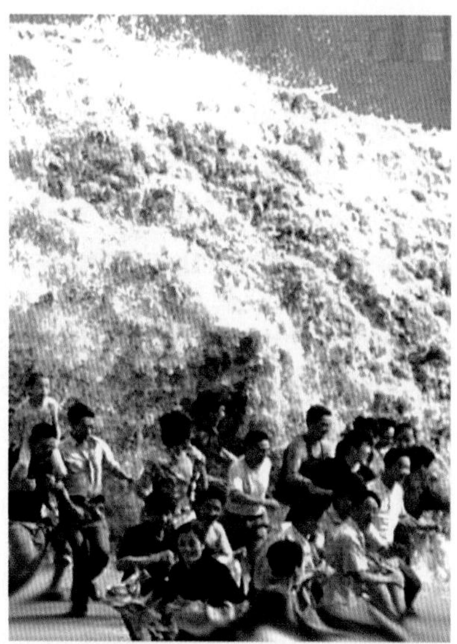

Fig. 9.5A: The most devastating Asian Tsunami, in December 2005, which killed lakhs of people across the world

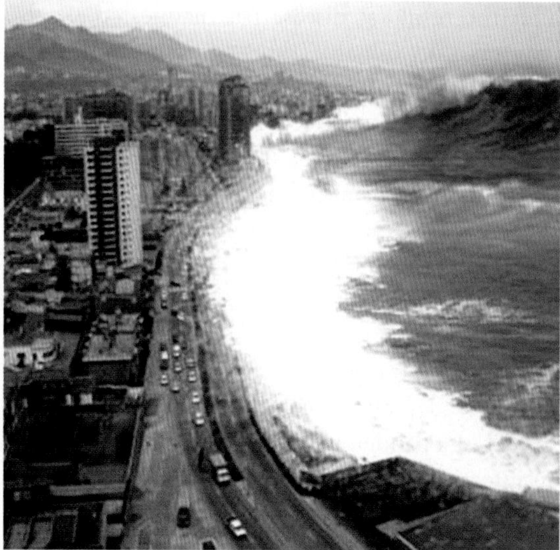

Fig. 9.5B: The photograph showing the killer waves of Tsunami

Forensic dentistry has provided victim identification in many different scenarios involving many different types and numbers of victims. As the result of a major highway accident in Spain in 1996, 28 victims were processed, and 16 of the victims were identified through dental records. The remaining 12 were not owing to extensive destruction of the dentition by fire or a lack of dental records.

The Ways a Dentist can be of Help in Case Need Arises in Disaster Management

The prime purpose of recruiting the assistance of dentists in responding to mass casualty incidents is to enable crisis managers to use scarce physician resources in the most effective manner possible by having some services they would ordinarily provide be successfully provided by dentists where possible. Local circumstances (i.e. the medical needs and resources of the community after a disaster and the nature of the disaster) determine how dentists can be of assistance. Some assigned duties do not tax the dentist's knowledge or experience (e.g. dispensing medications or immunizations), whereas others may require additional training or some supervision (e.g. providing basic medical care in quarantine situations). There are several general areas of response activity in which dentists can be helpful. These are:

1. Surveillance
2. Referral of patients
3. Diagnosis and monitoring
4. Triage
5. Immunizations
6. Medications
7. Infection control
8. Definitive treatment
9. Quarantine.

Surveillance: Some mass casualty events are distinct entities easily recognized and of easily defined duration and effect on a population (e. g. a severe weather event). Other disasters, particularly bioterrorism attacks and pandemics, often have relatively indistinguishable beginnings and ends and unpredictable effects on a population. Because of the variable incubation periods of infectious agents, the time of exposure can be estimated only after the resultant disease has manifested. It also may take up valuable time to determine that a population-wide problem actually exists. Dentists can be part of an effective surveillance network because they are scattered throughout a community much as the general population is and are visited by patients who are generally medically healthy and have not seen a physician. Observation of intra-oral or cutaneous lesions or both when they are present and the notification of public health authorities about these observations may facilitate the early detection of a bioterrorism attack or spread of a pandemic infection. Early detection of an infectious agent in a population may allow for reduction in the number of casualties by prompt initiation of preventive and therapeutic intervention.

Sales of over-the-counter medications are often monitored in the epidemiology community as a potential early warning of community-wide infections. Monitoring of unusual and unexplained "no show" patients in dental offices also may help provide an early warning.

Referral of patients: Patients who show early signs or symptoms of infectious diseases, have suspicious cutaneous lesions, or are suspected of having such diseases may be referred to a physician for a definitive diagnosis and appropriate treatment, if necessary. This referral may be important because early treatment or early initiation of prophylaxis can have a significant influence on the outcome of the patient's encounter with the disease. The clinical course of smallpox, for example, can be ameliorated by vaccination even after the patient has been infected.

Diagnosis and monitoring: After an infectious disease that causes mass casualties has been identified, dentists who are able to recognize the signs and symptoms of that disease may be able to identify afflicted patients. Dentists can collect salivary samples, nasal swabs, or other specimens when appropriate for laboratory processing that may yield valuable diagnostic information or indication of the progress of treatment, including the status of the patient's infectiousness.

Triage: In the effective response to any mass casualty event a system must be established to prioritize treatment among casualties, because immediate treatment for all casualties is not possible because of inadequate resources in personnel, facilities, and medical supplies. Dentists are able to assist in this important function with relatively little additional training. This assistance allows physicians to provide definitive care for patients most urgently in need rather than screening casualties. Dental offices could serve as triage centers if needed.

Immunizations: To limit the spread of infectious agents, whether from a natural pandemic, a deliberate bioterrorism attack, or contamination as a result of a local event, rapid immunization of great numbers of individuals may be required in a short amount of time. In major metropolitan areas, where the spread of communicable disease is facilitated, this effort may involve millions of people. Physicians and nurses may be unable to implement such a program in the critical time frame required. Dentists can participate in mass immunization programs with a minimum of additional training and may be the critical factor in the success of urgent programs. Dental offices can be used as immunization sites to minimize the concentration of potentially infected persons.

Medications: In mass casualty situations, particularly after a bioterrorism attack or the unfolding of a pandemic infection, the population may require medication to treat or prevent the manifestation of the infection being faced. Physicians, nurses, and pharmacists may not be able to effectively prescribe or dispense the medications necessary in the critical, appropriate time required. Dentists can be called on to prescribe and dispense the medications required after that determination has been made by the physicians and public health officials managing the disease outbreak. Dentists also can monitor patients for adverse reactions and side effects and refer patients who experience untoward effects from the medications to physicians for treatment, if necessary. Dentists also can be used as sources of information for patients concerning the medications they are using by communicating information on proper use, problems that may occur and their manifestation, and the need for compliance. Dentists can monitor the effectiveness of the treatment regimen.

Infection control: Dentists and dental auxiliaries practice sound infection control procedures in their offices on a daily basis. They are well versed and well practiced in infection control and can bring their expertise to mass casualty situations, particularly situations that involve infectious agents, to limit the spread of infection among individuals and between patients and responders who are rendering assistance. Decontamination of casualties from certain bioterrorism attacks in which contact with patient's clothing or skin surfaces may spread the agent to caregivers may be accomplished by dentists with some additional training. Dentists who are familiar with disaster mortuary activities can be useful in managing the remains of victims whose death is a result of the event, particularly infectious events. These remains most likely will be contaminated and require careful management to prevent further disease spread.

Definitive treatment: In addition to providing services that dentists ordinarily do, they may be able to augment or participate in the treatment provided by medical and surgical personnel. Dentists have training and experience in many areas that may be a part of casualty care in mass casualty events:

- Treating oral, facial, and cranial injuries
- Providing cardiopulmonary resuscitation
- Obtaining medical histories
- Collecting blood and other samples
- Providing or assisting with anesthesia
- Starting intravenous lines
- Suturing and performing appropriate surgery
- Assisting in patient stabilization
- Assisting in shock management.

Quarantine: During a pandemic or after a bio-terrorism attack with a communicable agent, strict quarantine restrictions may be imposed on the geographic area contaminated and its environs to help prevent or control the spread of the disease to other areas. The duration of the quarantine varies according to the incubation time of the agent and other factors. Before the existence of the area-wide contamination is established, primary care providers may become infected directly or through contact with patients seeking care. During the period of quarantine they may become disabled by the disease or even die. Dentists may not be similarly infected by patients because ill patients do not seek care from dentists and, if sufficiently ill, do not keep scheduled dental appointments, which minimizes intimate contact with infected persons. Dentists may be called on to provide some primary health care for people in the quarantined area.

How Dental Auxiliaries can Help

Confusion, disorganization, and lack of control are major barriers to an effective response to a mass casualty event. Experienced personnel are required to establish and maintain as orderly a process as possible for the immediate response to avoid public panic. Dental office clerical personnel are experienced in administrative functions, managing medical records, organizing patient flow, and maintaining communications between dentists and other health care providers. They can provide valuable assistance in those areas. Dental assistants can retain their role in assisting dentists, even expanding their function under supervision to help dentists in the new roles they may be asked to fill.

Dental hygienists can provide new clinical services with additional training, perhaps including administering immunizations in mass disaster immunization programs.

Preparation for Unfortunate Disasters and Protocols

Besides developing a disaster response plan for dentistry's response to mass casualty disasters, the profession itself must be made aware of the added responsibilities it may be asked to take on if traditional medical resources of the community are swamped by a surge in demand for care in the wake of a large-scale disaster. Additional education and training for dentists in specific areas of emergency response that build on the basic principles of medical care with which they are familiar can significantly expand the scope of services that dentists can provide effectively during these emergencies. Educational efforts should begin with dental students in during their undergraduate course curriculum education. The curriculum should be expanded to include more information on the management of large numbers of casualties, especially casualties generated by the intentional or non intentional spread of infectious agents. Dental students should understand the public health and emergency response communities and the control functions they provide in the event of an emergency. This material can be presented in separate dedicated courses or combined with appropriate existing course work. In either case it is advisable to have a separate course in the last year of dental school that pulls together all of the information taught during the preceding years as a summary.

In addition to the teaching of dental students, the existing profession needs similar education and training, which presents more of an educational challenge because of the practice responsibilities of dentists in the community and their ability to abstain from participation. As such, for the near future, most dentists who may be called on to assist in disaster response efforts most likely will not have received formal disaster training. The task of educating dental students falls primarily on dental schools. Educating and training dental practitioners is not as centralized as for dental students and must be accomplished by various means and from various sources, including dental schools, more than likely coordinated through the dental societies. There are opportunities for dentists who are interested in going beyond basic education and training in responding to mass casualty events through participation in various organizations sponsored by state and other government and NGO agencies.

Role of Dentists in Mass Disaster Forensics

Forensic interest in mass disasters centers on determination of the cause of the disaster and identification of the victims rather than preservation of life and limb. Historically, methods have included simple recognition, use of fingerprints, dental records, and skeletal identification using radiologic or anthropologic means. DNA analysis has become an essential tool in the analysis of samples in cases in which severe fragmentation of victims is involved. These methods in concert have led to the successful identification of thousands of victims of disasters such as earthquakes, floods, tsunami, or terrorist attacks. Each of these methods of identification has strengths and weaknesses that must be taken into account when evidence is collected. Proper preservation and storage of evidence is critical if analysis is to be accomplished in a reliable, efficient manner. Coordination of all analytical teams is also essential to provide a flow of evidence from section to section; all must work in concert to perform a task that can be of monumental proportion.

Evidence Protocols

Evidence processing, no matter what the disaster, is crucial to maintaining integrity of the collected evidence so that analytical results will stand up to scrutiny in the courts and provide closure for the families of the victims. The entire process in management of mass disaster should always follow a chain of events which is properly coordinated and executed in a phased manner so as to help out the victims and their families and not to unnecessarily complicate the situation further.

Phases of Response (Figs 9.6 A to F)

1st Responder

Any disaster whatever kind it may be is always first attended by Police, firefighter, and emergency medical services. The aim of all of these is to bring the situation under control, isolate the area, to prevent contamination from any hazardous substance, if located and to provide all feasible medical help to the survivors.

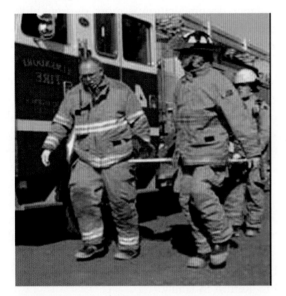

Fig. 9.6A: The various phases of response in events of mass disasters. Figure (A) shows the first emergency responders mainly medical and police personals

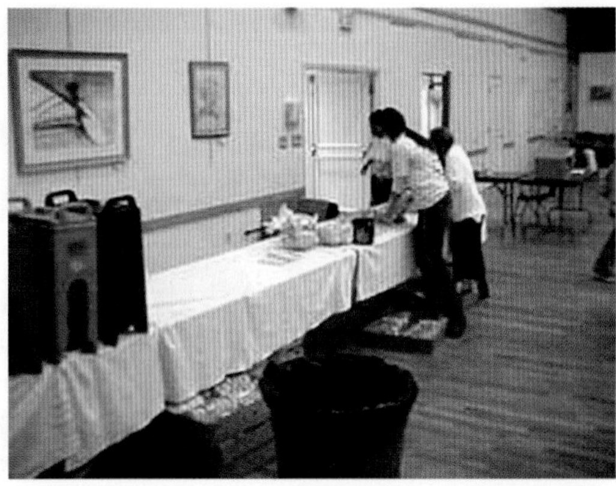

Fig. 9.6B: Arrangements made for the various procedures to be followed shortly after recovery of the remains of the disasters

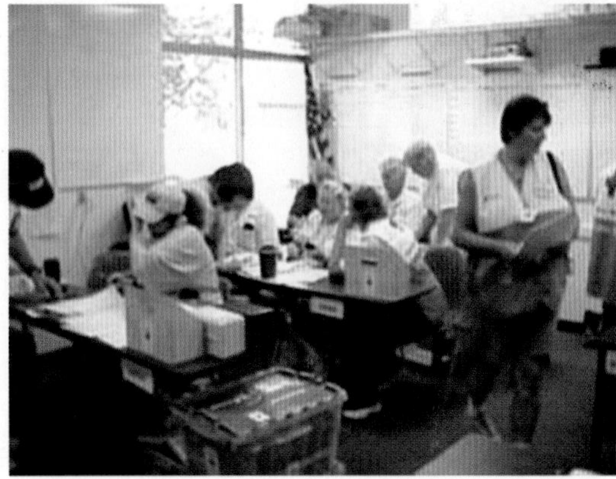

Fig. 9.6C: Team work showing the platform for collection and segregation of various records obtained from the family and relatives

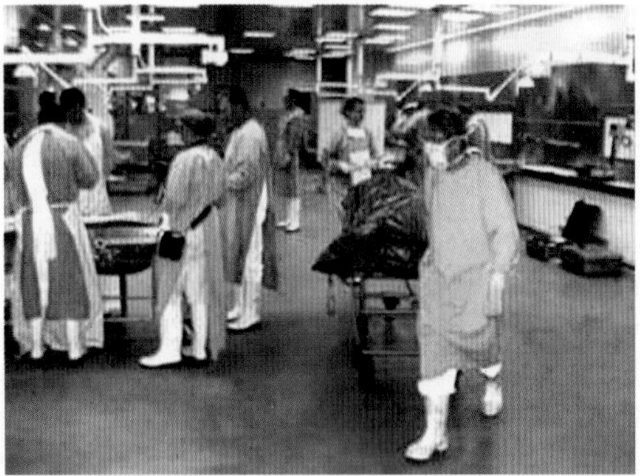

Fig. 9.6D: Various medical workers preparing for the process of postmortem examination and all investigations

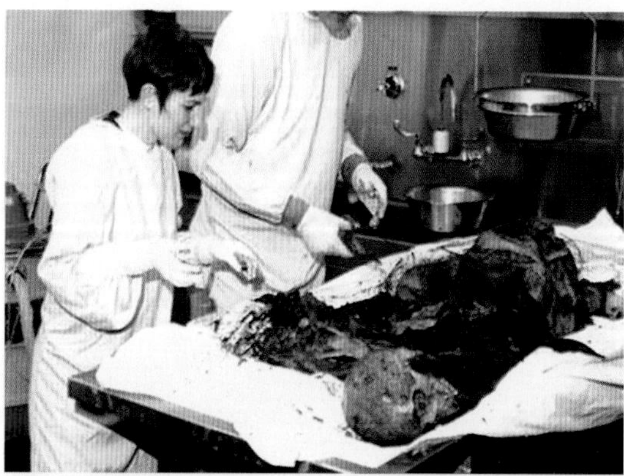

Fig. 9.6E: Medical personnel carrying out the process of autopsy and postmortem examinations

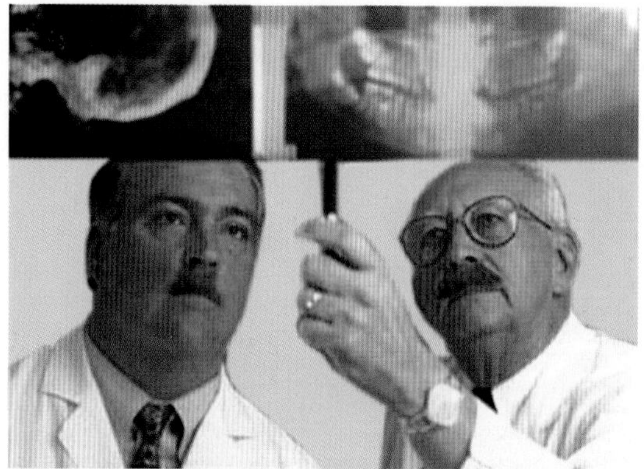

Fig. 9.6F: After collection of all antemortem and postmortem information, doctors compare them for the purpose of identification of the deceased

Stabilization

This phase of management starts with transportation of all the survivors to nearby medical facilities as soon as possible to save life, suppression of fire created (air crashes, fire disasters etc.). This is to be followed by removal of any hazardous substances like toxic chemicals, unburnt fuels or any other such substance to the responders and the public. Law enforcement for security is strengthened further, followed by the crime scene management. There should always be good communication to coordinate response, for resource management. A public information cell is also established to provide all the information about events and happenings along with the support services which are provided to the grieved families.

Resolution

After phase two ends, more complex events begins. These consists of removal and transport of human remains, control of environmental hazards and the morgue services.

Resolution of Site to Normal

This phase is taken care up by public health or environmental agencies, and also consists of resolution of responders to normal through critical incident stress debriefing counseling.

Identification center processing protocol is a continuous event of chain which takes place in the following schematic manner involving forensic odontologists at particular time. This collection begins with recovery of the evidence and processing in the site for analysis; without the time constraints imposed by the responsibility of patient care, evidence documentation is more rigorous. Each item of possible evidentiary value will undergo the following:

1. Recovery logged into temporary morgue
2. In processing to identification center chain of custody documentation
3. Photography, full body radiology, personal effects station
4. Fingerprints
5. Medical radiology
6. Pathology, cause and manner of death
7. Medical labs as directed (DNA)
8. Dental (AM/PM evidences)
9. Physical anthropology (age, sex, race, skeletal abnormalities)
10. Mortuary science, embalming
11. Return to family.

The medical response to a mass casualty incident will always be complicated. Providing quality care while understaffed, undersupplied, and possibly operating in an unfamiliar or inhospitable environment is not an easy task. The situation is further complicated when the mass casualty incident is the result of a terrorist act, which forces medical response to occur in conjunction with a federal criminal investigation. Although medical professionals and students commonly receive training on the recognition of terrorist events and appropriate interventions, legal aspects and evidence collection are rarely addressed in depth.

The Standard Operating Procedure

For all steps of the identification process, including antemortem record requests, fingerprint identification, forensic pathology and odontology, and DNA analysis, had to be agreed upon. Interpol took the lead in trying to coordinate data and institute standard operating procedures for physical evidence, but the legalities involved in obtaining medical records had to be negotiated. Interpol has also issued guidelines to help with the ante mortem records collection. The Interpol Victim Identification Guide, section 6.3.2.2, required all nations with possible missing citizens to provide all necessary records in an expedient manner; however, some countries took a conservative approach and gave estimated numbers of missing citizens, whereas others reported the numbers of citizens reported missing and presumed dead. This response inflated the number of records thought to be necessary in the identification process. The Interpol Victim Identification Guide also required original records in section 4.5.2.5; however, worldwide, the records that were sent varied greatly in quality, and many copies were substituted for original records. Even more crucial were the procedures necessary for the collection and preservation of evidence and the maintenance of the chain of custody of the evidence which would be used in the identification; speed was necessary due to the climate and the rapid decomposition of the bodies.

More personnel involved in the process can spread the work and relieve stress. The observed effects on health care professionals participating in mass disaster work have been documented to include distress while participating but also relief and satisfaction by making a positive impact in a disaster situation. Support gained through the other professionals in the work group adds to the positive feelings that can be derived through successful work in a mass disaster. Further documentation indicates that persons who participate in mock disaster drills feel they are better prepared to participate in authentic events. Additional personnel in conjunction with increased training opportunities should help reduce the stress on involved personnel and aid in faster analysis times.

Chain of Custody

Once an item of evidence has been seized or is located on a patient, care must be taken to record the whereabouts and access to the item in writing; the more susceptible the item is to contamination or tampering, the more closely it should be monitored. For example, an article of clothing with a distinctive logo would be more readily recognizable than a small piece of shrapnel removed from a wound. Medical records can serve as a chain of custody between providers throughout care to establish the time, location, and status for objects of interest that are not removed from the patient on scene but hours or days later. Items that are discovered and collected in the field should be labeled (name of patient, name of practitioner, date, time) and preferably stored in an area with limited public access until they are collected and signed for by a law enforcement officer; inconsistencies in delivery and receipt conditions could lead to the suppression of evidence.

Evidence Collection and Preservation

Overall, medical professionals should attempt to the best of their ability to store evidence in a manner that will facilitate future analysis.

First, one should avoid cutting through holes in patient clothing that were created before their arrival for care. Maintaining holes intact will help forensic specialists recreate the scene, corroborate the size and force of an object that penetrated the victim, and give guidance for tests to determine the presence or absence of trace evidence. Cutting through the hole causes permanent distortion to the fabric (especially in the case of knitted fabrics) and can contaminate the surface of the fabric with metal or other debris from the scissors that might not be distinguishable from pertinent evidence.

Second, one should avoid sealing items while they are still damp. Wet items may grow mold or mildew that will contaminate the evidence and make further analysis more difficult. If the possibility exists, the item should be allowed to dry before sealing the container.

Third, one should avoid the use of plastic bags when possible. Plastic can cause the degradation of biologic and chemical evidence and can lead to a moist environment inside the bag. All evidence, regardless of nature or origin, should be handled with gloved hands to protect it from trace damage (such as fingerprints) and to protect medical professionals from exposure to toxic chemicals or other agents. Although these measures may sound tedious, they have been practiced by sexual assault nurse examiners in hospital settings for over many years.

The forensic odontology team will be highly involved in many of the steps; their work will be suspect without proper in-processing and documentation. Dental ID team can be divided into several different sections, based on its mission—Vale and Noguchi.

A. Recovery team: If called upon for disaster protocol.
B. Antemortem section: As told by the Morlang, this is supposed to be the most difficult section for dental teams, involving hardships and a lots of communication.
C. Postmortem section: It consists of examination of all dental structures, photographic documentation of remains, reconstruction and stabilization of fragmented or burned remains, excision of jaws—if needed, charting of all injuries, anomalies, restorations.
D. Comparison section: After all the neded AM/PM information is obtained, the next step is to compare the obtained records in the same manner as that for any other forensic dental identification.

Dental Records and Mass Disasters

In many instances, such as when victims are severely burned, traditional forensic techniques do not provide conclusive means of identification. Pathologic conditions noted in dental records, treatments, and prosthetic devices may survive fires when identifying markings and DNA may not. Dental records are among the most readily available ante mortem information that can be accessed by disaster emergency response teams. As such, forensic odontology continues to be a crucial element in nearly all mass disasters whether natural, accidental, or intentional. At the onset of a disaster, various teams of dentists will be established to start collecting ante mortem data based on lists of missing persons, a task that relies heavily on the nature of victims (e.g., military versus civilian). Once these records have been compiled, forensic odontologists can begin comparisons between remains and ante mortem records. Traditionally, overlays have been used in many disaster situations, even before the 1980s. These overlay procedures have been simplified with time and still serve local coroner or medical examiner offices that may not have the volume or resources to maintain a database; however, the number of victims in a mass disaster situation makes simple comparison unacceptable.

Overlays have given way to computerized matching software. Data comparison systems such as computer-assisted postmortem identification (CAPMI), WinID, Plass, and DAVID software have enabled rapid entry of ante mortem records and post mortem data into a database capable of completing rapid comparison of huge amounts of data. Each program has allowed new levels of detail and greater operator control leading to increased suggested match accuracy; however, all suggested matches are verified by members of the mass disaster team. Other information beyond the description of dentition can be used in the forensic odontology field, such as labeled dental prostheses. Victims possessing all or most of their dentition have physical characteristics necessary for their identification, whereas those missing all of their teeth lack such information.

Identification from prosthetics has been around since the 1800s. Markings on prosthetic devices should be able to establish the identity of the patient or victim, be easily and quickly applied, and be fire resistant or placed in such a manner that they are protected by the tongue. The marking should not interfere with the function of the device and be unobtrusive, and the appearance should be acceptable to the patient. Some of the simplest marking techniques involve surface marks inscribed by scalpels, pencil marks that are covered by dental polymer, and inscribing the cast from which the device was made. More recently, markings have been enclosed in the prosthetic device using polymethyl methacrylate to ensure permanency. Metal identification bands have been enclosed in compartments within the device, which are completely invisible when completed and cosmetically appealing but readily recognizable during radiologic examination.

Radiofrequency identification (RFID) tags have been developed that are small enough to be implanted into a prosthesis or a prepared molar. This technology originally served the veterinary field but is easily transferred to human use. Identification would be accomplished through the use of an interrogator that triggers a power surge in the RFID chip which responds by providing information to the reader. This method could, if implemented, ease the work involved in the identification of victims of a mass disaster; however, there will be some time lapse before such devices are frequently seen in the overall population.

Man Made Disasters

Forensic Techniques and Evidence Sources in Specific Scenarios

Intentional man-made events are generally broken down into five major categories: chemical, biologic, nuclear/radiologic, and explosive (CBRNE). Each of these categories can be divided further into specific agents or patient characteristics. To best serve medical responders, for each major category, enlisted here in are description of standard analysis, an overview of emerging detection and forensic techniques, possible scenarios in which medical professionals may discover evidence, and measures to protect the integrity of the evidence while ensuring personal safety. In any investigation, the bulk of physical evidence is collected by law enforcement professionals or specially trained military units. Detailed analysis is performed in a laboratory setting that is determined by the nature of the incident. Nevertheless, there is a chance that medical responders may discover evidence that will be pertinent to an investigation. Specific items that may be of interest to investigators are covered in detail under each scenario.

Chemical Scenario

The specific forensic techniques use in the investigation of a chemical event will vary based on the nature of the agent; however, certain facts will require resolution for the state to build a sufficient case for the prosecution of suspects. The verified agent identity, proof of victim exposure to agents, and the ability of suspects to synthesize and disseminate the agent will be of particular interest to those involved in prosecution. Preliminary agent identification will likely come as victims present with symptoms associated with toxic exposure (e.g. dyspnea, rhinorhea, ocular pain, dizziness, vomiting). Intelligence related to possible terrorist threats in the area might also support the preliminary agent identification. The support of hazardous material (HAZMAT) teams will provide more information; hand held detectors and manual testing will confirm the presence of an agent class (e.g. nerve agent versus sulfur mustard). Improvements in the reliability and range of detectable agents are being explored with the use of different forms of spectrometry (such as Fourier transform infrared spectroscopy), photometry, and chip-based sensors based on carbon nano-tubes.

As part of the detailed analysis, scientists will also note the impurities and precursors found in the sample. Few chemical reactions provide 100 percent yield in every step; in the Tokyo subway attack, **(Fig 9.7A and B)** the liquid sampled on the train was only 30 percent sarin. The other 70 percent of the substance provided clues as to the synthetic protocol used, allowing law enforcement officials to narrow the search to facilities/business entities that had purchased these chemicals recently. The sophistication of the synthetic model and the purity of the product will also indicate the type of facility and personnel that would likely be associated with the agent production. Examinations of organic and aqueous extractions of samples using instrumentation routinely used in forensic investigations, such as gas chromatography/mass spectrometry and liquid chromatography/mass spectrometry, have proven sufficient to identify most agents, especially when coupled with pre-concentration techniques and tandem mass spectrometry.

Most chemical agents are either non-persistent (vapor) or require wet decontamination. Because life and limb supersede a forensic investigation, samples will not be taken before decontamination or medical intervention, even if personnel were able to take samples on scene. As an alternative to immediate or superficial collection, biophysical changes specific to agent exposure can be determined through blood analysis. Raman spectroscopy also shows promise as a noninvasive means to determine exposure to chemical and

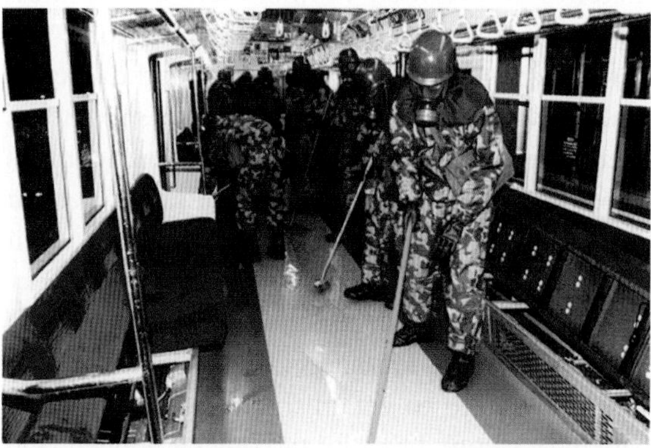

Fig. 9.7A: The train in Tokyo subway passage where a chemical attack of Sarin gas was deployed

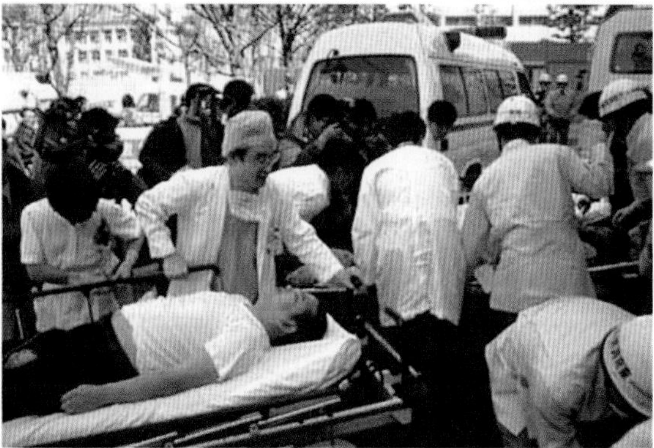

Fig. 9.7B: Picture showing the casualties in Tokyo train attack

biologic agents. At the time of an attack, it is highly likely that intelligence gathering will have narrowed the field of suspects. Through interrogation and investigative work, it is also possible that a facility or dissemination device will be located. Chemical events are particularly dangerous to medical responders, especially for those operating in the "cold zone". Many chemical agents can be absorbed through the skin (or latex gloves), leaving responders vulnerable to secondary contamination.

By the time a dental responder is on scene, the nature of the agent will be at least preliminarily confirmed, and the manner of decontamination will have been decided. With this in mind, observing a patient's attempt to avoid decontamination (which will require removal of clothing) should be considered highly suspicious, and law enforcement officials should be notified of this behavior. If when monitoring patients triaged as minimally injured, several patients exhibit a sudden onset of more severe symptoms simultaneously, the medical responder should notify medical team leaders and law enforcement. The sudden onset may be caused by a secondary device or by proximity to the dissemination device. In both instances, the authorities should be notified, and all personnel should prepare to undergo decontamination measures. If the agent is persistent, the medical responder should report any objects found in the patient's possession or in the treatment area that appear oily or greasy but should not attempt to handle the item, even with gloved hands.

Biologic Agents

The investigation of a biologic agent is the most challenging CBRNE event. Although an outbreak of an unusual nature (such as smallpox) **(Fig. 9.8)** would trigger an immediate response and investigation, most biologic agents act slowly within a population, and patients present with nondescript ailments in many locations over an extended period of time (days or weeks as opposed to minutes or hours in a chemical attack). The core questions of agent identity, patient exposure, and agent production require investigation. In the best case scenario, agents will be detected before an infection occurs. The persistence of biologic agents and the necessity of relatively high concentrations of biologic agents for infection to occur are used to the advantage of law enforcement and public health officials. Various federal efforts to create sentinel detectors, aim to provide identification of agents as they are released into the environment through continuous sampling at a static location; however, these technologies rely on the airborne presence of the agent, which may not occur in cases of food-borne dissemination.

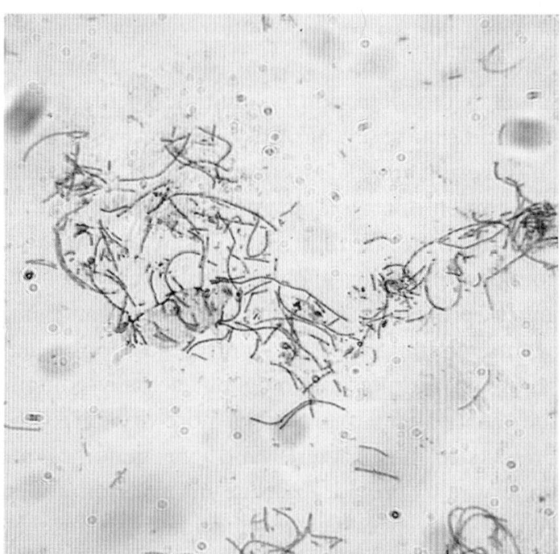

Fig. 9.8: Biological attacks, showing the Anthrax spores in the US postal departments

Currently, sentinels are not ubiquitous; therefore, a real possibility remains that the first warning of an attack will occur when citizens become infected. Agent identity will initially be established through common histologic procedures performed at hospitals, public health laboratories, or specialized facilities. Analytical techniques are being refined to offer faster and more accurate agent characterization that can be used for any type of agent and to more readily recognize hoaxes. Microchip based technologies allow for simultaneous detection of multiple agents in the field and clinical settings The prevalence of genetic engineering may also contribute to a delayed recognition of a biologic attack.

Techniques widely used in academic and commercial settings allow scientists to control the genetic properties and abilities of bacterial and viral agents, meaning that an agent could "look" like salmonella during screening but actually contain the genetic ability to produce a more virulent toxin. Projects to map bacterial and viral genomes are underway to provide baseline information about genetic differences between and among strains that are currently found in the environment so that the future release of a laboratory cultured agent will be more readily apparent. Unlike chemical agents, the production of biologic agents does not require regulated chemical precursors. The equipment and chemicals necessary to replicate or modify a bacteria or virus have many benign uses and are ubiquitous in biologic and genetic laboratories, enhancing the possibility of "dual use" facilities. Several businesses are devoted solely to the creation of DNA sequences to order and do not always screen these sequences against the DNA sequences of known biologic agents; therefore, the possibility exists that a major part of production did not even occur within a facility. Nevertheless, intelligence suggesting that this method was used to orchestrate a biologic attack would allow law enforcement to trace involved parties through billing records of a sequencing company. Rather than focusing on the specific location or ability to produce the parent agent, a link to the equipment used in the replication of the agent might be established.

DNA analysis of samples found in a suspected facility could be compared with the DNA analysis of samples taken from the scene and from victims, and statistical models derived from genome mapping projects could allow probabilities of association to be extrapolated, much in the same manner that DNA analysis of bodily fluids can yield a probability of association with an individual.

A medical provider may contribute to an investigation in two likely ways:

1. By recognizing and reporting a person of interest or
2. By recognizing a device that was part of the dissemination of the agent.

During any sort of epidemic (natural or intentional), populations are affected at different times and at different rates; a patient presenting with a more developed infection than anyone else in the area is a person of interest. This individual may have come into contact with the agent before anyone else in the community (perhaps as a result of travel) or may have had involvement in the synthesis or dissemination of the agent. In both cases, this person will assist public health and law enforcement authorities in pinpointing the origins of the outbreak and will provide useful information in the case of an outbreak.

The second possibility is the discovery of a dissemination device in the possession of a patient. Items such as vials, medicine droppers, test tubes, and other containers would be of interest to law enforcement officials, particularly if these containers were concealed but provided easy access, such as being taped to the wrist. Another item of interest would be architectural plans, especially if they include details of a heating, ventilating, and air conditioning system. Handling items potentially contaminated with biologic agents should be performed while using the recommended personal protective equipment associated with the particular agent.

Nuclear/Radiologic Event (Fig. 9.9)

A radiologic event will require immediate evacuation (much like a chemical event) and the intervention of specially trained teams, in detection, characterization, and recovery efforts. If recently suggested guidelines are adopted, an area of 500 m (approximately 0.31 miles) will be evacuated and

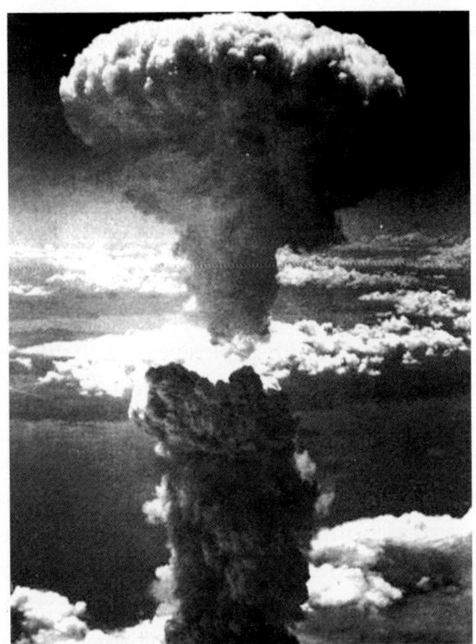

Fig. 9.9: The site of nuclear explosion in Japan during the Atomic bombings in Hiroshima and Nagasaki, Japan

considered the "hot" zone where radiation levels are considered too high to operate without appropriate protection and medical oversight. Information discovered by these teams could be used at the launch of a police investigation. For example, the specific isotope discovered on scene will indicate whether the material was likely to have been derived from industrial or medical instrumentation and will lead to the cross-check of those facilities for reports of stolen or damaged equipment. Detector technology based on neutron generation and gamma ray spectra interpretation offers the ability to characterize unexploded ordnance.

As the threat of radiologic exposure diminishes, information about the device can be sought similar to the investigation of an explosion, especially in the case of a radiologic dispersion device or "dirty bomb." Emerging technologies are capable of detecting and classifying explosives from a distance, making it possible for information to be gathered while minimizing the chance of injury. Again, forensic scientists will focus on the explosives and the contaminants to link the device with a facility and a perpetrator. The most probable circumstance for medical volunteer involvement would be in response to a radiologic dispersion device. If a patient presents with symptoms associated with high levels of radiation exposure but shows no sign of trauma or gross external contamination or if he or she presents with only burns to the hands or forearms, the patient would be a person of interest to law enforcement because they may have been involved in the preparation or transport of the device. Patients close to the explosion site may receive penetrating injuries from shrapnel. Facilities on scene and operating procedures may not allow for the removal of the foreign body, but a note on the nature of the shrapnel, patient information, and destination hospital (if known) would be useful to the investigation. If the foreign body is removed (if it is blocking the airway), provider information, the time, date, and patient information should be noted on the bag and the item placed away from traffic flow until law enforcement officials are able to retrieve it. In the radiologic dispersion device scenario, the amount of particulate matter on a single piece of shrapnel is not likely to cause a health risk.

Explosive Events

Bombings are the most common form of terrorist action **(Fig. 9.10)** to date. Hundreds of events have occurred internationally causing countless fatalities and casualties. As a result, law enforcement agencies are relatively prepared for the necessary analyses following an explosive event; most forensic laboratories have sections devoted to arson and explosive investigations. Some police forces cross-train officers in urban search and rescue to allow forensic investigators early access to the crime scene in the safest manner possible. As is true in the other scenarios, the goal of the forensic investigation is to characterize the agent (through recreation of

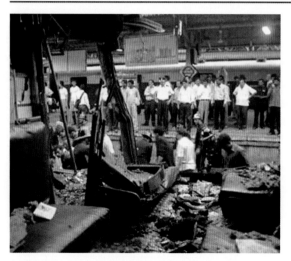

Fig. 9.10: The picture showing the terrorists evoked explosion of the Mumbai local trains resulting in hundred of casualties

the device and the chemical composition of the explosives), link the agent to an individual or group, and prove that an individual or group planted the device in a specific location.

To prove the existence of an explosive device (as opposed to an accidental explosion), investigators seek evidence of the four required components of an improvised explosive device: A power source, initiators, explosives, and switches. A fifth component, which is not necessary but can provide useful information, is fragmentation and shrapnel such as ball bearings, nuts, and screws included as part of the device to inflict greater damage and increase the likelihood of secondary blast injuries. Bringing these components together can give officers an idea of the level of sophistication of the device and the level of training of the offenders and can provide a possible connection between crimes.

For example, the use of home-manufactured rather than commercially machined screws was a trademark of explosives in the Unabomber cases, and the use of a Big Ben alarm clock was consistent among all of the devices planted by Eric Rudolph (the Olympic Park bomber). Also, if several devices were used in the same attack, evidence of these necessary components would confirm the number of devices used and whether specific design characteristics were shared among the devices. Characterization of the actual explosive will begin with an examination of the physical characteristics of the device fragments. Low explosives deflagrate, that is, they propagate energy through thermal conductivity; therefore, the discovery of fragments that are warped or charred would be indicative of a low explosive. High explosives detonate, which is the propagation of energy through a pressure wave at supersonic speeds; fragments that have sharp edges and limited signs of heat exposure would indicate the possible use of a high explosive. If physical components are not immediately recovered, surrounding structures and damaged objects can be swabbed and tested for the presence of explosive residue. Currently, colormetric tests are employed to determine whether to sample an area or object for more specific analysis. Such tests rely on a chemical reaction between the explosive and an introduced agent that results in a color change.

Studies of the use of photo-luminscent techniques that use laser excitation to improve visualization in the field have been developed and are undergoing validation and testing. In specialized laboratory settings, explosive identification may also be achieved through re-crystallization and observation under polarized light. Some of the handheld monitors used for chemical detection can also detect the presence of explosives; however, more sensitive and accurate instrumentation based on Raman spectrometry is emerging that is capable of detecting explosive mixtures at a distance. Neutron interrogation devices have demonstrated the ability to characterize explosives (and other substances) by reading the gamma ray signatures released by an object following excitation by neutrons released by the detector. This testing is especially useful in the determination of the fill of unexploded or buried devices. Further confirmation can be achieved with laboratory-based analysis, which is made necessary by the fact that most improvised explosives are derived from commonly used, commercially available products with benign uses.

For example, a nitrate-based fertilizer mixed with diesel fuel creates an explosive material (ammonium nitrate fuel oil). The presence of nitrates or the presence of diesel fuel is insufficient to definitively characterize the nature of the explosive; both substances could be detected by chance in a given area. Analytical techniques that reveal more information about the specific structure or molecule complex are more useful in characterizing explosives. Sensitivity is further improved with concentration techniques such as solid phase extraction before analysis, as well as the use of artificial neuronal networks, a form of enhanced software to modulate the separation conditions according to the specific needs of the sample. Recently, success has been reported in extracting DNA from skin cells left on the surface of exploded pipe bombs; therefore, genetic analysis could also prove that an individual handled a specific device.

The aim of the primary investigation of a suspect is to connect the individual or a group with the explosives used in an event. Police officers will likely use preliminary techniques on scene, such as colormetric tests, to determine the presence of explosives and will use the results as probable cause to detain a suspect pending further investigation. Explosive residues are readily collected from nonporous surfaces, skin, and fabric. Studies have shown that hair has the ability to concentrate vapors from some military explosives and that concentrations can be linked to exposure time and still be traced after washing or environmental exposure. In the laboratory setting, characteristics of trace elements associated with the explosive, such as sulfur, can be analyzed to associate the explosive material with a suspect or may be found in the suspect's possession (even in trace form) with explosive material recovered from the scene.

The nature of an explosive event provides the greatest opportunity for a medical responder to recover evidence or identify persons of interest. The most dangerous situation would be the discovery of an undetonated device on the body of a patient. This situation might occur in a suicide bombing in which multiple bombers planned to attack a site, one or more perpetrators carried devices that did not detonate, and the suspects sustained injury as a result of the proximate blast, or if the device was intended to detonate upon removal from the patient by medical personnel. In the event of such a discovery, one should notify law enforcement immediately. Do not attempt to remove the device or move the patient any more than absolutely necessary. Evacuate the surrounding area rather than attempting to move the device (or the patient it is attached to). Other persons of interest may be less severely wounded patients who act nervous rather than panicked, particularly if the individual seems focused on police activities. Law enforcement officials may not be readily available for interrogation, but a detailed description of the individual including identifying characteristics and contact information should be provided to investigators, along with any transport information.

Penetrative injuries of varying severity are common in bombings; recorded injuries range from hardware to bone fragments from a suicide bomber. Because fragmentation evidence can be useful in device reconstruction or trace analysis, police knowledge of the removal of such fragments from patients is useful. Fragments associated directly with the device are important; objects that resemble batteries, springs, electronics (e.g. wires, transistors, microchips, cellular phone components), or plastic tubing should be noted. If the items are removed in the field, one should package and store shrapnel following the guidelines presented previously, making sure to wear gloves and a mask to prevent DNA contamination. In the more likely circumstance that the patient is transported with the shrapnel still embedded, the medical responder should make note of the patient's name, identifying characteristics, the nature of the shrapnel, and the transport hospital (if known) and should provide this information to law enforcement officials. In an explosive event that creates extreme structural damage, clothing removed from patients evacuated from the scene could be of use. Evidence collection will always run secondary to engineering concerns such as structure stability. The ability to start the investigation by conducting an initial analysis on articles of clothing will save a great deal of time, because safety concerns may disallow evidence collection from the explosion site for hours or days. One should store items of clothing as described earlier.

Dental Radiography in Mass Disasters

Field Equipment for Mass Disasters

In mass disasters involving multiple bodies in remote sites or under compromised conditions, radiographs are often made on location. A tripod-mounted portable dental X-ray unit such as the Min-X-ray is used. A power source is provided by a generator. Proper shielding is needed. Considering the workload and urgency in a mass disaster, one does not have the luxury of waiting for ante-mortem radiographs. All bodies and recovered dental fragments should be X-rayed. Full-mouth radiographs are preferred but when individual periapical views are too time-consuming and jaw removal is permitted, occlusal-sized film can include the entire posterior dentition in two to four exposures. Double film packets should be used. The films can be processed with an automatic dental X-ray film processor equipped with a daylight loading hood. If incoming antemortem films are being duplicated, a second processor should be used to avoid mix ups. If a processor is not practical, there is Polaroid TPX radiographic film, an 8 × 10 inches film with self-contained chemistry for instant processing.

X-ray film mounts, folders, and labels must be on hand to keep radiographs separate and identifiable back to their source. A computer at the mass disaster site can electronically digitize and export radiographic images for rapid com-parison.

Commingled, Skeletonized, Carbonized, and Mutilated Remains

When human remains appear to be missing jaws or teeth or when scattering and displacement has occurred, it is worthwhile to make flat plate radiographs with location grids of the entire body or recovered rubble in search of teeth or surviving prostheses. Such dispersion and destruction occurs in some house fires, skeletonized remains, and in mass disasters when bodies are mutilated or commingled. Skeletonized teeth are fragile and brittle. They tend to fracture, usually at right angles and with smooth cleavage through both enamel and dentin. These wedges of fractured tooth structure can be glued in place with Duco® cement or cyanoacrylate cement. Specimens can be preserved so as to prevent fracture by boiling, bleaching in Clorox, then dipping in a solution of polyvinyl acetate resin. The bones and teeth are then coated and permeated with a clear, thin, invisible preservative. The effect of intense flash fires upon teeth is to cause boiling of the pulp and explosion of the crowns which then break off at the gumline, leaving roots within their sockets. Heat which develops more slowly causes exfoliation of enamel, leaving dome-shaped mounds of charred coronal dentin. These teeth are easily lost from their sockets. Recovered conical roots should not be forced back into sockets because of their fragility. Rather, they should be guided in and checked radiographically. Generally, if a charred root has a gray (ashed) surface and a black (carbonized) surface, the gray side is labial (indicating higher heat and more complete combustion) and the black side is lingual. Carbonized and ashed teeth and bone are friable and can crumble with the slightest touch or movement. Teeth might disintegrate when the jaws are removed. These teeth can be stabilized with spray acrylic, cyanoacrylate, polyvinyl acetate, or Duco® cement. Spray acrylic is easiest to apply *in situ*. Polyvinyl acetate is acceptable, but most time-consuming.

Despite its delicateness, conflagrated mineralized tissue retains its radiographic characteristics although some shrinkage occurs. Lowered kVp is recom-mended as the specimens require less X-ray penetrating ability. In remains where teeth have been lost postmortem, the shape of the roots can be reconstructed by filling the empty sockets with radiopaque material (dental alginate impression material mixed with barium sulfate) before making postmortem radiographs.

Summary

As the role of the oral health professional as a medical responder becomes more widely accepted throughout the country, the probability of a dental emergency responder responding to a terrorist event (a de facto crime scene) will increase. As part of continuing education, oral health professionals interested in pursuing a role in disaster response should seek out opportunities to enhance their knowledge of rules of evidence in the states in which they practice and obtain knowledge of operating procedures and technical capacities specific to their city, county, and state. This knowledge will help the dental emergency responder distinguish physical evidence that is most likely to be of analytical value.

Bibliography

1. Albert H Guay. The role dentists can play in mass casualty and disaster events. Dent Clin N Am. 2007;51:767-778.
2. Alfano MC. Bioterrorism response. J Am Dent Assoc. 2003;134(3):278-80.
3. Assael LA. Readiness and response: the oral and maxillofacial surgeon's role in disaster. J Oral Maxillofac Surg. 2005;63(11):1565-6.
4. Beveridge AD, Payton SF, Audette RJ, et al. Systematic analysis of explosive residues. J Forensic Sci. 1975;20(3):431-54.
5. Brannon RB, Connick CM. The role of the dental hygienist in mass disasters. J Forensic Sci. 2000;45(2):381-3.
6. Brannon RB, Morlang WM. The USS Iowa disaster: success of the forensic dental team. Journal of Forensic Sciences. 2004;49(5):1067-8.
7. Colvard MD, Lampiris LN, Cordell GA, et al. The dental emergency responder: expanding the scope of dental practice. J Am Dent Assoc. 2006;137(4):468-73.
8. DeValck E. Major incident response: collecting ante-mortem data. Forensic Sci Int. 2006;159(1):S15-9.
9. Flores S, Mills SE, Shackelford L. Dentistry and bioterrorism. Dent Clin North Am. 2003;47:733-44.
10. Guay AH. Dentistry's response to bioterrorism: a report of a consensus workshop. J Am Dent Assoc. 2002;133(9):1181-7.
11. Valenzuela A, Martin-de las Heras S, Marques T, et al. The application of dental methods of identification to human burn victims in a mass disaster. Int J Legal Med. 2000;113:236-9.
12. Valenzuela A, Martin-de las Heras S, Marques T. The application of dental methods of identification to human burn victims in a mass disaster. Int J Legal Med. 2000;113:236-9.

Chapter 10

Child Abuse, Neglect and Domestic Violence: Role of a Dentist

Abhishek Singhania, Shikha Atreja

Chapter Overview

- Definitions
- Child abuse in India and Indian statistics
- Bruises
- Pathogenesis of contusions and factors affecting the development and appearance of a bruise
- Characteristic bruises
- Conditions that may be confused with abusive bruising
- Legal matters regarding child abuse and neglect
- Recognizing child abuse/neglect
- Reporting child abuse or neglect
- Critical steps in investigating and interviewing the possible victim
- Photo documentation
- Techniques to help visualize bruising
- Dating bruises and associated misconceptions and limitations
- Domestic violence and battered women

INTRODUCTION

Before 1950, it was thought that the incidents of family violence were isolated. This idea arose in part because of the prevailing attitude that men had right to discipline their wives and to use corporal punishment on their children i.e. "spare the rod and spoil the child" attitude.

In the 1960s, movements began that increased awareness of child abuse and in 1970s, activities followed that were aimed at preventing abuse of women and elderly person.

Child abuse is a state of emotional, physical, economic and sexual maltreatment meted out to a person below the age of eighteen and is a globally prevalent phenomenon. However, in India, as in many other countries, there has been no understanding of the extent, magnitude and trends of the problem. The growing complexities of life and the dramatic changes brought about by socio-economic transitions in India have played a major role in increasing the vulnerability of children to various and newer forms of abuse.

Child abuse has serious physical and psycho-social consequences which adversely affect the health and overall well-being of a child. According to WHO: "Child abuse or maltreatment constitutes all forms of physical and/or emotional ill-treatment, sexual abuse, neglect or negligent treatment or commercial or other exploitation, resulting in actual or potential harm to the child's health, survival, development or dignity in the context of a relationship of responsibility, trust or power."

Definitions

The term 'Child Abuse' may have different connotations in different cultural milieu and socioeconomic situations. A universal definition of child abuse in the Indian context does not exist and has yet to be defined. According to WHO:

Physical Abuse: Physical abuse is the inflicting of physical injury upon a child. This may include burning, hitting, punching, shaking, kicking, beating or otherwise harming a child. The parent or caretaker may not have intended to hurt the child. It may, however, be the result of over-discipline or physical punishment that is inappropriate to the child's age.

Sexual Abuse: Sexual abuse is inappropriate sexual behavior with a child. It includes fondling a child's genitals, making the child fondle the adult's genitals, intercourse, incest, rape, sodomy, exhibitionism and sexual exploitation. To be considered 'child abuse', these acts have to be committed by a person responsible for the care of a child (for example a baby-sitter, a parent, or a daycare provider), or related to the child. If a stranger commits these acts, it would be considered sexual assault and handled solely by the police and criminal courts.

Emotional Abuse: Emotional abuse is also known as verbal abuse, mental abuse, and psychological maltreatment. It includes acts or the failures to act by parents or caretakers that have caused or could cause, serious behavioral, cognitive, emotional, or mental trauma. This can include parents/caretakers using extreme and/or bizarre forms of punishment, such as confinement in a closet or dark room or being tied to a chair for long periods of time or threatening or terrorizing a child. Less severe acts, but no less damaging, are belittling or rejecting treatment, using derogatory terms to describe the child, habitual tendency to blame the child or make him/her a scapegoat.

Neglect: It is the failure to provide for the child's basic needs. Neglect can be physical, educational, or emotional. Physical neglect can include not providing adequate food or clothing, appropriate medical care, supervision, or proper weather protection (heat or cold). It may include abandonment. Educational neglect includes failure to provide appropriate schooling or special educational needs, allowing excessive truancies. Psychological neglect includes the lack of any emotional support and love, never attending to the child, substance abuse including allowing the child to participate in drug and alcohol use.

Child Abuse in India and Indian Statistics

Nineteen percent of the world's children live in India. According to the 2001 Census, some 440 million people in the country today are aged below eighteen years and constitute 42 percent of India's total population i.e. four out of every ten persons. This is an enormous number of children that the country has to take care of. While articulating its vision of progress, development and equity, India has expressed its recognition of the fact that when its children are educated, healthy, happy and have access to opportunities, they are the country's greatest human resource. A recent study in India revealed that more than 50 percent children suffer from one or another kind of child abuse. Seeing that 40 percent of our population comprises children/adolescents, the number of victims can be over 20 millions.

It is young children, in the 5 to 12 years group, who are most at risk of abuse and exploitation.

The State of Andhra Pradesh, Assam, Bihar and Delhi have almost consistently reported higher rates of abuse in all forms physical and sexual as compared to other states.

Following are the statistics as determined in the 207 page studies on Indian children from various states titled "Study on Child Abuse India 2007" by ministry of health and family welfare (**Fig. 10.1**), government of India, regarding incidence of various kinds of child abuse in rural and urban India. It has very clearly emerged that across different kinds of abuse, it is young children, in the 5 to 12 years group, who are most at risk of abuse and exploitation.

Physical Abuse

1. Two out of every three children were physically abused.

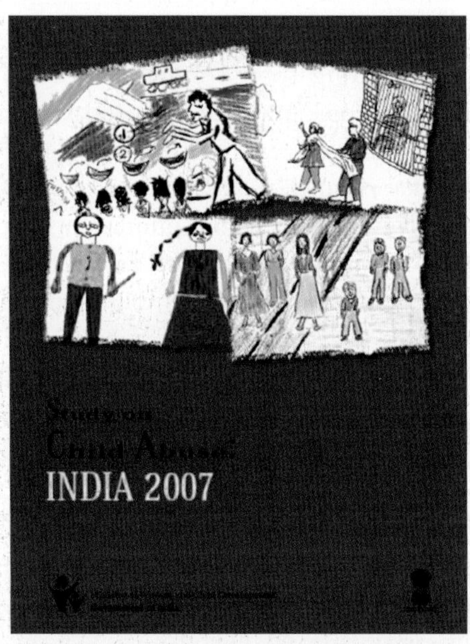

Fig. 10.1: Picture showing the cover page of the the project work "study on child abuse- INDIA 2007", by Ministry of Health and Family Welfare, Government of India

2. Out of 69 percent children physically abused in 13 sample states, 54.68 percent were boys.
3. Over 50 percent children in all the 13 sample states were being subjected to one or the other form of physical abuse.
4. Out of those children physically abused in family situations, 88.6 percent were physically abused by parents.
5. 65 percent of school going children reported facing corporal punishment i.e. two out of three children were victims of corporal punishment.
6. 62 percent of the corporal punishment was in goverment and municipal school.
7. The State of Andhra Pradesh, Assam, Bihar and Delhi have almost consistently reported higher rates of abuse in all forms as compared to other states.
8. Most children did not report the matter to anyone.
9. 50.2 percent children worked seven days a week.

Sexual Abuse

1. 53.22 percent children reported having faced one or more forms of sexual abuse.
2. Andhra Pradesh, Assam, Bihar and Delhi reported the highest percentage of sexual abuse among both boys and girls.
3. 21.90 percent child respondents reported facing severe forms of sexual abuse and 50.76 percent other forms of sexual abuse.
4. Out of the child respondents, 5.69 percent reported being sexually assaulted.
5. Children in Assam, Andhra Pradesh, Bihar and Delhi reported the highest incidence of sexual assault.
6. Children on street, children at work and children in institutional care reported the highest incidence of sexual assault.
7. 50 percent of abusers are persons known to the child or in a position of trust and responsibility.
8. Most children did not report the matter to anyone.

Emotional Abuse and Girl Child Neglect

1. Every second child reported facing emotional abuse.
2. Equal percentage of both girls and boys reported facing emotional abuse.
3. In 83 percent of the cases parents were the abusers.
4. 48.4 percent of girls wished they were boys

Bruises

Bruises are a very much neglected branch of injuries. These words were originally delivered in a 1938 address to the Medico-Legal Society of Great Britain by Sir Bernard Spilsbury. More than half a century later in 1991, Langlois and Gresham quoted these same words and observed that "little has changed since then". Remarkably, in 2006, the words of Sir Spilsbury continue to be true; bruises remain a very much neglected branch of injuries.

Bruising is one of the earliest, most common, and easily recognizable signs of physical child abuse and can signal escalating interpersonal violence within a household. Early detection of abuse through recognition of bruising coupled with appropriate intervention can help to prevent future and potentially more severe physical assaults. Bruising is also an occurrence of accidental injury and results from normal childhood activity. It is important to note that bleeding beneath an intact skin surface can occur from medical conditions and an absence of bruising does not mean that an abusive injury did not occur.

Differentiating between inflicted and non-inflicted injury mechanisms can be complex and challenging, especially in cases of mobile children. The age and developmental status of a child in combination with the number and the location of bruises are important factors in determining whether a bruise resulted from an accidental or inflicted mechanism. Appropriate identification of injury etiology is critical to ensure the safety of the child.

Pathogenesis of Contusions and Factors Affecting the Development and Appearance of a Bruise

A contusion, or bruise, may be defined as bleeding beneath the intact skin at the site of blunt impact trauma. The use of the term contusion should be limited to those circumstances in which an examiner has concluded that blunt impact occurred at the site of discoloration. A contusion differs from an ecchymosis in pathogenesis, and these terms should not be used interchangeably. An ecchymosis may be defined as blood that has dissected through tissue planes to become visible externally. An ecchymosis may be visible in an area that was never subjected to trauma. A classic example of an ecchymosis that becomes visible in an area free of blunt trauma is the Battle sign **(Fig. 10.2)**. The area of discoloration over the mastoid process that is associated with basilar skull fractures involving the middle fossae. Another example of ecchymosis is the development of bilateral periorbital ecchymoses **(Fig. 10.3)** (often referred to as "raccoon eyes"). A contusion is a form of hematoma, but not all hematomas are contusions. A hematoma may be defined as blood that has extravasated from the vascular system into the body. A hematoma

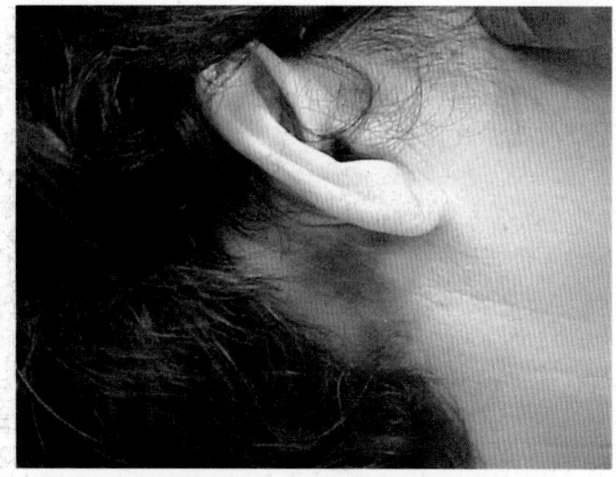

Fig. 10.2: Battle sign, typically present behind the pinna of the ear

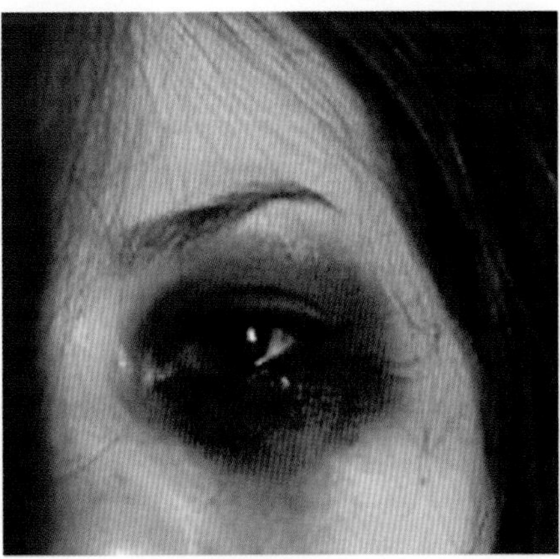

Fig. 10.3: Raccoon eyes presenting as periorbital ecchymosis and edema

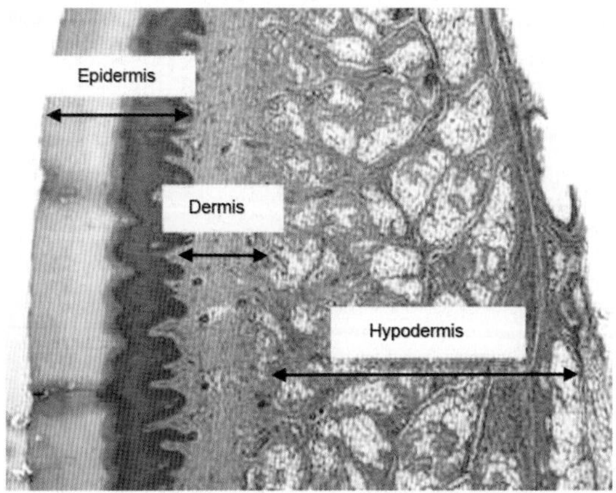

Fig. 10.4: Histological picture showing the three prominent layers of the skin viz. epidermis, dermis and hypodermis

may or may not be associated with trauma. Hematomas may develop in the presence of natural disease processes in the absence of trauma. Physicians working in the field of child physical abuse must remember that each and every word within a medical record may become part of a criminal court proceeding. These physicians are cautioned to be precise and accurate in terminology; loose use of terms and medical slang should be avoided.

The skin is generally composed of three main layers (**Fig. 10.4**) epidermis, dermis, and subcutaneous tissues. The epidermis is a compact and firm outer layer that is not easily damaged by crushing forces. The dermis is the middle layer composed of a superficial capillary network and a fibrous structure that is capable of stretching under force and returning to its original form without damage. The subcutaneous tissues comprise the innermost layer, which is rich in capillaries and fat and may be easily deformed. The capillary networks of the two inner layers of the skin are the structures most affected during injury with the majority of hemorrhage occurring in the subcutaneous tissue. Blood leaks into the perivascular tissues when damage occurs to blood vessels either through impact or a pressure increase that exceeds the injury threshold of the vessel wall. This extravasation without the loss of the integrity of the skin surface is known as bruising or contusion and may be evident as discoloration.

Petechiae represent blood that has extravasated from the tiniest branches of the vascular system; they are characterized by pinpoint or pinhead-size hemorrhages beneath intact overlying skin or mucous membranes. Petechiae may range up to two mm in diameter. The color, shape, and location of a bruise changes as hemoglobin is broken down and resorbed. The time that it takes for a bruise to appear is dependent on many factors, including: type of injuring force, depth of the injury, diffusion of the blood through the damaged tissue, and the type(s) of tissue injured. The skin varies in relative tissue composition and thickness throughout the body to meet the functional requirements of the different body parts. As a consequence of the skin's structural differences, some body regions bruise more readily, whereas others require the application of greater force for bruising to result. The extent of injury associated with a bruise may not be apparent from the appearance of the overlying skin. A superficial bruise may discolor the skin immediately, whereas deep bruising may take days to appear or may never become apparent externally.

The biochemical processes that occur in the skin and underlying tissue during the stages of repair result in changes in the appearance of the injury, which is the reason photographic documentation is critical. Bruising may be caused by brief sudden contact with a blunt object or continually applied pressure. Direct blunt impact injuries may result from the body moving toward the blunt object (e. g. a fall into a piece of furniture) or the blunt object moving toward the body (e.g. being struck with an object). Pinching or gripping at the body with the hand or an implement is an example of applications of continual pressure that may also result in characteristic bruising.

Factors Affecting the Development of a Bruise

Factors affecting the development of a bruise include properties of:

1. The impacting object (or surface),
2. Force of impact, and
3. Properties of the body region impacted, including
   a. Vascularization of the tissue bed at the impact site,
   b. Tightness of the skin,
   c. Presence or absence of tissue planes,
   d. Presence of underlying bone such as in the area of the iliac crest and the zygomatic arch,
   e. The state of the coagulation system of the patient (e.g. has disseminated intravascular coagulation developed?), and
   f. Medications that may affect the patient's clotting cascade and ability to form a clot.

A severe bruising force may crush and tear subcutaneous fat, fascia, muscle, blood vessels, nerves, and periosteum, or these tissues may be gradually compressed as local swelling occurs. Bruising may be more readily apparent in regions in which there is greater vascularization and locations where the tissue is loose compared to areas where the skin is more strongly supported. The presence or absence of multiple tissue planes may influence the area and size of bruising as the tissue planes may allow the blood to track to sites remote from the initial impact.

In addition, there will be differences in the development of a bruise depending upon the duration of impact. If there is a rapid application of force, then the applied pressure is brief allowing immediate extravasation of blood, which may be evident externally in the form of a bruise. If there is an application of pressure without forceful impact—If the same amount of force is applied more slowly, then there may be no rupture of blood vessels, and thus an absence of bruising.

Characteristic Bruises

Distinctive bruising patterns result from different injury mechanisms.

Grip/Grabmarks: Bruises from a continually or forcefully applied grip are often relatively round and may coincide with 2 to 4 fingertips. Frequently, a thumb bruise may also be noted on the opposite side.

Closed-fisted Punch: Punches generally result a series of 2 to 3 bruises that are relatively round, with each bruise corresponding to a knuckle on the hand of the assailant. This bruising pattern is sometimes observed on the abdomen of children who have suffered physical abuse. However, it should be remembered that more than 40 percent of children dying from abusive blunt abdominal trauma have no contusions visible on the external abdominal wall.

Slap or Impact with Solid Cylindrical Object: Tramline bruising is a common pattern characterized by parallel linear bruises with regions of sparing between them. This specific bruising pattern is created when a relatively light object impacts the skin surface rapidly. A classic example is the pattern left on a cheek from an open-handed slap mark. The pattern often consists of 3 parallel linear contusions with central sparing. The width of the central sparing roughly corresponds to the width of the fingers. This pattern of linear contusions with central sparing develops as the tissues along the edge of the impact site undergo the greatest deformation. The impacts from the individual fingers are of insufficient force to cause an underlying crushing injury.

Other Objects or Household Implements: Often during an assault, the pattern of either the impacting object or something lying between the impacting object and the skin, such as the textile pattern of the clothing, is imprinted into the skin resulting in a pattern bruise. Such patterned bruising may also occur intradermally. Patterned bruises in the shape of instruments may be diagnostic of physical abuse. Belts and electrical cords are common examples of household instruments that leave distinctive patterns.

Bites: The typical bite mark is a series of aligned contusions in a round or oval ring-shape consisting of 2 arches (**Figs 10.5 A and B**). For more details on bite marks and their appearences, readers are advised to please see the chapter on the Bite Marks.

The various types of abuses maybe categorized as follows (**Table 10. 1**).

Conditions that may be Confused with Abusive Bruising

Some common conditions including Mongolian spots, cultural remedies, phyto-photo-dermatitis, and bleeding disorders may be confused with contusions in children. These conditions do not preclude abuse, but should be considered in children presenting with areas of discoloration and no other injuries on physical exam or imaging. Mongolian spots are areas of blue or blue-black discoloration usually located on the lower back or buttocks. They are also common in the more superior midline of the back, sometimes noted over the thoracic or cervical region, and may be present just about anywhere on the body. They are seen more commonly in African-American and Asian children, and usually fade by 5 years of age. If an examiner is unsure whether a particular area of coloration is a Mongolian spot versus a contusion, re-examination after 10 days or so will resolve the issue. A bruise will show fading in 1 to 2 weeks time, whereas Mongolian spots remain relatively unchanged in the short term. Indeed, some people retain them into adulthood. Coining and cupping are folk remedies using coins with oil or a heated cup applied to the skin for healing purposes. Although these are usually painless procedures, they can cause extravasations of blood into the perivascular tissues that appear as bruises.

A

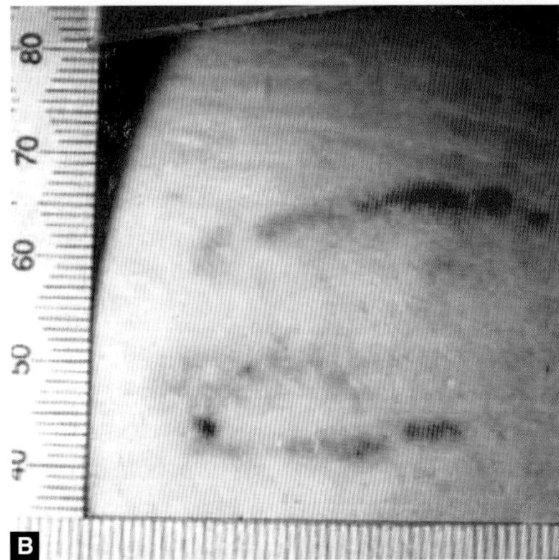

Figs 10.5A and B: Typical bite mark on the arm of a child presenting as ring, shaped of two ovals representing two arches

Phytophotodermatitis occurs after contact of the skin with certain vegetables or fruit (e.g. celery, limes) and then sunlight **(Fig. 10.6)**. The skin becomes hyperpigmented, which can mimic a bruise. Often, a caretaker will have the agent on his/her hands and touch the child. The resulting lesion will appear as a finger or handprint. A thorough history of contact with these agents is necessary.

Henoch-Schonlein purpura is a form of vasculitis that involves the small blood vessels and commonly occurs in children after an upper-respiratory tract infection or other illness. The purpuric skin rash may appear as bruising **(Figs 10.7A and B)** and most generally affects the buttocks and lower extremities.

Bleeding disorders such as platelet disorders, idiopathic thrombocytopenic purpura **(Fig. 10.8)**, Von Willebrand disease, or leukemia can cause easy bruising. Consequently, children will present with unusual or numerous bruises and little history to

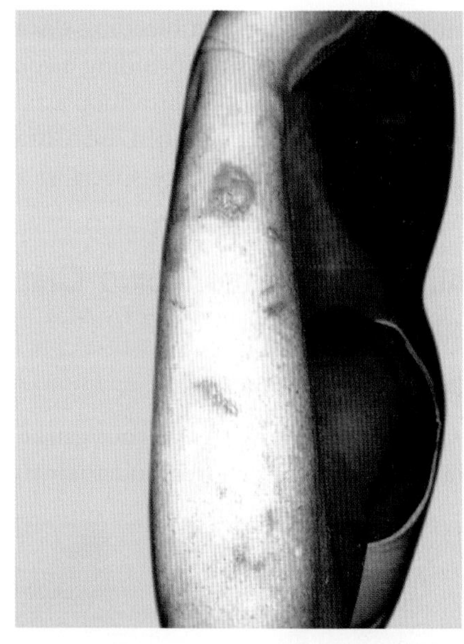

Fig. 10.6: A case of photodermatitis of the forearm, which may be mistaken for any abusive phenomenon

Table 10.1: Showing the summary of various types of abuse

Physical Abuse	*Sexual Abuse*	*Emotional Abuse*	*Gild Child Neglect*
• Slapping/kicking • Beating with stave/stick • Pushing • Shaking	Severe forms: • Sexual assault • Making the child fondle private parts • Making the child exhibit private body parts • Exhibiting private body parts to a child • Photographing a child in the nude Other forms: • Forcible kissing • Sexual advances during travel situations • Sexual advances during marriage situations • Exposure: Children forced to view private body parts • Exposure: Children forced to view pornographic materials	• Humiliation is the lowering of the self esteem of the child by harsh treatment, ignoring, shouting or speaking rudely, name calling and use of abusive language • Comparison in between siblings and with other children	• Lack of attention to girls as compared to brothers • Less share of food in the family • Sibling care by the girl child • Gender discrimination

account for the bruising. If a bleeding disorder is suspected, laboratory testing including a complete blood count, activated partial thromboplastin time, and prothrombin time should be obtained; consultation with a hematology specialist should also be considered.

Legal Matters Regarding Child Abuse and Neglect

The Constitution of India

The Constitution of India recognizes the vulnerable position of children and their right to protection. Following the doctrine of protective discrimination, it guarantees in Article 15 special attention to children through necessary and special laws and policies that safeguard their rights. The right to equality, protection of life and personal liberty and the right against exploitation are enshrined in Articles 14, 15, 15(3), 19(1) (a), 21, 21(A), 23, 24, 39(e) 39(f) and reiterate India's commitment to the protection, safety, security and well-being of all it's people, including children.

Article 14: The State shall not deny to any person equality before the law or the equal protection of the laws within the territory of India.

Article 15: The State shall not discriminate against any citizen on grounds only of religion, race, caste, sex, place of birth or any of them.

Article 15 (3): Nothing in this article shall prevent the State from making any special provision for women and children.

Article 19(1) (a): All citizens shall have the right to freedom of speech and expression.

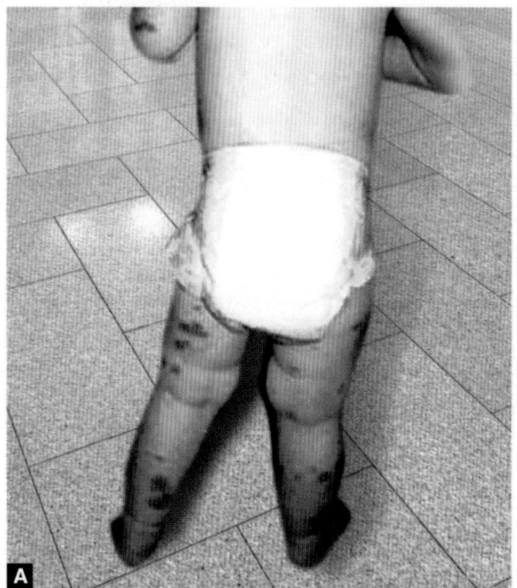

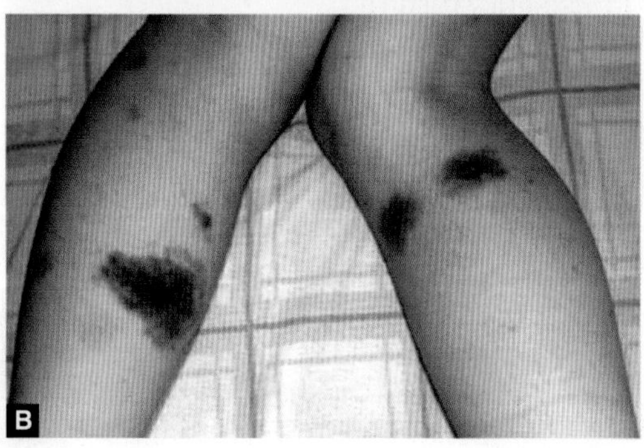

Figs 10.7A and B: Henoch-Schonlein Purpura on the legs of a child patient, mimicking an abusive inflicted injury

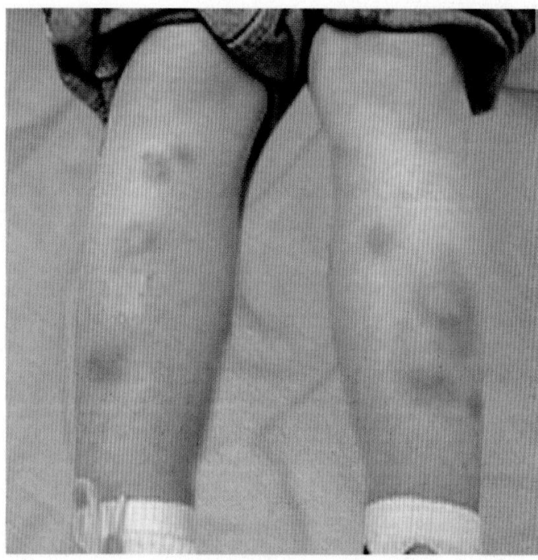

Fig. 10.8: An yet another disease, Idiopathic Thrombocytic Purpura (ITP), which may also be mistaken for an abusive injury

Article 21: Protection of life and personal liberty—No person shall be deprived of his life or personal liberty except according to procedure established by law.

Article 21A: Free and compulsory education for all children of the age of 6 to 14 years.

Article 23: Prohibition of traffic in human beings and forced labor (1) Traffic in human beings and beggars and other similar forms of forced labour are prohibited and any contravention of this provision shall be an offence punishable in accordance with law.

Article 24: Prohibition of employment of children in factories, etc. No child below the age of fourteen years shall be employed to work in any factory or mine or engaged in any other hazardous employment.

Article 39: The state shall, in particular, direct its policy towards securing:

a. That the health and strength of workers, men and women, and the tender age of children are not abused and that citizens are not forced by economic necessity to enter vocations unsuited to their age or strength.
b. That children are given opportunities and facilities to develop in a healthy manner and in conditions of freedom and dignity and that childhood and youth are protected against exploitation and against moral and material abandonment.

International Conventions and Declarations

India is signatory to a number of international instruments and declarations pertaining to the rights of children to protection, security and dignity. It acceded to the United Nations Convention on the Rights of the Child (UN CRC) in 1992, reaffirming its earlier acceptance of the 1959 UN declaration on the Rights of the Child, and is fully committed to implementation of all provisions of the UN CRC. In 2005, the Government of India accepted the two optional protocols to the UN CRC, addressing the involvement of children in armed conflict and the sale of children, child prostitution and child pornography. India is strengthening its national policy and measures to protect children from these dangerous forms of violence and exploitation. India is also a signatory to the International Conventions on civil and political rights, and on economic, social and cultural rights which apply to the human rights of children as much as adults. Three important international instruments for the protection of child rights that India is signatory to, are:

Convention on the Rights of the Child (CRC) adopted by the UN General Assembly in 1989, is the widely accepted UN instrument ratified by most of the developed as well as developing countries, including India. The Convention prescribes standards to be adhered to by all State parties in securing the best interest of the child and outlines the fundamental rights of children, including the right to be protected from economic exploitation and harmful work, from all forms of sexual exploitation and abuse and from physical or mental violence, as well as ensuring that children will not be separated from their families against their will.

Convention on the Elimination of All Forms of Discrimination against Women (CEDAW) is also applicable to girls under 18 years of age. Article 16.2 of the Convention lays special emphasis on the prevention of child marriages and states that the betrothal and marriage of a child shall have no legal effect and that legislative action shall be taken by States to specify a minimum age for marriage.

SAARC Convention on Prevention and Combating Trafficking in Women and Children for Prostitution emphasizes that the evil of trafficking in women and children for the purpose of prostitution is incompatible with the dignity and honour of human beings and is a violation of basic human rights of women and children.

Recognizing Child Abuse/Neglect

Dentists are positioned uniquely to detect signs of child abuse. According to statistics, 50 percent to 65 percent of all physical trauma associated with abuse occurs in head, face or neck. Following is a list of head, face and neck injuries that should alert dentists to possibility of abuse and neglect. Besides the list, any injury to the head, face, neck or mouth that is burns caused by specific objects, such as an iron, curling iron, kitchen implement or cigarette, patterned injuries recognizable as caused by an object, such as belt buckle and adult human bites, may be added to the list.

The common sites that are frequently seen as a result of abuse are **(Figs 10.9A and B)**:

Head: Skull injuries, bald spots (traumatic alopecia), bruises behind ears (Battle's sign)

Eyes: Retinal hemorrhage, blackened eyes (raccoon eyes)

Nose: Fractures, displacement

Lips: Bruises, Lacerations, angular abrasions (gag marks)

Intra-oral: Frenum tears, palatal bruising, residual tooth roots

Maxilla/Mandible: Fractures/improperly healed fractures, Malocclusion from previous fractures

Teeth: Fractured, mobile, avulsed or discolored teeth, untreated rampant caries, untreated, obvious infections or bleeding.

Detecting Child Abuse in the Dental Office

Case History

When a child presents for examination, particularly if there is an injury involved, the history may alert the dental team to the possibility of child abuse. Indeed, the history may be the single most important source of information. Because legal proceedings could follow, the history should be recorded in detail. While one should always realize that there are other possible explanations, the possibility of child abuse or neglect should be considered whenever the history reveals the following:

1. The present injury is one of a series of injuries that the child has experienced.
2. The family offers an explanation that is not compatible with the nature of the injury. For

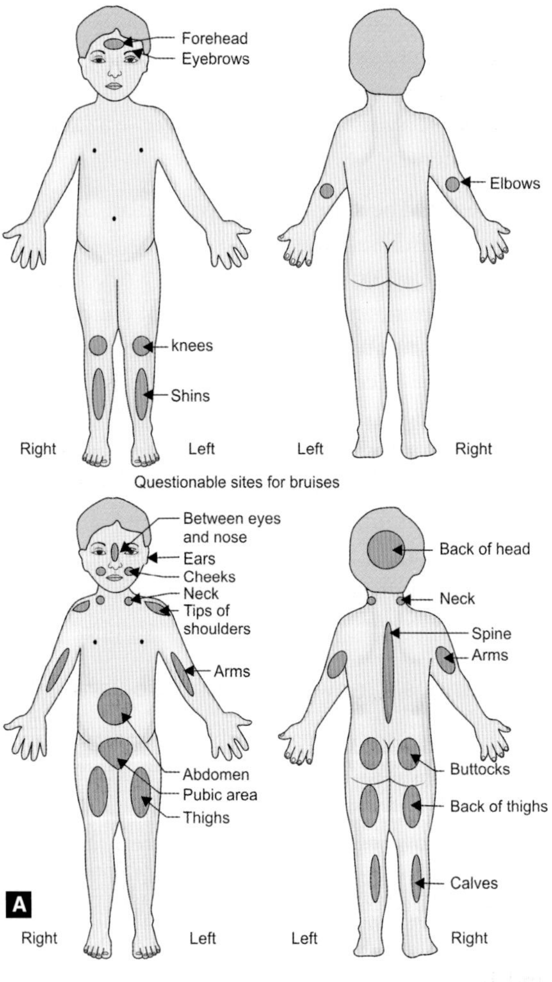

Fig. 10.9A:

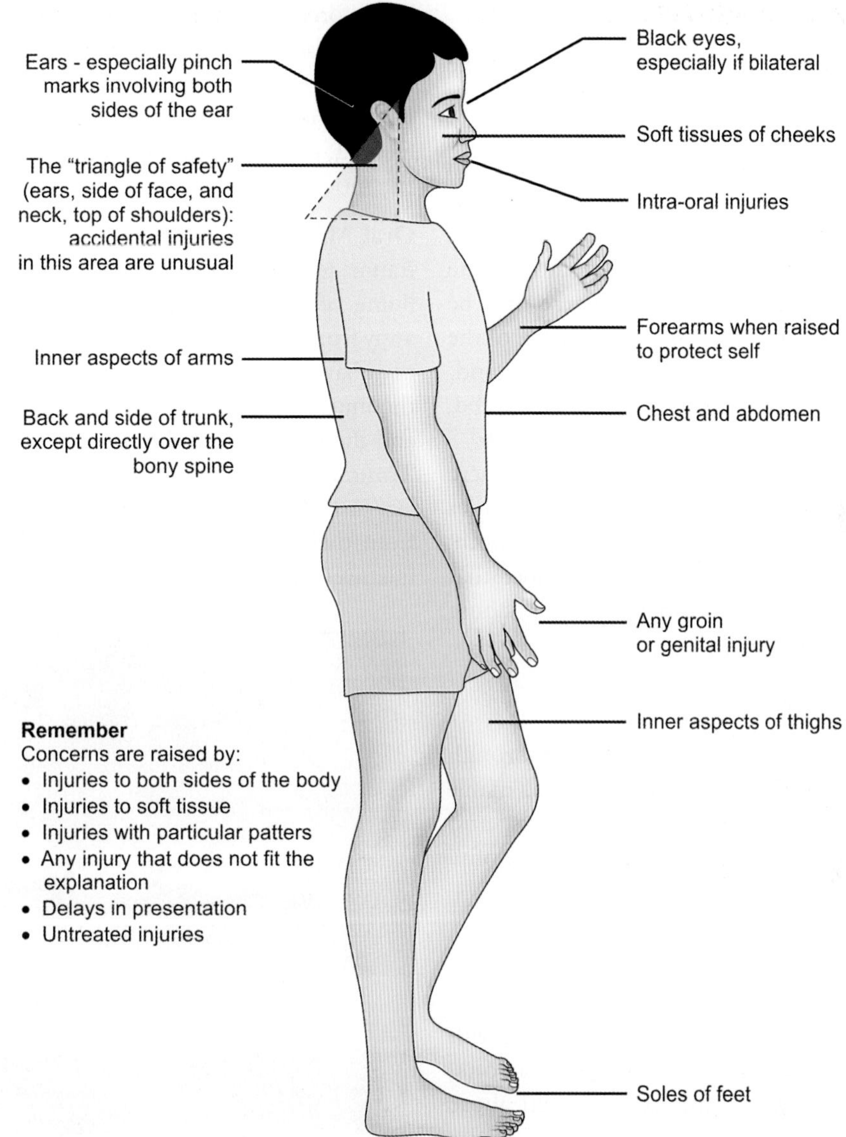

Figs 10.9A and B: The graphical diagrams showing the most common site of the injuries in case of the child abuse

example, one notable author recalls a case in which an effort was made to explain away a clearly identifiable human bite mark as a scrape caused by the edge of a diving board.

3. There has been an extraordinary delay in seeking care for the injury.
4. The family does not want to discuss the circumstances of the injury. While the above findings are by no means conclusive, they should cause the examiner to look further for possible signs of abuse, and to consider this among the possibilities to be confirmed or eliminated.

General Physical Findings

Before examining the mouth, alert members of the dental team may note general physical findings that are consistent with child abuse or neglect:

1. The child's nutritional state is poor and growth is subnormal.
2. Extraoral injuries are noted: They may be in various stages of healing, indicating the possibility of repeated trauma. There may be bruises or abrasions that reflect the shape of the offending object, e.g. belt buckle, strap, hand.
3. Cigarette burns or friction burns may be noted, e.g. from ligatures on wrists, gag on mouth.
4. There may be bite marks, bald patches (where hair has been pulled out), injuries on extremities or on the face, eyes, ears, or around the mouth.

As always, the examiner must remember that there may be explanations other than child abuse for some of these findings.

Findings on Dental Examination

Examination of dental injuries includes thorough visual observation, radiographic studies, manipulation of the jaws, pulp vitality tests, and percussion. Transillumination may also be helpful.

Typical Oral Lesions

Both oral and facial injuries of child abuse may occur alone or in conjunction with injuries to other parts of the body. The oral lesions associated with child abuse are usually bruises, lacerations, abrasions, or fractures. Suspicion of child abuse should be particularly strong when new injuries are present along with older injuries. Thus scars, particularly on the lips, are evidence of previous trauma and should alert the investigator to the possibility of child abuse. As noted earlier, further investigation is required when the explanation for the injuries does not justify the clinical findings.

Torn Frenums: Tears of the frenula, particularly the labial frenum, are frequently seen in child abuse cases **(Fig. 10.10)**. These injuries may result from blunt force trauma. For example, the labial frenum may be torn when a hand or other blunt object is forcibly applied to the upper lip to silence the child. Injuries of this type may also occur in forced feeding, as a result of the bottle being forced into the mouth.

Oral Mucosa Torn from Gingival: Blunt force trauma to the lower face may also cause the mucosal lining of the inner surface of the lip to be torn away from the gingiva. A forceful slap, for example, may have this effect. The location and extent of the injury will depend on the magnitude of force and the location and direction of the blow.

Trauma to the teeth: Severe trauma to the lower face may loosen teeth, completely displace them from their alveolar sockets, and/or cause dental fractures **(Fig. 10.11)**. It is not uncommon for

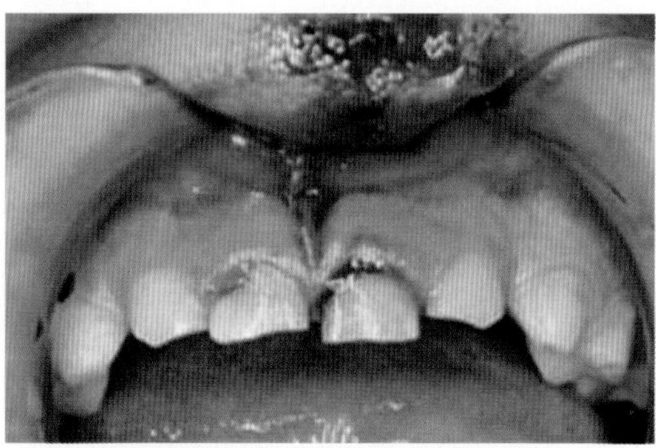

Fig. 10.10: Torn maxillary labial frenum

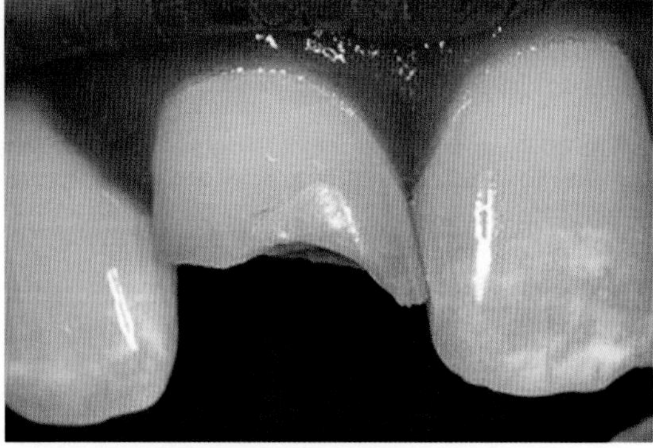

Fig. 10.11: Fractured maxillary central incisor in case of child patient reflecting some sort of traumatic injury

root fractures to occur, but this finding may be missed unless the radiographs are examined carefully. These injuries, as well as most other traumatic injuries, may be accidental rather than abusive. Therefore, one must always determine whether the injury is compatible with the explanation given. If the dental injuries resulted from a fall, for example, one would usually expect to also find bruised or abraded knees, hands, or elbows. When these additional injuries are not present, further inquiry is appropriate.

In evaluating and reporting dental injuries, it may be helpful to use Andreasen's classification, based on a system adopted by the World Health Organization. It is summarized below:

Crown Infraction: Incomplete fracture (crack) of enamel with loss of tooth substance.

Uncomplicated Crown Fracture: Confined to enamel or enamel and dentin, pulp not exposed.

Complicated Crown Fracture: Involves enamel and dentin, pulp is exposed.

Uncomplicated Crown-root Fracture: Involves enamel, dentin, and cementum, but does not expose pulp.

Complicated Crown-root Fracture: Involves enamel, dentin, cementum, and exposes pulp.

Concussion: Injury to supporting structures without abnormal loosening or displacement of the tooth, but with marked reaction to percussion.

Subluxation (loosening): Injury to supporting structures with abnormal loosening, but without displacement of the tooth.

Intrusive luxation: Tooth displaced into alveolar bone, injury accompanied by comminution or fracture of alveolar socket.

Extrusive luxation: Tooth partially displaced out of its socket.

Lateral luxation: Tooth displaced in a direction other than axially, with comminution or fracture of alveolar socket.

Exarticulation (complete avulsion): Tooth completely avulsed from socket. Comminution of alveolar socket: crushing and compression of alveolar socket, found with intrusive and lateral luxation.

Fracture of alveolar socket wall: Fracture confined to the labial or lingual socket wall.

Fracture of mandible or maxilla: Involves the base of mandible or maxilla and often the alveolar process, may or may not involve alveolar socket.

Laceration of gingiva or oral mucosa: Shallow or deep wound in mucosa resulting from tear, and normally produced by sharp object.

Contusion of gingiva or oral mucosa: Bruise usually caused by blunt object, no break in mucosa, usually causes small submucosal hemorrhage.

Abrasion of gingiva or oral mucosa: Superficial wound produced by rubbing or scraping mucosa, leaving raw, bleeding surface.

Discolored Teeth: The tissues of the dental pulp receive their primary blood supply through the apical foramen. When the tooth receives a concussion, the apical blood vessels may be severed, or hematoma or edema may occlude the blood vessels as they enter the tooth. As a consequence, the pulp may become necrotic and nonvital. Necrosis of the previously pink pulp tissues will usually cause a noticeable darkening of the tooth (**Fig. 10.12**). In some cases of dental trauma, the dental pulp's response to the injury may be to deposit additional secondary dentin in the pulp chamber. This may continue until the entire pulp chamber is filled in, or obtunded. Again, the loss of the hollow pulp chamber with its normally pinkish contents is likely to cause a change in the color of the tooth.

It is important to remember that both of the processes described above occur over a period of weeks, or even months. Consequently, when a child presents with current dental trauma and also has one or more dark teeth unrelated to caries, it is probable that the child has experienced previous trauma. Further inquiry to determine the nature of the trauma should be undertaken.

Previously Missing Teeth: In examining a child who has experienced recent trauma, it may be noted that one or more teeth has been lost prior to the present incident. The etiology of this earlier tooth loss should be investigated. If it was due to "an accident", a pattern of repeated trauma has been established. This pattern needs to be evaluated, and child abuse is one of the possibilities to be considered.

Trauma to the Lip: It is not uncommon to find contusions, lacerations, burns, or scars on the lips of abused children. Bruises to the lip may result from forced feeding. Burns on the lip, as well as burns on the face or tongue, may be signs of physical punishment. Bruises at the angles of the mouth may result from efforts to gag or silence a child.

Trauma to the Tongue: The tongue of an abused child may exhibit abnormal anatomy or function due to scarring. This may result from a burn or other trauma.

Other Soft Tissue Injuries: Trauma to the mouth may also cause ulceration of the palate or uvula. Additionally, lacerations are sometimes found in the floor of the mouth, which may be caused by forced bottle feeding.

Severe Injury to Jaws and Associated Structures: Fractures of the maxilla, mandible, **(Fig. 10.13)** and other cranial bones may be found in cases of child abuse. If the radiologic study shows signs of old as well as new fractures, a pattern of repeated trauma has been found, and needs to be investigated with reference to possible child abuse. The examination for maxillofacial fractures is performed within the concept of overall patient care, including airway maintenance, control of hemorrhage, and neurologic examination. In a significant number of jaw fractures there is also damage to associated structures, including the cribriform plate, nasal, and zygomatic bones. Intracranial lesions and skull fractures may also be present. The diagnosis of fractures of the jaws is made primarily on the basis of clinical and radiographic findings.

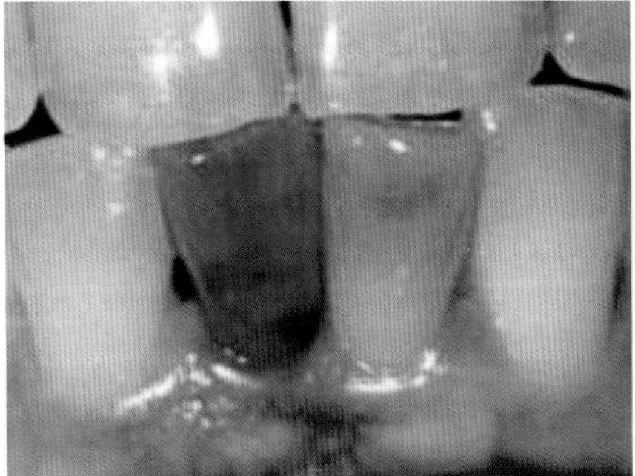

Fig. 10.12: Discolored mandibular anterior teeth, reflecting a previous episode of trauma to the area in question

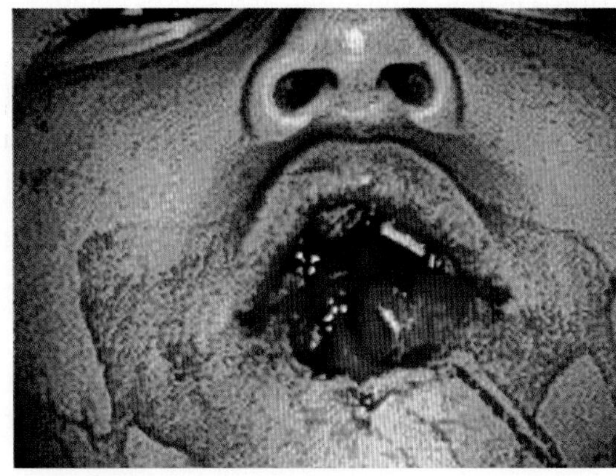

Fig. 10.13: Severely fractured jaws in a case of child patient

The clinical examination includes both extraoral and intraoral palpation. Bilateral palpation is helpful to detect asymmetry. Swelling or ecchymosis in the lower face is suggestive of fractures of the mandible. Fractures should also be suspected if there is an abrupt change in the occlusal level of the teeth. This may be associated with open bite, difficulty in opening the mouth, and facial asymmetry. Other signs and symptoms include abnormal mobility of bony structures, or the ability to move the mandible beyond its normal excursion in any direction. Dingman and Natvig suggested supporting the angle of the mandible and pressing the anterior mandibular region up and down to detect fractures of the body of the mandible.

Crepitation and deviation of the midline on closing may be diagnostic signs, as well. Pain in the area of the temporomandibular joints may suggest fractures in this region. The medical practitioner who observes dental trauma is well advised to seek consultation with a dentist experienced in dental injuries to children. This might be a pediatric dentist, oral and maxillofacial surgeon, or general dentist. This added expertise is important, not only to care for the present injury, but also to help evaluate previous trauma.

Bruises Resulting from Physical Child Abuse

An absent, vague, or implausible history is often associated with cutaneous injuries resulting from physical abuse. Frequently, bruising is an incidental finding, unrelated to the reason why the patient presents for medical care. All children, especially infants and young children, who present to the emergency department for any symptom, should be undressed, and the skin should be carefully examined. All cutaneous injuries should be documented for location, size, pattern, and color, as well as the presence of pain and swelling. A child presenting with bruising to multiple planes **(Fig. 10.14)** or body surfaces (e.g. left and right side), without plausible explanation, should be concerning for abuse. This distribution indicates that the body has sustained forces severe enough to cause bruising from multiple directions.

This pattern of injury does not typically result from minor household accidents. Pierce et al observed that stair falls involving multiple contacts between the body and the stair surface resulted in two or fewer bruises. If bruises are present on multiple planes, typically, the injuries on one plane result from an initial impact between the body and an object or hand, and the injuries on the opposite plane result from a secondary impact between the body and another object. For example, if a child is struck by an assailant and the force of the strike causes the child to impact with a piece of furniture, then bruises may appear on the plane of the body on which the child was initially struck and on the plane of the body that impacted the furniture.

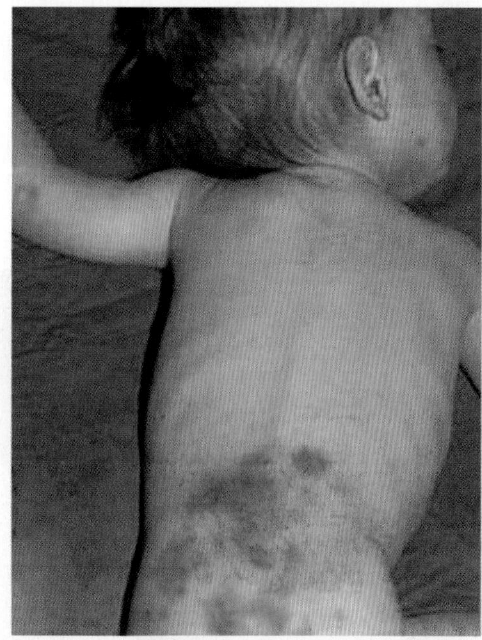

Fig. 10.14: A severely injured kid with multiple marks of assaults over his body

Subtle differences in bruising location within a given body region may raise concerns and affect the plausibility of the stated injury mechanism. In addition, studies indicate that the distribution of bruises may be indicative of injury etiology.

In infants and young children, bruises to the head (with the exception of the forehead), neck, ears, and torso including chest, abdomen, genitourinary region, back, and buttocks rarely result from accidental injury mechanisms. Therefore, bruising on infants or young children in these regions, without an appropriate history, should be concerning for abuse and appropriate medical evaluation and testing should follow. Bruising to the pinna and helix is rarely accidental and is concerning for inflicted injury, especially if present bilaterally. Unilateral, non-accidental ear injury is predominantly left-sided resulting from blows by a right-handed assailant. Ear bruising **(Fig. 10.15)** may be subtle and children should be examined carefully for such injuries. Feldman described four pediatric cases, each with petechial hemorrhages on the top of the pinnae resulting from abuse. It is believed that the apex of the ear is folded on itself and crimped against the head by a blow resulting in capillary injury. The auricular injuries in each case exemplify bruising conforming to the anatomic lines of stress rather than the shape of the injuring object.

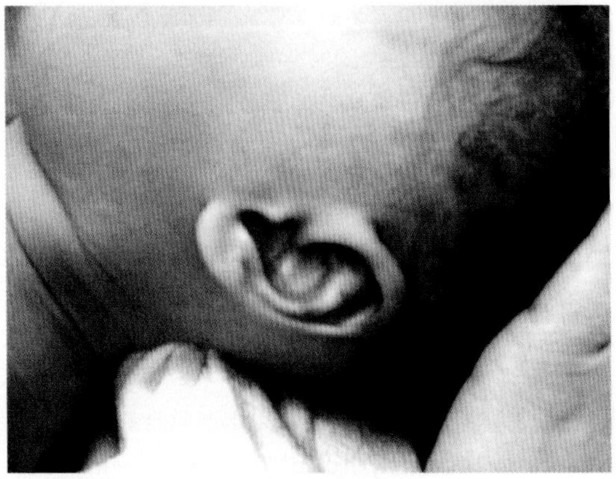

Fig. 10.15: A child with abusive injuries on the pinna of the ear

When a young child presents with bruising to the head or face without a documented and plausible trauma history, head imaging should be strongly considered. Ear bruising may be an indication of increased morbidity and mortality. Tin ear syndrome, characterized by distinct unilateral ear bruising, radiographic evidence of ipsilateral cerebral edema with obliteration of the basilar cisterns, and hemorrhagic retinopathy, results from rotational acceleration produced by blunt trauma to the ear. This triad of injuries is concerning for child abuse. Genitourinary bruising may occur from straddle injuries as a result of bicycle and playground accidents or falls. In such situations, the highly vascularized tissue is compressed against the underlying osseous tissue, and the majority of wounds are superficial. Non-penetrating straddle injury mechanisms typically result in minor trauma to the external genitalia; this includes superficial lacerations to the scrotum or penis in boys and lacerations or abrasions of the labia in girls, with the labia minora being the most frequently injured structure. Accidental straddle injuries may occur either anterior or posterior to the posterior hymenal border. However, more injuries occur anteriorly because the tissues are more likely to be compressed by the bony prominence. Minor injuries to the posterior fourchette have been documented in children presenting with a history of non-penetrating straddle injury. Hymenal trauma is associated with a history of penetrating injury and is concerning for abuse. Bruising to the penis can be seen in cases of physical abuse, especially in situations surrounding toilet training.

The caregiver may inflict injuries as a result of unrealistic expectations. If bruising to the penis occurs from an accidental situation such as becoming caught in a zipper or slammed in the toilet seat, the appropriate history should be available. Genital bruising accompanied by a vague or absent history is concerning for an abusive injury. Strangulation may cause petechiae or bruising along the neck and/or cephalad petechiae including the mucous membranes and the periorbital regions. Subconjunctival hemorrhages may also be seen. Ligatures may cause linear bruising over the wrists and lower extremities. These marks may not be bilateral or completely circumferential. Forceful hair pulling results in the scalp being lifted off of the calvarium. When this occurs, a large hemorrhage can result which tracks down over the forehead and face, and appears as widespread bruising over these areas. The discoloration often evolves over a few days. In addition, loss of clumps of hair is often seen and may be mistaken for tinia capitis.

Reporting Child Abuse or Neglect

It is absolutely vital that photographs of the child be taken as soon as possible after the child has been brought to the doctor. Any person may report abuse/neglect. Reporting is not accusation; it is a request for assistance, investigation and protection. If it seems child is in immediate danger, police should be called. Before reporting, one should have all records of suspicion along with patient's full detail. Prevent abuse and neglect through dental awareness coalition.

When one suspects child abuse, it is important to document the findings thoroughly. This record of the evidence is crucial for whatever legal proceedings may follow. Documentation may involve written notes, photographs, and radiographs. In some cases videotapes or audiotapes may be helpful. If the child requires medical attention, referral should be made to the proper resource. Even if immediate medical care is not required, if a pediatrician is readily available the dentist may wish to consult regarding the suspected child abuse prior to reporting. However, the absence of consultation does not relieve the dentist from the responsibility to promptly report suspected abuse.

To illustrate the reporting requirement, California law requires that any child-care custodian, health practitioner, nonmedical practitioner, or employee of a child protective agency who has knowledge of, or who observes a child whom he or she suspects has been the victim of child abuse, report to a child protective agency immediately or as soon as possible and send a written report within 36 hours of learning of the incident. The definition of health practitioner includes dentist resident, dental hygienist, and other licensed individuals, which includes the registered dental assistant. The report can be made to the local police agency or welfare department.

Critical Steps in Investigating and Interviewing the Possible Victim

Investigators must overcome the unfortunately frequent social attitude that "babies are less important than adult victims of homicide and that natural parent would never intentionally harm their own children". When battered child syndrome is suspected, investigators should always express concern towards type and severity of injuries. Ask child if he feels safe at home and whether injuries were intentional and given by whom. Collect information about the "acute" injury that led the person or agency to make the report. Conduct interviews with the medical personnel who are attending the child and review medical records. Interview all persons who had access to or custody of the child during the time in which the injury or injuries allegedly occurred.

Always interview the caretakers separately as joint interviews can only hurt the investigation. Do not be surprised if parents deny or frame situations to explain, particularly when they change explanation to match questions. Parent/caretaker should be reassured about confidentiality of talks. If only one caretaker is suspected of abuse, the non-abusive caretaker may need to sign for release of the records. If both are suspected, then there are provisions that override normal confidentiality rules in the search for evidence of child abuse. Caretaker's changes in explanations often mean investigators must visit the home or the scene of the injury more than once.

The ideal time to obtain such evidence is immediately after the child's injury is reported, before caretakers have an opportunity to tamper with the scene. If the child apparently suffered cigarette burns, collecting cigarette butts found in the home may facilitate analysis of the burn patterns. If the case involves a combination of sexual and physical abuse, collecting the child's clothing and bedding may allow identification of what happened and who was involved.

If the child shows evidence of bite marks, saliva swabbing should be done to allow positive identification of the biter. If the child has suffered a depressed skull fracture, any objects the approximate size of the fracture should be seized for appropriate analysis.

If a bite mark is present or suspected, it is important to collect trace evidence as well as photographic documentation; it is often possible for an expert to determine the identity of the specific biter. Procedures for collection of trace evidence should be developed after consultation with the local crime laboratory for advice based on methods and services available at that particular laboratory. Some investigators suggest the "double swab" technique in which the skin surface is first swabbed with a sterile cotton tipped applicator moistened with sterile saline. This first swab is followed by a dry swab. Both swabs should be allowed to completely air-dry before being placed in individual envelopes that are then sealed with tape. Chain of custody, with written documentation thereof, must be maintained for all evidence collected. Information necessary for the chain of custody form includes the names of persons collecting or receiving evidence, the type of evidence collected or received, and the date of receipt. If possible, a forensic dentist should be consulted at the earliest stages of the evaluation. The forensic dentist can help with identification of the bite type, pattern variations, identification of the biter, and may perform additional types of photographic documentation.

Photo Documentation

It is important that skin findings are well documented from the earliest stages of medical care, especially if there is concern for abuse. Quality photographs provide critical documentation and may be helpful later for legal purposes. A 35-mm or high-resolution digital camera may be used. Photographs taken in either format will become part of the patient's permanent medical and legal record. Images must be stored in a secured medium and certified as being the original image. When non-genital injuries are photographed, the first picture should be of the victim's face (an identification label with patient number may be included) and other photographs should follow in a systematic order. A minimum of two photographs of each cutaneous finding are recommended. The first photograph should be an orientation photograph that shows the injury in the context of the body region involved as well as the anatomical orientation of the injury. The second photograph should be a close-up of the injury with a scale in the picture. In some jurisdictions, it may be standard practice to take a third photograph. This third photograph is a close-up image taken without a scale to show that nothing is being concealed. Many forensic examiners use a standard L-shaped scale recommended by the American Board of Forensic Odontology. The scale should be placed in close proximity to and in the same plane as the injury being photographed to avoid perspective distortion, which may alter the size or contour of the wound pattern relative to the scale. If an American Board of Forensic Odontology ruler is not used, a circular scale, such as a coin, may be used to document size. Photographs should be taken in the film plane meaning the camera is positioned parallel to the injury, with the lens at a 90° angle relative to the injury. If the injury is a bite mark, the documentation sequence is modified as follows for the preservation and collection of genetic evidence on the wound: initial photograph (to demonstrate the untampered appearance, location, and orientation), salivary trace evidence collection, and comprehensive photo documentation. All photographs should be taken with the bite mark parallel to the film plane and in the orientation in which the bite was inflicted. If the bite marks are located on curved surfaces of the body, each arch may have to be photographed separately to keep the wound parallel to the film plane and prevent distortion. Adequate lighting should be used for all photographs. A ring flash may help to decrease washout that occurs with a regular electronic flash.

Techniques to Help Visualize Bruising

When light strikes human skin, it is either reflected, transmitted to deeper layers, scattered, or absorbed. Different wavelengths of light vary in ability to penetrate human skin, and the various biologic components that comprise the skin have varying absorptive and fluorescent properties. The spectrum of normal skin is dominated by the summed absorbances of hemoglobin and melanin, with small contributions from fibrous protein, collagen, and fat. When a bruise is present, there are increased amounts of hemoglobin at the injury site followed by bio-compositional changes resulting from the healing process. These changes affect the absorbance and fluorescence curves of the skin. Using alternative light sources, which deliver wavelengths of light outside of the visible spectrum of 400 to 700 nm, can aid in better visualizing trauma, patterned injury, and disease. This is due, in part, to differences in the degrees of absorption and fluorescence by the different biologic components in the illuminated region. Wavelengths from 10 to 400 nm are defined as ultraviolet (UV) and those greater than 700 nm are defined as infrared (IR). Ultraviolet radiation penetrates human skin only a few microns into the epidermal tissue. This shallow penetration results in less scatter of the reflected rays and a great degree of definition of surface detail; the shorter the wavelength, the greater the resolution. Infrared light has deeper penetration of up to 3 mm and allows injuries below the surface of the skin to be visualized. Because UV and IR wavelengths are outside the visible spectrum, it is impossible to see the details of an injury as they appear in UV or IR radiation with the unaided eye. Photographic techniques with specialized film and filters sensitive to the UV and IR wavelengths may be used to capture an image of the injury, which can then be seen with the unaided eye. However, these reflective UV and IR photography techniques have limitations in emergency department settings and for use with children; specifically, high cost, specialized and fragile equipment for multiple users, and requiring children to hold still due to long exposure times.

Ultraviolet illumination is another technique that may help to visualize regions of abnormality on the skin and may be better suited for pediatric emergency care. With this technique, a source of incident radiation stimulates electrons to higher energy levels. As the electrons return to stable orbit, energy is released, often in the form of light, which is known as fluorescence. When induced with incident radiation, many biologic compounds exhibit fluorescence and have characteristic absorption spectra. Vogeley et al used a Wood's lamp as a source of UV illumination and a digital camera to improve bruise detection. With the accessibility of a Wood's lamp in most pediatric facilities, and the elimination of the specialized filters, lenses, and films required by reflective photography, UV illumination is a more pragmatic and less expensive technique for the clinical setting.

In addition, use of a digital camera eliminated the need for low lighting conditions, long exposure times associated with the 35 mm format, and, ultimately, the requirement for children to be still for extended periods. The UV illumination has allowed enhanced visualization of faint bruises and those that were not otherwise visible. Further work and studies with children are needed in this area.

Ultraviolet and IR lighting techniques are not used routinely in the documentation of contusions in most medical examiner offices. Evidence visualized via these methods may not be admissible in court unless it has been shown to be scientifically recognized and clinically accepted by the scientific/ medical community. Acceptance may include publication in a peer-reviewed journal. To date, the best technique for documentation of contusions remains the complete and accurate examination and documentation of findings using good light in a controlled environment such as the medical examiner office or the hospital exam room. All findings should be documented in multiple formats, including photographic, diagrammatic, and written forms.

Dating Bruises and Associated Misconceptions and Limitations

Often, there is a need to date when a bruise occurred for child protective or legal purposes. Consequently, various techniques have been used in attempts to assess the age of bruises; these are described in an article by Langlois and Gresham. Among these techniques, visual assessment has been a commonly used method to age bruises; however, it is a process that remains notoriously inexact. Forensic pathology textbooks and texts focused on physical abuse of children have attempted to describe changes in bruise color over time, and although there does appear to be some evolution of color, there is no clearly predictable order. In addition, most research related to the color evolution of bruises is based on adult cadavers and these findings may not be translatable to living children. Some of the inherent difficulties in dating bruises include the amount of bleeding, depth of injury, bruise location, skin color, ambient light at the time of examination, and chronicity of bruising.

Stephenson and Bialas photographed accidental bruises of known ages in children. The photographs were reviewed by a blinded observer asked to describe the colors present in the bruise and estimate the age of injury. Age estimations were incorrect in 20 of 44 cases, and accuracy was unrelated to the age of the child, presence of a fracture, or bruising site. The study showed that multiple colors can be present within a single bruise and bruises can change color at very different rates. The study concluded that aging bruises from photographic evidence is imprecise. Bariciak et al investigated whether it was possible to accurately estimate the age of a bruise on direct clinical examination and found physician estimates, despite level of clinical training or experience, to be highly inaccurate within 24 hours of actual age of injury and not much better than chance alone.

Munang et al found the practice of relying on color, including yellow, to age bruises to be imprecise and flawed because of inter-and intra-observer variations in describing color.

Hughes et al conducted a study to understand the perception threshold for the color yellow and determine how consistently observers perceived the presence of yellow. They found variability in the threshold for the perception of yellow color among the general population and a declining ability to perceive yellow coloration as the observer's age increased.

These studies demonstrate that caution must be used when offering opinions on the age of a bruise. The estimated age (and presence) of a bruise should never be the sole criteria for a diagnosis of child abuse. Instead, the diagnosis should be determined by incorporating the findings of a careful history of the injury, past medical history, family history, associated risk factors, physical examination, and appropriate laboratory testing and imaging.

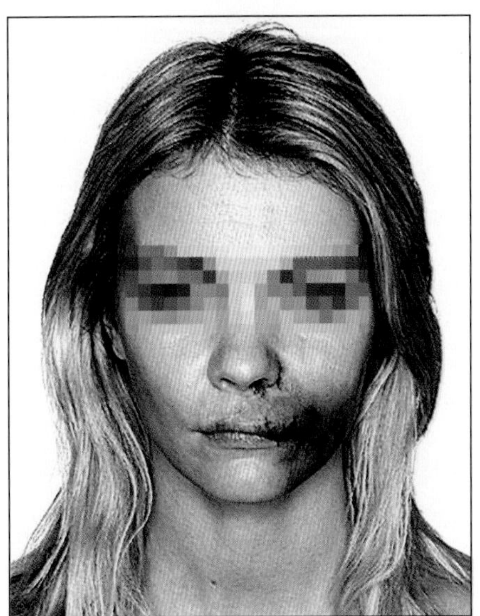

Fig. 10.16: Women patient with injuries on her face and lips, pointing towards some sort of abusive trauma

Domestic Violence and Battered Women

Battered Women Syndrome: It has been defined as a symptom complex occurring as a result of abusive actions directed against a woman by her male partner. It has been reported in approximately 15 percent of male-female relationships. Because of injuries to the head/neck, **(Fig. 10.16)** dentists treating injuries of head and neck might be 1st to examine and treat such patients.

Laskin counseled oral surgeons to be aware of non-accidental trauma. These injuries may include—fractures of nasal bones, jaws, orbital complex, fractured, avulsed, subluxated teeth or lacerations/contusions. Muelleman et al indicated that facial abrasions and contusions were most common form of injury patterns.

Summary

Bruising is one of the earliest and most common signs of physical child abuse. All infants and young children should have a careful skin examination when presenting for medical care. Multiple factors must be taken into account to distinguish accidental and inflicted etiologies, including bruise location and pattern, additional injuries or medical findings, developmental capabilities of the child, and the plausibility of the stated injury mechanism. Bruises resulting from normal activity generally occur over bony prominences on the front of the body, most commonly on the lower leg and forehead. Bruising is rare in preambulatory infants. Bruises to the torso, head (with the exception of the forehead), neck, ears, and multiple planes of the body are concerning for abuse. Children with disabilities or significant motor delay may have different bruising patterns because of their unsteady gait or assistive devices. Proper written and photographic documentation of cutaneous injuries is critical.

Bibliography

1. K Kaczor et al. Bruising and physical child abuse, Clin Ped Emerg Med. 7:153-60.
2. Kacker L, Kumar SVD. Study on Child Abuse: INDIA 2007 Ministry of Women and Child Development Government of India.
3. Kenney JP. Short communication, Domestic violence: A complex health care issue for dentistry today. Forensic Science International. 2006;159S S121-S125.
4. Langlois NE, Gresham GA. The ageing of bruises: a review and study of the colour changes with time. Forensic Sci Int. 1991;50:227-38.
5. Roberton DM, Barbor P, Hull D. Unusual injury? Recent injury in normal children and children with suspected non-accidental injury. BMJ. 1982;285: 1399-1401.
6. West MH, Barsley RE, Hall JE, et al. The detection and documentation of trace wound patterns by use of an alternate light source. J Forensic Sci. 1992;37:1480-8.
7. Wright F. Photography in bite mark and patterned injury documentation-part 1. J Forensic Sci. 1998;43:881-7.

Annexure I

Forensic Dentistry Kit

Various instruments required for a preliminary forensic investigation must include the following.

List of Various Materials and Instruments

- Reference material
- Tape recorder
- Paper pads
- Manilla envelopes for case records
- Identification forms
- Tags with string or wire
- Masking tape
- Staplers with staples
- Felt tip pens
- Large felt tip markers
- Plastic denture bags
- Pencils
- Clip boards
- Plastic cups
- Fatigues/work clothes
- Boots
- Work gloves
- Scrub suits
- Rubber aprons or surgical gowns
- Surgical gloves
- Surgical masks
- Portable dental X-ray
- Dental X-ray
- Film badge monitor system
- Automatic film processor with daylight loading hood
- Dental X-ray film mounts
- Dental X-ray film envelopes
- X-ray light view boxes
- Processor chemicals
- Lead shielding
- 35 mm camera
- 35 mm film
- Modeling clay
- Boxing wax
- Fiberoptic lights or flashlights
- Striker saw or hand saw
- Straight and curved retractors
- Scalpel handles
- Scalpel blades
- Large scissors
- Large hemostats
- Mouth props
- Tongue blades
- Cotton applicators
- Mouth mirrors (front surface)
- Explorers
- Periodontal scalers
- Cutting pliers
- Stratight pliers
- Mallet
- Millimeter rule
- Disclosing solution
- Hydrogen peroxide solution
- Sodium hypochlorite solution
- 4 × 4 sponges
- Toothbrushes
- Computer/equipment
- Computer paper
- Computer forms
- File cabinet
- Batteries

Annexure II

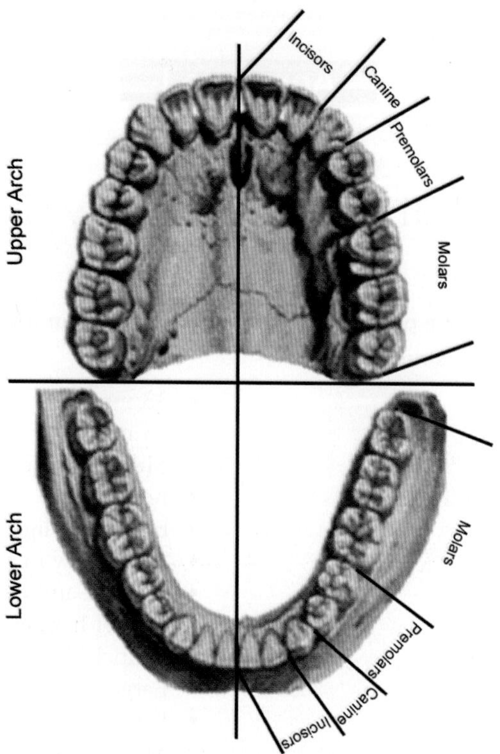

The upper (Maxilla) and lower jaw (Mandible), with the teeth

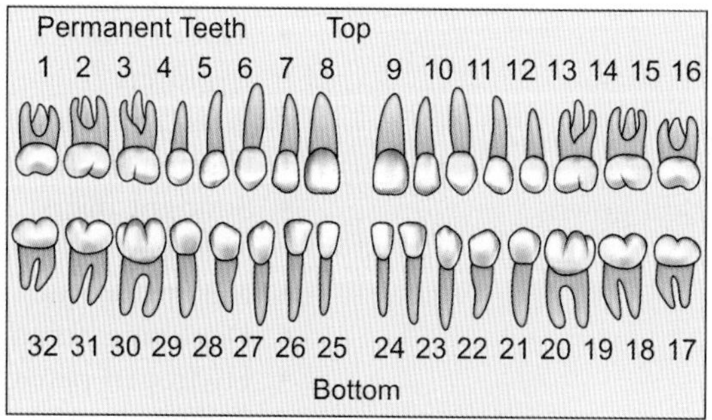

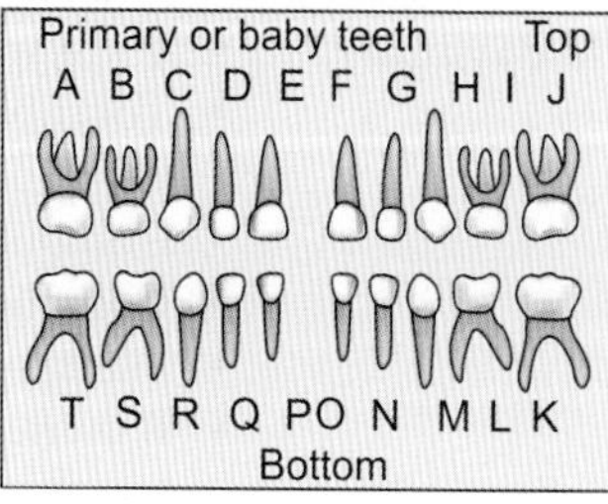

The universal numbering system for both deciduous and permanent teeth

Annexure III

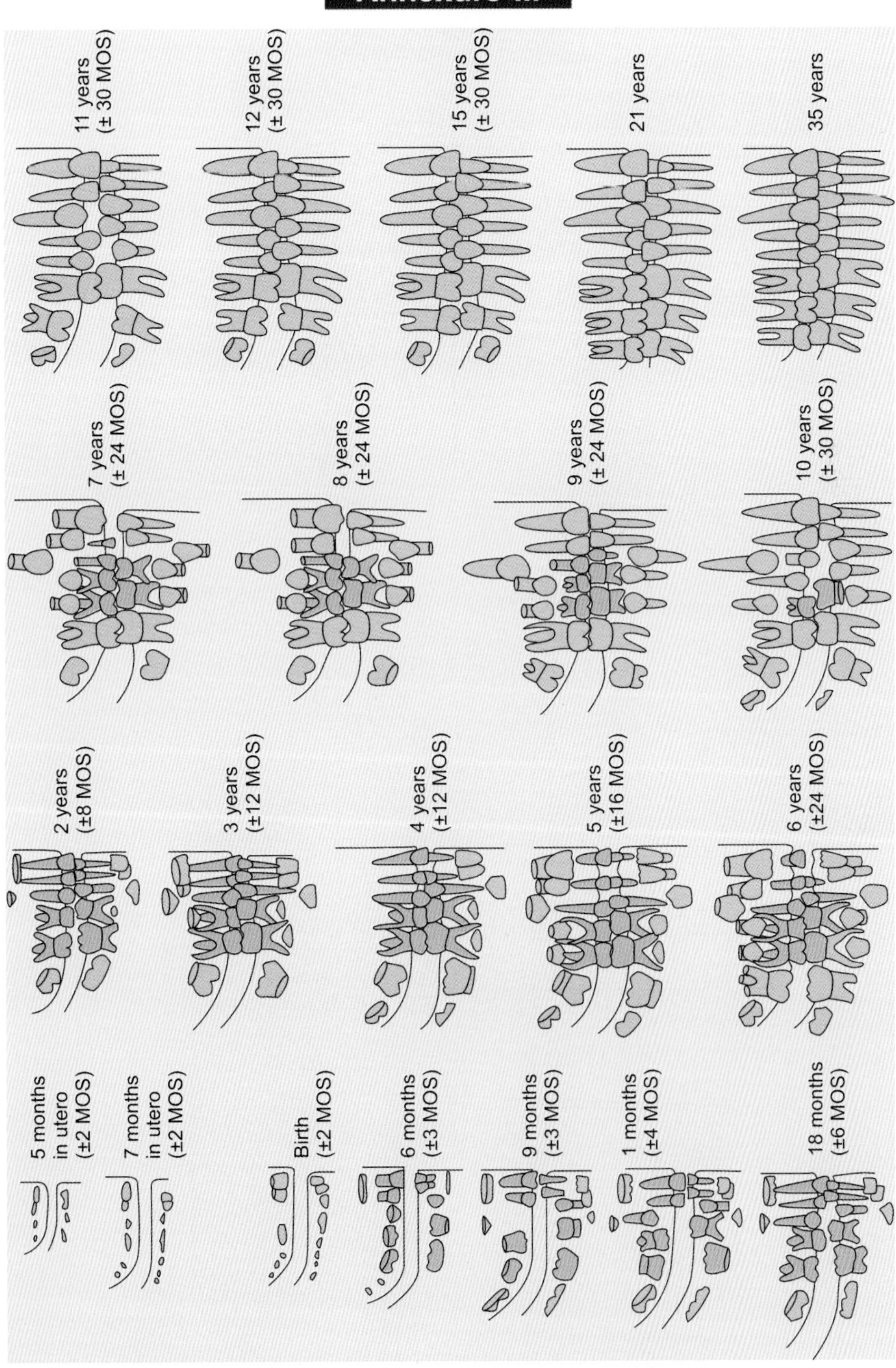

The dental age depending upon the eruption status of the teeth in the oral cavity

Index

Page numbers followed by *f* refer to figure and *t* refer to table

U

V

W

X